ATLAS OF COLOR
DOPPLER ECHOCARDIOGRAPHY

ATLAS OF COLOR
DOPPLER ECHOCARDIOGRAPHY

Navin C. Nanda, M.D.
Professor of Medicine and Director
Heart Station and Echocardiography-Graphics Laboratories
University of Alabama at Birmingham
Birmingham, Alabama

Lea & Febiger Philadelphia • London
1989

Lea & Febiger
600 Washington Square
Philadelphia, PA 19106-4198
U.S.A.
(215) 922-1330

Library of Congress Cataloging-in-Publication Data

Nanda, Navin C. (Navin Chandar), 1937–
   Atlas of color Doppler echocardiography.

   Includes bibliographies and index.
   1. Doppler echocardiography — Atlases.   2. Heart —
Diseases — Diagnosis — Atlases.   3. Heart — Valves —
Diseases — Diagnosis — Atlases.   I. Title. [DNLM:
1. Echocardiography — atlases.   2. Heart Diseases —
diagnosis — atlases.   WG 17 N176a]
RC683.5.U5N35   1988   616.1′207543   88-8994
ISBN 0-8121-1078-1

Printed and bound in Hong Kong
Produced by Mandarin Offset

DEDICATION

This book is dedicated to my parents, Mrs. Maya Vati Nanda and the late Dr. Balwant Rai Nanda; my wife, Dr. Kanta Nanda; and our children, Nitin, Anita, and Anil.

FOREWORD

Through this Atlas, Dr. Navin C. Nanda has provided readers with a portion of the expertise which he has developed in the exciting field of color Doppler echocardiography and has used here at the University of Alabama at Birmingham for nearly 5 years. There can be no doubt that surgeons and cardiologists have been tremendously aided in decision-making before and during cardiac surgery by this expertise.

Technologic advances are certainly the basis of modern cardiovascular medicine and surgery. Without the expertise of experienced physicians, however, technologic advances cannot be translated into clinical progress. We consider ourselves fortunate to have Dr. Nanda in our institution to aid and lead us in this regard. In this Atlas, he offers others his personal knowledge and expertise to assist them as well. I feel honored to be able to recommend this Atlas to you.

John W. Kirklin, M.D.
Professor of Surgery
Division of Cardiovascular/Thoracic Surgery
University of Alabama at Birmingham
Birmingham, Alabama

PREFACE

The tremendous popularity of color Doppler flow imaging which has led to its widespread use in a relatively short period has encouraged me to prepare this **Atlas** for physicians, technologists, and others interested in this exciting and innovative noninvasive diagnostic modality. It encompasses my experience with this technique since its first introduction in this country in our Echocardiography Laboratory at the University of Alabama at Birmingham over 4½ years ago. The aim of this book is to provide a comprehensive state-of-the-art review of this new field in an atlas type of format to facilitate demonstration of the various types of flow patterns observed in both acquired and congenital cardiac disease.

The **Atlas** is organized into 11 sections. The first section explains the basic concepts of color Doppler echocardiography in a simple manner, avoiding complex mathematical formulas and equations. The second section covers comprehensively normal flow patterns observed in various two-dimensional echocardiographic planes; numerous anatomic drawings are included in this section. The third section, which deals with lesions involving the mitral valve, extensively illustrates the various color Doppler findings noted in mitral stenosis and regurgitation. The next section demonstrates the usefulness of color Doppler echocardiography in the evaluation of aortic valve stenosis, aortic regurgitation, and both dissecting and nondissecting aortic aneurysms. Color Doppler findings in disease processes involving the tricuspid and pulmonary valves are demonstrated in the next two sections. Section 7 demonstrates the utility of color Doppler echocardiography in the functional evaluation of various types of mechanical and tissue prosthetic valves; differentiation of normal from abnormal flow patterns is comprehensively covered. The next two sections demonstrate various types of flow patterns seen in hypertrophic cardiomyopathy, as well as in ischemic heart disease, and their clinical significance. A large section of the **Atlas** is devoted to congenital heart disease, classified as shunt lesions (atrial septal defects, ventricular septal defects, patent ductus arteriosus, coronary fistulas), obstructive lesions, and complex lesions. Detailed coverage of the usefulness and limitations of color Doppler in various congenital lesions is provided in this section. The last section of the book covers miscellaneous lesions.

Each section of the **Atlas** begins with an introduction which delineates and explains the color Doppler findings of the lesions covered in that section. The numerous color Doppler illustrations in each section are supplemented by detailed anatomic drawings and pictures of tissue specimens, most of them in color also. The illustrations exemplify fine points in technique and diagnosis as well as avoidance of pitfalls during a color Doppler examination. A special attempt has been made to make the figure legends as comprehensive and detailed as possible. The references listed at the end of each section provide additional background reading material for the reader, and acknowledge the work of many investigators who have contributed to the advancement of Doppler and color Doppler echocardiography.

I hope and expect that this **Atlas,** with over 1600 anatomic and color Doppler illustrations from several commercially available machines, will represent the most detailed, definitive, and comprehensive work in this field to date. Practically all color Doppler illustrations were taken from studies performed personally by me. Care was taken to write the text in an easy-to-understand, uniform style, using simple language and a direct, straightforward, and concise approach. The book should therefore benefit the beginner as well as the more experienced echocardiographer. The **Atlas** is also expected to be useful to the Preceptorship Teaching Program at the University of Alabama at Birmingham in echocardiography and color Doppler. This program, begun in 1984, has so far been of use to more than 300 physicians and over 300 technologists from 34 states. In addition, 65 physicians and technologists from 20 overseas countries have learned this technique in our laboratory.

This **Atlas** is supplemented by a **Textbook of Color Doppler Echocardiography,** which consists of 33 chapters contributed by outside experts as well as our Echocardiography Laboratory staff. In addition, a **Video Tape of Color Doppler Echocardiography** about two hours in length, consisting of interesting color Doppler case material from our laboratory, has been prepared to supplement both the **Atlas** and the **Textbook.**

I am most grateful to several individuals in the University of Alabama at Birmingham Hospital who have directly or indirectly contributed to the growth and de-x

velopment of the Echocardiography Laboratory. First and foremost, Dr. Gerald Pohost, Director, Division of Cardiovascular Disease, has enthusiastically supported and encouraged all the activities of our laboratory and was directly instrumental in helping us obtain color Doppler equipment. We are grateful to many other members of the Division of Cardiovascular Disease, especially those of the Cardiac Catheterization Laboratory, for providing us with full clinical support and facilitating access to hemodynamic data for correlation with color Doppler findings. Dr. James Moon, University of Alabama Hospital Administrator, and his associates have also taken an active interest and given us extraordinary support in terms of space, personnel, and equipment needs as our laboratory expanded rapidly over the past 4 years. We are most grateful to the Division of Cardiovascular Surgery, especially Drs. John W. Kirklin, Albert D. Pacifico, James K. Kirklin, and George L. Zorn, Jr. for actively referring patients to our laboratory and for providing us with surgical correlation in the patients operated upon by them. The remarkable growth and expansion of our laboratory would not have been possible but for the enthusiastic support and encouragement given by the above individuals.

Dr. Ricardo Ceballos, Professor of Pathology, and Dr. Benigno Soto, Professor of Radiology and Director of the Division of Cardiac Radiology, provided us with illustrations of pathological specimens for use in the **Atlas**. I also appreciate the help of Dr. James B. Caulfield, Professor of Pathology, in this regard. I am thankful to Dr. Edward V. Colvin, Assistant Professor, Division of Pediatric Cardiology, and Dr. Ajit P. Yoganathan, part-time Associate Professor of Medicine at the University of Alabama at Birmingham, for their support in the preparation of this **Atlas**. Samuel Collins of the Veterans Administration Medical Center, Birmingham, Alabama, and Rod Powers and Luiz Pinheiro de Melo Filho, working in Dr. Jorge Moll's Echocardiography Laboratory in Rio de Janeiro, Brazil, did all the art work for the **Atlas**. Their help and contributions are gratefully acknowledged. I am also thankful to Photography and Instructional Graphics of the University of Alabama at Birmingham; the Audiovisual Division of the Veterans Administration Medical Center, Birmingham, Alabama; and Dr. Jorge Moll, Rio de Janeiro, Brazil,

for their support and help. I would also like to thank Acuson Computed Sonography, Advanced Technology Laboratories, Aloka Company Ltd., Biosound, Inc., Corometric Medical Systems, Hewlett Packard, Interspec–Vingmed Company, Kontron Electronics, Siemens Medical Company, and Toshiba Medical Systems for providing access to their systems, and for their advice and support in the preparation of the **Atlas**.

Fellows from the Echocardiography-Graphics Laboratories and the Division of Cardiovascular Disease have actively assisted in clinical as well as research efforts, and it was while teaching them that I became aware of the need for a book of this type. The present and former Research Fellows and Echocardiographic Associates who helped in the preparation of the **Atlas** are Drs. Ming C. Hsiung, Frederick Helmcke, Rajendra Goyal, Isidre Vilacosta, Po-Hoey Fan, Kanwal Kapur, and Krishan Aggarwal. Drs. Hsiung, Helmcke, Kan, Fan and Kapur helped photograph the still-frame color Doppler images for use in the **Atlas**. In addition, Dr. Fan helped in the preparation of the references. The help given by Sally Moos, our Technical Director; John Cooper, Assistant Technical Director; and technologists Gladys Cloud, Lapraydia King, Connie Mays, and Octavia Storey, is also deeply appreciated. Elizabeth Philpot, Echocardiography Laboratory Staff Engineer; Lindy Chapman, Administrative Assistant; and my wife, Dr. Kanta Nanda, provided expert editorial assistance. Elizabeth Philpot also made major contributions to the preparation of Section 1. Marcy Ashburn, Barbara Black, Delores Carlito, Alice Hanvey, and Karla Herrman helped in the typing of the manuscript. It would not have been possible for me to complete this project were it not for the dedicated assistance and whole-hearted support given by these individuals.

Finally, I am grateful to my family—my mother, Mrs. Maya Vati Nanda; my wife, Kanta; and our children, Nitin, Anita, and Anil for good-naturedly (for the most part) putting up with my absences from home during weekends, and late evening and early morning hours during which time the majority of the work connected with the preparation of this **Atlas** was accomplished.

Birmingham, Alabama   Navin C. Nanda, M.D.

CONTENTS

STANDARD ABBREVIATIONS

AA	Ascending aorta	LVO, LVOT	Left ventricular outflow tract
ACC	Acceleration	MF	Mitral flow
AL	Aliasing	MP	Mitral prosthesis
AO	Aorta	MPA	Main pulmonary artery
AP	Aortic prosthesis	MR	Mitral regurgitation
AR	Aortic regurgitation	MS	Mitral valve stenosis
AS	Aortic valve stenosis, Atrial septum	MV	Mitral valve
ASD	Atrial septal defect	PA	Main pulmonary artery
AV	Aortic valve	PDA	Patent ductus arteriosus
B	Baseline	PMR	Paravalvular mitral regurgitation
BF	Backflow	PR	Pulmonary regurgitation
CA	Coronary artery	PRF	Pulse repetition frequency
CS	Coronary sinus	PS	Pulmonary valve stenosis
CW	Continuous wave	PV	Pulmonary valve, Pulmonary vein
DA	Descending thoracic aorta	RA	Right atrium
DMR	Diastolic mitral regurgitation	RAA	Right atrial appendage
EV	Eustachian valve	RCA	Right coronary artery
FA	Flow acceleration	REG	Regurgitation
FF	Forward flow	RPA	Right pulmonary artery
FL	Flow	RV	Right ventricle
HV	Hepatic vein	RVO, RVOT	Right ventricular outflow tract
ILTG	Intraluminal tube graft	SVC	Superior vena cava
IS	Infundibular septum	TP	Tricuspid prosthesis
IVC	Inferior vena cava	TR	Tricuspid regurgitation
L	Liver	TS	Tricuspid valve stenosis
LA	Left atrium	TV	Tricuspid valve
LAA	Left atrial appendage, Left atrial area	2D	Two-dimensional
LMCA	Left main coronary artery	V, VEG	Vegetation
LPA	Left pulmonary artery	VMR	Valvular mitral regurgitation
LV	Left ventricle	VS	Ventricular septum
LVH	Left ventricular hypertrophy	VSD	Ventricular septal defect

Note: Other abbreviations appear in figures and are explained in accompanying legends.

<h1>Section 1</h1>

<h1>BASICS</h1>

M-mode echocardiography, the earliest noninvasive technique used to diagnose cardiac function, gives a real-time one-dimensional display of cardiac function. It can be used to accurately time intracardiac events such as valve closure, provide dimensional measurements of small cardiac structures such as the mitral valve, and detect small movements inside the heart such as valve fluttering. To obtain a larger and clearer view of the heart, two-dimensional (2D) echocardiography has been developed. It displays the anatomical structure of the heart in two dimensions, allowing detection of structural abnormalities.

Conventional pulsed and continuous wave Doppler echocardiography expand the capabilities of M-mode and 2D echocardiography by providing additional flow information. Pulsed Doppler is used to locate blood flow on the 2D image created by 2D echocardiography and to record the velocities in that flow. Pulsed Doppler, however, has limited ability for measuring high velocities. This limitation can be overcome by the use of continuous wave Doppler. Both of these techniques are based on the physical principles of wave phenomena. Specifically, high frequency sound waves are transmitted from a transducer into the heart. At these high frequencies, sound waves travel along a straight line, which is referred to as the transmission beam. These waves are then deflected after they hit moving entities such as red blood cells and the heart valves. The deflected waves return to the transducer at a lower frequency or longer wavelength and, thus, with waveforms out of phase with the original transmitted waves or with the occurrence of the maximum and minimum of the waveforms offset as compared to the original waveforms. The change in frequency between the transmitted and received waves or the Doppler frequency shift is recorded. The Fast Fourier Technique (FFT), a digital technique, then estimates the distribution of the Doppler frequency shifts recorded, and the Doppler equation is used to calculate the velocities in the flow sample.

The resultant frequency and phase shifts between the transmitted and received waves depend on the angle of incidence or the angle between the ultrasonic beam and the direction of the flow in the sample (Fig. 1-1). When this angle is approximately equal to zero or the ultrasonic beam is aligned parallel to the direction of the flow in the sample, all of the deflected waves will be received by the transducer. In addition, the velocities in the flow will be measured directly and their measured values will not need to be angle-corrected. This alignment generates the most reliable flow information. When the angle is large, some of the deflected waves bypass the transducer because the deflected waves are randomly directed rather than directed towards the transducer. Also, an incorrect alignment causes the direction of the flow not to be aligned directly with the beam. This causes the velocity in the flow to be underestimated, and to find the actual magnitude of the velocity in the flow, the measured velocity must be angle-corrected. Angle correction, however, does not work if the incident angle is very large.

With the pulsed Doppler technique, the sound waves are transmitted only one at a time at a variable rate. This rate is referred to as the pulse repetition frequency or PRF. The PRF determines the depth at which these signals can travel and the maximum measurable velocity, called the Nyquist limit. For example, a lower PRF allows the examination of a deeper depth, but the maximum measurable velocity is decreased. When the velocity is higher than the maximum measurable velocity, aliasing or the continual presence of both positive and negative Doppler frequency shifts is observed. Aliased flow has often been misinterpreted as turbulent flow because of the observation of both the positive and negative Doppler frequencies. The flow in which aliasing is observed, however, may be laminar.

In addition, the velocity can be measured only in a small area or, in other words, a sample volume using pulsed Doppler (Fig. 1-2). This sample volume is positioned in the expected area of flow on the 2D image and the Doppler frequency shift is recorded and the velocity

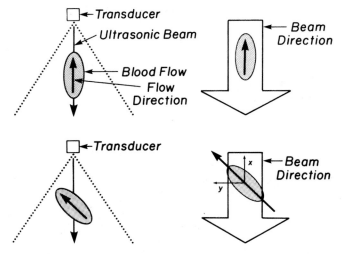

Figure 1-1 Angle of incidence. The angle between the direction of the flow in the sample and the ultrasonic beam generated by the transducer is referred to as the angle of incidence. This incident angle determines the direction of the deflected waves and the directional component of the velocity variable that is measured. The most reliable information is obtained when this angle is approximately equal to zero, because all of the deflected waves are received by the transducer and the measured velocity, which in this case has only one directional component with respect to the beam, does not have to be angle-corrected (top). When the angle is significant, some of the deflected waves bypass the transducer because the deflected waves are randomly directed rather than directed towards the transducer. In addition, the velocity can be considered as having both an x and y direction or vectorial components with respect to the beam (bottom) and, to find the actual magnitude of the velocity in the flow, the measured velocity must be angle-corrected. When the incident angle is very large, however, angle correction does not work, and the true velocity cannot be assessed.

profile of the flow in this region is calculated. The size of this sample volume depends significantly on the conventional Doppler system used and its instrumental settings.

The initial pulsed Doppler systems were single-gated systems; that is, they had only one electronic "gate" to allow the transmission of the sound waves. To overcome the limitations of single-gated pulsed Doppler, the small sample volume and the limited maximum measurable velocities, multi-range gated (MRG) pulsed Doppler were developed. MRG pulsed Doppler uses a number of single "gates" with different time delays to allow transmission of the sound waves at different times and for different sampling sites. Thus it generates a significant amount of flow information that must be reduced by averaging the data for each sampling point to make the data manageable.

Continuous wave Doppler can send and receive sound waves continuously because the transducer consists of two crystals, which serve separately as a transmitter and receiver, rather than one, which must have both functions as in the pulsed Doppler transducer. Because of the continuous transmitting and receiving of signals, the Doppler frequency shifts are recorded for all of the moving entities along the transmission beam, and no measurable velocity limitations exist.

Color Doppler echocardiography, the newest tech-

nique, is based on principles similar to those of multi-range gated pulsed Doppler echocardiography (Fig. 1-2). It is clearly superior to pulsed Doppler, however, and overcomes the limitations of the latter because it displays the actual flow patterns occurring in the heart. In general, these flow patterns are color-coded, based on the calibration of the color bar, and are superimposed on the 2D image displayed by 2D echocardiography, virtually generating a 2D display of real-time flow information.

To produce a "moving" color picture of the flow occurring in the heart, the transducer emits a fixed number of ultrasonic beams at a specified rate of PRF to interrogate a large number of sample volumes along the transmission beam. The direction of the transmission beam is then changed so that another group of sample volumes can be analyzed. This continues until the entire flow picture is created and the analysis begins again. This change in direction occurs sequentially in either the left or right direction, and the number of different directions in which the transmission beam is steered is predefined. The term "scan line" or "sector line" is used by most color Doppler manufacturers to designate each of these directional lines, and the term "frame rate" is used to specify the time required to create this image. The depth that the transmission beams can interrogate, the PRF, the number of scan lines, and the frame rate are interdependent, and thus the optimal combination of these settings must be found to obtain the most accurate flow information. The available combinations of these parameters and the results from these combinations, however, vary with each commercial color Doppler system. Therefore, each examiner must be fully knowledgeable about his system so that the optimal combinations of the various parameters can be determined and the maximum amount of accurate flow information obtained.

Theoretically, these parameters also affect the resolution of the final displayed image. For example, a short

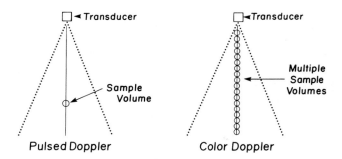

Figure 1-2 Pulsed and color Doppler sample volume. At any given time, the measurements obtained using pulsed Doppler are assessed only in a small area called the sample volume. This sample volume is positioned in the expected area of flow on the 2D image and the flow information is recorded. The size of this sample volume depends significantly on the conventional Doppler system used and its instrumental settings. Color Doppler generates the same type of flow information, but produces a "moving" color picture of the flow occurring in the heart by the ultrasonic beam interrogating a large number of sample volumes along successive transmission beams.

examination depth causes a sharply detailed image of the flow patterns occurring, but in many patients, especially large adults, a short examination depth cannot be used, and the flow patterns may be less clear. In clinical practice, however, these considerations do not presently pose a significant problem.

To generate the desired flow information from the large number of sample volumes along the transmission beam, the signals from the sample volumes must be filtered, but the usual filters such as the high pass filters require constant inputs instead of irregular inputs as used for the transmission of the ultrasonic beams. Therefore, a moving target indicator (MTI) filter must be used (Fig. 1-3). It filters out the strong slow-moving or often stationary echoes generated by the tissues and allows the weaker high-velocity echoes produced by the blood flow to pass.

The data to form these images is then generated from the analysis of this flow information using the autocorrelation technique, because the large number of samples cannot be analyzed in a short time using the FFT technique. As discussed previously, when a transmitted wave from the transducer hits a moving entity, it returns to the transducer at a lower frequency or longer wavelength, and thus with a waveform out of phase or offset with the original transmitted wave. The autocorrelation technique analyzes the resultant phase shift rather than the frequency shift between the original transmitted and resultant received waveform to detect moving flow and to generate a modal frequency, which can be used in the Doppler equation to calculate mean flow velocities and display the flow. The quantitative value of the mean velocity at each pixel, which is the smallest picture element coded with color, can be determined both off-line and on-line using a color image analyzing system, and for laminar or nonturbulent flows, the value of this mean velocity is approximately equal to the value of the peak velocity (Fig. 1-4).

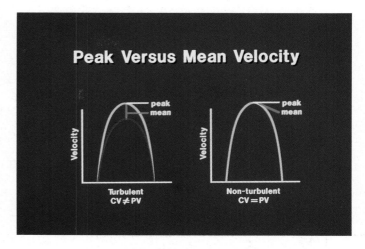

Figure 1-4 Comparison of mean and peak velocities in laminar flow. For laminar or nonturbulent flows, the value of the mean velocity measured at each color pixel (smallest picture element coded with color) is approximately equal to the value of the peak velocity. For turbulent flows, however, these velocities as shown are not equal. CV = color velocity, PV = pulsed Doppler velocity.

The color flow image is displayed using three basic colors: red, blue, and green. Additional colors may also be observed, but they result from the mixing of these three colors (Fig. 1-5). The colors red and blue are used to indicate directional information. In general, blue represents flow away from the transducer and red represents flow toward the transducer. Green is often added to the colors red and blue to represent the velocity or variance and the amount of turbulent or disturbed flow present, depending on the color map used for the selected commercial color Doppler system. Each color Doppler system displays specified flow information by

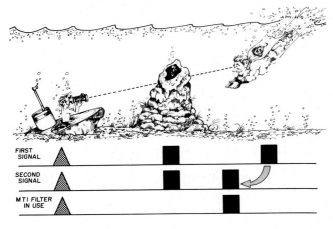

Figure 1-3 Moving target indicator (MTI). An MTI filter must be used to filter out the pulsed signal inputs generated by color Doppler to obtain the desired flow information. This filter removes the strong slow-moving or often stationary echoes generated by the tissues and passes through the weaker high-velocity echoes produced by the blood flow.

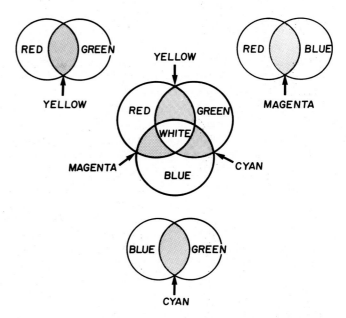

Figure 1-5 Color combinations. Red, blue, and green are the three basic colors used to display the color flow image. Other colors such as cyan, magenta, yellow, and white may also be observed, but these result from the mixing of the three primary colors.

using different combinations of the primary colors and the properties of color such as hue (the amount of a primary color contained), saturation (the amount of white contained), and intensity (brightness). A 2D calibration or color bar is displayed on each color map to show the color and color property combination selected for displaying the flow information. This bar provides a reference for determining the flow information from the displayed signals. The flow information to be displayed is selected by the examiner using a specific color map available on his color Doppler system.

As discussed previously, aliasing occurs when the flow measured has velocities higher than the maximum measurable velocity or the Nyquist limit. When velocity is calibrated in terms of intensity, nonaliased or primary flow is shown with the brightest color or the highest velocities in the center of the flow and the darkest colors or the lower velocities in the outer portion of the flow. Aliased or secondary flow is shown when low-velocity signals or the darkest color is surrounded by high-velocity signals or the brightest color. This reversed flow pattern results because the velocities are indicated by the reversed colors or, in other words, a complete "wrap-around" of the color or calibration bar has occurred (Fig. 1-6). A second "wrap-around" of the color bar occurs when the color Doppler displays flow patterns with velocities greater than twice the Nyquist limit. In this case, the higher velocities or brightest colors appear inside the aliased portion of the flow and correspond to the color intensities that indicate the high and low velocities in the primary flow.

The use of either the velocity or power mode also allows selected flow information to be displayed. The power or amplitude mode, which is available on only some commercial color Doppler systems, is used to enhance the display of information about the number of red blood cells contained in the flow or, in other words, the display of amplitude flow information. The velocity mode is used to display information about the velocity and variance in the flow. The power mode displays more information about low-velocity flows than the velocity mode and therefore is used to help detect these flows. This is because the power mode displays a large number of red blood cells with low velocities with brighter and thus more easily distinguishable colors. The velocity mode detects the higher velocities much better than the lower velocities because the low-velocity signals are not easily distinguished from noise and artifact signals.

The superiority of color Doppler to pulsed Doppler echocardiography can be demonstrated in the evaluation of various regurgitant lesions. For example, tricuspid regurgitation (TR) signals using color Doppler can be examined in multiple planes over a much shorter time than pulsed Doppler echocardiography, which requires the complete interrogation of the entire right atrium (RA) using small sample volumes. This interrogation by pulsed Doppler may also not be accurate, because the longer time required by this technique allows for more

influence on the resultant flow information from patient movement. In fact, patient movement can change the imaging plane being examined. There is also the problem of examiner fatigue.

In addition, when high velocities must be recorded, continuous wave Doppler still provides the most accurate results. Color Doppler, however, by displaying the flow patterns, provides a reference for the placement of the continuous wave Doppler cursor in the flow signals, unlike pulsed Doppler. This improves the speed and accuracy at which the continuous wave Doppler examination can be conducted.

Color Doppler does have limitations in displaying the flow patterns occurring in the heart. Care must be taken to view the flow patterns in multiple imaging planes to

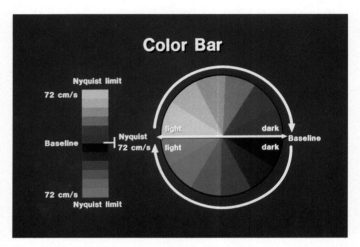

Figure 1-6   The color bar and color aliasing. The color or calibration bar is divided into different levels of color brightness when velocity is calibrated in terms of intensity. The brightest step is assigned the maximum measurable velocity or the Nyquist limit, and the lowest velocity or no velocity is assigned to the color black or no color. The velocities lower than the Nyquist limit are then assigned to a color brightness level between the brightest step and no color, depending on the number of brightness levels used by that specific color Doppler system. In general, when the flow has velocities lower than the Nyquist limit, the brightest color or the highest velocities are displayed at the center of the flow, and the darkest colors or the lower velocities are displayed in the outer portion of the flow. When the flow is aliased or has velocities higher than the Nyquist limit, low velocity signals or the darkest colors are displayed surrounded by high velocity signals or the brightest colors. This reversed flow pattern results because the velocities are indicated by the reversed colors or, in other words, a complete "wrap-around" of the color or calibration bar has occurred. This "wrap-around" is better understood by looking at this pattern in terms of a circle. A circle of colors can be formed by taking the colors forming the color bar and matching colors at the end of the bar together as shown. The direction of the flow, either toward or away from the transducer, determines the direction to move around the circle, and the color depicting the displayed velocity is determined by moving around the color circle to the color scaled for that velocity. If the velocity is greater than the Nyquist limit, the color depicting that specific velocity is found by moving more than halfway around the circle of colors into the opposite sequence of intensities. A second "wrap-around" of the color bar or a complete cycle around the color circle occurs when the color Doppler displays flow patterns with velocities greater than twice the Nyquist limit. In this case, the higher velocities or the brightest colors appear inside the aliased portion of the flow and correspond to the color intensities that indicate the high and low velocities in the primary flow. This results in a flow pattern with the brightest colors surrounded by the darkest colors, which are surrounded in turn by the brightest colors.

obtain a three-dimensional estimate of the size and shape of a given flow jet. Also, the transducer must be positioned as parallel as possible to the flow direction to reduce the incident angle and allow more reliable flow information to be obtained.

The color Doppler display depends on the sector angle used to spatially display the flow information and the analysis of the scan lines to form this image. The scan lines partitioning the sector image indicate the directions of the ultrasonic transmission beams used to develop the image and the angles between the flow direction and the ultrasonic beam (Fig. 1-7). These incident angles vary across the sector image, and the direction used to analyze the scan lines varies. These varying angles cause a uniform velocity flow jet to be erroneously depicted by Doppler color flow mapping as having different velocities at various positions in the flow. An ideal color Doppler system must be developed to display the true flow velocities during a real-time study by internally angle-correcting the velocities along each individual scan line in the sector image.

The techniques of color Doppler echocardiography are mastered by first gaining expertise in 2D echocardiography, and second, obtaining a good understanding of the basic Doppler principles and acquiring experience with conventional pulsed and continuous wave Doppler echocardiography. After these are achieved, the echocardiographer is ready to learn the principles of color Doppler and then to develop expertise and experience in recognizing various normal and abnormal cardiac flow patterns. In addition, the echocardiographer must know the capabilities of his color Doppler system to find the optimal instrument setting combinations that provide the most accurate and reliable flow information.

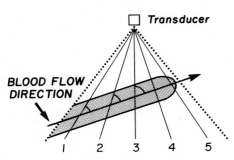

Figure 1-7 Effect of the ultrasonic beam scanning on uniform flow velocity. The color Doppler display depends on the sector angle used to spatially display the flow information and the analysis of the scan lines to form this image. The scan lines partitioning the sector image indicate the directions of the ultrasonic transmission beams used to develop the image and the angles between the flow direction and the ultrasonic beam. These incident angles vary across the sector image as shown by the angles subtended by the flow direction and the lines 1 through 5, and the direction used to analyze the scan lines varies. When the incident angle is approximately equal to zero or the ultrasonic beam is aligned parallel to the direction of the flow in the sample (i.e., as for line 1), the flow information is measured directly and their measured values do not need to be angle-corrected. When the angle is large (i.e., as for line 3), an incorrect alignment causes the direction of the flow not to be aligned directly with the beam. This causes the flow information such as the velocity in the flow to be underestimated, and to obtain the actual magnitude of the velocity of the flow, the measured velocity must be angle-corrected. Angle correction, however, does not work if the incident angle is very large. These varying angles and analysis directions cause a uniform velocity flow jet to be erroneously depicted by color Doppler flow mapping as having different velocities at various positions in the flow. An ideal color Doppler system must be developed to display the true flow velocities during a real-time study by internally angle-correcting the velocities along each individual scan line in the sector image.

REFERENCES

1. Baker, D.W.: Pulsed ultrasound Doppler blood-flow sensing. I.E.E.E. Trans. Son. Ultrason. su-17:170, 1970.
2. Baker, D.W., Rubenstein, S.A., and Lorch, G.S.: Pulsed Doppler echocardiography: Principle and application. Am. J. Med. 63:69, 1977.
3. Brandestini, M.A., Howard, E.A., Weile, E.B., Stevenson, J.G., and Eyer, M.K.: The synthesis of echo and Doppler in M-mode and sectorscan. Proc. Ann. Mtg. Am. Inst. Ultrasound in Med. 125, 1979.
4. Angelsen, B.A.J., and Kristoffersen, K.: On ultrasonic MTI measurement of velocity profiles in blood flow. I.E.E.E. Trans. Biomed. Eng. BME-26:665, 1979.
5. Namekawa, K., Kasai C., Koyano, A.: Imaging of blood flow using auto correlation. Ultrasound Med. Biol. 8(Supp. 1):138, 1982.
6. Miyatake, K., Okamoto, M., Kinosita, N., Izumi, S., Owa, M., Takao S., Sakakibara, H., and Nimura, Y.: Clinical applications of a new type of real-time two-dimensional flow imaging system. Am. J. Cardiol. 54:857, 1984.
7. Kasai, C., Namekawa, K., Koyano, A., and Omoto, R.: Real-time two-dimensional blood flow imaging using an autocorrelation technique. I.E.E.E. Trans. Son. Ultrason. SU-32:458, 1985.
8. Bommer, W.J.: Basic principles of flow imaging. Echocardiography 2:501, 1985.
9. Durrell, M., and Nanda, N.C.: Doppler color flow mapping. In N.C. Nanda (ed): Doppler Echocardiography, New York, Igaku-Shoin, p. 515, 1985.
10. Omoto, R., and Kasai, C.: Basic principles of Doppler color flow imaging. Echocardiography 3:463, 1986.
11. Tamura, T., Yoganathan, A., and Sahn, D.J.: In vitro methods for studying the accuracy of velocity determination and spatial resolution of a color flow mapping system. Am. Heart J. 114:152, 1987.
12. Gesserk, J.M., and Moore, G.W.: Color flow imaging display modes and data acquisition parameters. Echocardiography 4:375, 1987.
13. Lobodzinski, S.M., Loevenskiold, T., Gjevra, K., Ginzton, L., and Laks, M.M.: Computer processing of color Doppler images. Conference on color Doppler flow mapping, October 1987.
14. Aggarwal, K.K., Philpot, E.F., Moos, S., Yoganathan, A.P., and Nanda, N.C.: Color Doppler flow mapping: Intra and inter-machine variability for low flow velocities in an in vitro model (Abstract). J. Am Coll. Cardiol., 11:98A, 1988.
15. Aggarwal, K.K., Nanda, N.C., Moos, S., Philpot, E.F., Helmcke, F., Kandath, D., and Yoganathan, A.P.: Comparison of amplitude and velocity modes in low flow states by color Doppler (Abstract), Ibid.
16. Schott, J.R., Moos, S., Raqueno, R., Ghosh, A., and Nanda, N.C.: Feasibility analysis of 3-dimensional reconstruction of color Doppler flow velocities (Abstract). J. Am. Coll. Cardiol.:165A, 1987.
17. Ghosh, A., Schott, J.R., Moos, S., and Nanda, N.C.: Merging color Doppler imaging with 4-dimensional echocardiogram reconstruction (Abstract). J. Am. Coll. Cardiol. 9:111A, 1987.

Section 2

NORMAL

NORMAL COLOR DOPPLER EXAMINATION

For comprehensive assessment of normal color Doppler flow patterns, echocardiographic examination must be conducted using the optimal instrument settings for imaging and analysis in multiple planes on the available color Doppler systems. These optimal instrument settings provide the maximum amount of flow information, and the imaging in multiple planes gives a complete 3D picture of the flow patterns occurring in the heart. This helps the examiner to evaluate cardiac lesions in a comprehensive manner. This section describes the flow patterns observed in a normally functioning heart. The examiner must understand these flow patterns to detect any abnormalities in their appearance that would indicate the presence of a cardiac lesion.

A 2D echocardiographic examination conducted in a healthy individual using the standard parasternal long axis view shows flow signals during diastole moving from the left atrium (LA) through the mitral valve (MV) into the left ventricle (LV) and turning toward the left ventricular outflow tract (LVOT). During systole, flow signals are observed moving from the LV into the aorta through the open aortic leaflets. No signals are seen moving into the LA through the closed MV. Aliasing can sometimes be observed when the Nyquist limit is lower than the maximum velocity in the flow. For example, if the peak velocity during systole is 0.60 m/sec and the Nyquist limit for that particular study is only 0.39 m/sec, aliasing will occur. When the transducer is angled slightly, the pulmonary venous inflow into the LA also can sometimes be delineated.

Depending on the orientation of the cardiac structure in the imaging plane, the flow signals will appear either as red or blue in color. The red color signifies that the flow is moving towards the transducer and the blue color means that it is moving away. For example, with a low parasternal imaging plane, flow signals moving into the aorta and the LVOT are blue during systole because of the posterior orientation of the aorta and the LVOT. With a standard long axis plane, the flow signals in the LVOT are red during systole and blue during diastole because the aorta and the left ventricular outflow (LVO) are oriented anteriorly during systole and posteriorly during diastole.

Short axis views at the level of the aortic root often display red signals moving from the RA into the right ventricle (RV) (and toward the transducer) through the open tricuspid valve (TV) during diastole. Careful angulation of the transducer allows the examiner to see the inferior vena cava (IVC) and red signals moving from it into the RA. During atrial systole, blue signals may be seen moving from the RA into the IVC (and away from the transducer). Blue signals can also be observed moving from the right ventricular outflow tract (RVOT) into the pulmonary artery through the open pulmonary valve leaflets during systole. With further angulation of the transducer, blue antegrade flow signals can be seen moving into the proximal left and right branches of the main pulmonary artery during systole. The pulmonary vein openings are not easily delineated by 2D examination using the short axis view, but flow moving from these veins into the LA can be seen in this imaging plane, helping to define their openings into the LA. An examination of both the right and left atrial appendages may show flow signals entering these areas during ventricular systole and exiting into the body of the respective atrium during atrial systole. In some patients, flow signals may be shown in the right main coronary artery, in the entire extent of the left main coronary artery, and in the proximal left anterior descending and circumflex branches. Relatively high-velocity signals of flow acceleration may be visualized in the aortic root directly opposite the orifices of both the right and left main coronary arteries. These flow acceleration signals represent a localized area of high velocity flow near where a considerably smaller vessel branches off from a larger vessel or where the flow moves into another chamber through a relatively narrow orifice or channel (Fig. 2-1). These signals in this imaging plane may help in detecting the origin of the right or left main coronary artery. Care must be taken in using this plane not to mistake superimposed flow from the adjacent main pulmonary artery for coronary artery blood flow.

A diastolic short axis view at the level of the MV may show flow signals in the open mitral orifice and the RV. Transducer angulation to obtain the right ventricular inflow plane may reveal prominent flow signals moving from the coronary sinus into the right heart during diastole.

The apical 4-chamber view is useful to view flow signals moving from the atria through the atrio-ventricular valves into both ventricles. These flow signals tend to appear first in the RV and then in the LV during diastole because the TV opens a little earlier than the MV. This may not always be evident on color 2D examination because of the use of slow frame rates, which cause inaccuracies in timing flow events. In general, during diastole, flow signals turn red in color as they move from the atria into the respective ventricles (and toward the transducer). In late diastole, the flow signals tend to swirl superiorly in the direction of the aortic root and thus turn blue in color. During ventricular systole, the flow signals in the LV also move medially and superiorly toward the outflow tract and hence turn blue in color. Similar findings are observed in the apical long axis view except that blue flow signals are clearly seen entering the aortic root during systole.

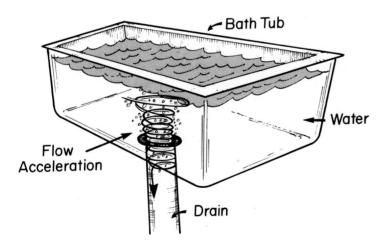

Figure 2-1 Flow acceleration. A simple example of the generation of flow acceleration can be shown by observing the draining of water from a household bathtub. Flow acceleration or a localized area of high velocity develops as the large body of water moves toward the "hole" or opening in the bottom of the tub through which water flows into the drain. Adjacent to the "hole," the area of flow acceleration becomes smaller and tends to take the shape and size of the circular "hole." This finding has clinical significance. For example, in a patient with mitral regurgitation, inspection of the size and shape of the flow acceleration present adjacent to the mitral valve (MV) may provide a good estimate of the size of the anatomical defect in the MV through which the regurgitation is occurring.

The subcostal imaging plane is used to define the flow patterns in the hepatic veins (HVs) and the IVC. Antegrade blue signals are seen moving from the hepatic veins into the RA during ventricular diastole and systole. During atrial systole, however, retrograde flow is observed moving from the RA into the IVC and the HVs. Angling the transducer to the left from the IVC position causes the abdominal aorta to be visualized. Prominent pulsatile flow signals are seen within its lumen during systole. The subcostal 4-chamber view shows flow signals moving away from the atria into the respective ventricles during diastole and flow signals moving from the LV posteriorly toward the aortic root during systole. In patients with a good subcostal window, the subcostal right ventricular inflow-apical-outflow plane can be used to observe flow signals in the right heart. This imaging plane shows flow signals moving from the RA to the RV and then through the pulmonary valve into the main pulmonary artery. Flow signals in the right ventricular apex can also be observed. The transducer can be angled in this view to visualize flow signals moving from the superior vena cava (SVC) into the RA.

A suprasternal examination performed with the transducer placed in the suprasternal notch or supraclavicular region in a patient placed supine with the head turned to one side is useful in visualizing flows in the great vessels. In the suprasternal long axis plane, prominent flow signals are seen moving superiorly into the ascending aorta and arch and then directed inferiorly into the descending aorta. Branches of the aortic arch are also visualized, and prominent flow signals can often be seen moving into them with appropriate transducer angulation. The neck vessels are easily detected using the suprasternal or supraclavicular color Doppler examination because flow signals in these vessels can be seen even though the vessels themselves are not clearly outlined by 2D imaging. After these prominent flow signals have been detected, the transducer can be angled in various directions to outline the vessel's walls and the lumen more completely. In the suprasternal short axis plane, the aortic arch, right pulmonary artery, SVC, and flow signals in these vessels are clearly visualized. Pulmonary venous flow is also visualized in the LA. Transducer manipulation may show flow signals moving in the main and left pulmonary arteries and flow signals moving from the azygos vein into the SVC. Antegrade flow in the ascending aorta is observed moving toward the transducer as red signals, while antegrade flow in the descending aorta is directed away from the transducer and hence is blue in color.

The right parasternal examination, performed with the patient in the right lateral decubitus position, provides one of the best views, especially in adults, of the entrance of the SVC into the RA. This entrance can also be delineated in children and adults with good subcostal windows using the subcostal view. Flow in the IVC can be seen using the right parasternal imaging plane entering into the RA often through the Eustachian valve. Manipulation of the transducer also allows the examiner to visualize flow signals entering into the LA from all the pulmonary veins, even though the pulmonary vein openings are not clearly delineated. Two discrete red jets representing anteriorly directed flow are observed entering the LA from the left superior and inferior pulmonary veins and two discrete blue jets representing posteriorly directed flow are observed moving from the right superior and inferior pulmonary veins into the LA. Identification of these four jets originating from the four pulmonary veins excludes the presence of anomalous pulmonary venous drainage. The atrial septum (AS), clearly visualized in this view, can be seen extending from the entrance of SVC into the RA to the entrance of the IVC. This allows any defect in the sinus venosus, fossa ovalis, or basal portion of the AS to be delineated. In addition, the flow signals moving through a septal defect tend to be parallel to the ultrasound beam using this view. This results in a more reliable assessment of the defect. The coronary sinus and flow signals moving from it into the RA can also be observed by angling the transducer in this plane. The LV may also be viewed in this plane in some patients, and all three leaflets of the TV can be viewed in short axis view in this plane by rotating the transducer to obtain a short axis view of the RV.

Large left pleural effusion, thoracic descending aortic aneurysm, or mediastinal masses may displace the lungs, allowing acoustic access to various cardiac structures and chambers from the posterior aspect. Therefore, in these patients, the transducer can be positioned in the posterior intercostal spaces with the patient turned in the left or right lateral decubitus position to examine the cardiac structures through the back wall.

The described flow patterns have been characterized as they would appear using the velocity mode on available color Doppler systems. The power mode can be also used to observe flow occurring in a heart, especially low-velocity flows such as occur in the LA. These low-velocity flows may be visualized more clearly using this mode by decreasing the reject setting and increasing the gain setting. This setting change, however, may introduce noise into the examination, making the flow signals hard to distinguish. The power mode is available only on some commercial color Doppler systems.

Normal cardiac flows cannot be accurately timed by 2D color Doppler because of its slow frame rate. Color M-mode, however, is ideal for this because of its rapid frame rate. Timing the flow events requires a fast frame rate because a slower frame rate may cause overlapping of the flow events. A color M-mode examination is conducted by placing the cursor through the observed flow signals and then evaluating the flow occurring along the cursor using an autocorrelation technique. This has been found useful in accurately assessing the timing of flow signals in cardiac chambers and vessels such as both the left and right coronary arteries and the SVC and IVC.

REFERENCES

1. Omoto, R. (ed): Color Atlas of Real-time Two-dimensional Doppler Echocardiography. Philadelphia, Lea and Febiger, 1984.
2. Miyatake, K., Okamoto, M., Kinoshita, N., Izumi, S., Owa, M., Takao, S., Sakakibara, H., and Nimura, Y.: Clinical application of a new type of real-time two-dimensional Doppler flow imaging system. Am. J. Cardiol. 54:857, 1984.
3. Schoenfel, M.R.: Color-coded, real-time, two-dimensional Doppler echocardiographic mapping of intracardiac blood flow. J. Cardiovasc. Ultrason. 4:3, 1985.
4. Sahn, D.J.: Real-time two-dimensional Doppler echocardiographic flow mapping. Circulation 71:849, 1985.
5. Switzer, D.F., and Nanda, N.D.: Doppler color flow mapping. Ultrasound Med. Biol. 11:403, 1985.
6. Switzer, D.F., and Nanda, N.C.: Color Doppler echocardiography: The new frontier. Cardiol. Prod. News 5:1, 1985.
7. Stewart, W.J., Levine, R.A., Main, J., and King, M.E.: Initial experience with color-coded Doppler flow mapping. Echocardiography 2:511, 1985.
8. Nanda, N.C. Case Studies in Color Doppler Echocardiography. New York, Igaku-Shoin Medical Publishers, Inc., 1985.
9. Switzer, D.F., and Nanda, N.C.: Color-coded Doppler flow mapping. CARDIO 3:18, 1986.
10. DeMaria, A.N., Smith, M., Branco, M., and Kwan, O.L.: Normal and abnormal blood flow patterns by color Doppler flow imaging. Echocardiography 3:475, 1986.
11. Perry, G.P., and Nanda, N.C.: Color Doppler echocardiography. Int. J. Cardiac Imaging (in press, 1988).
12. Nanda, N.C., Hsiung, M.C., Helmcke, F., Goyal, R.G., Kan, M.N., and Cooper, J.: Color Doppler detection of flow in coronary arteries (Abstract). Clin. Res. 35:308A, 1987.
13. Kyo, S., Takamoto, S., Matsumura, M., Yokote, Y., and Omoto, R.: Color flow mapping visualization of coronary blood flow using transesophageal transducer (Abstract). Proceedings of the 49th Meeting of the Japan Society of Ultrasonics in Medicine, 247, 1986.
14. Recusani, F., Valdes-Cruz, I.M., Sahn, D.J., and Hoit, B.: Detection of coronary flow by pulsed Doppler and color Doppler flow mapping and its differentiation from pulmonary insufficiency (Abstract). J. Am. Coll. Cardiol. 7:14A, 1986.

SECTION 2 NORMAL

Normal color Doppler flow patterns in various echo planes (left parasternal, apical, subcostal, right parasternal, and suprasternal/supraclavicular) are demonstrated in this section.

Figure N-1 **Long axis view.** (A–D) Flow signals (red) are visualized moving from the LA into the LV through the MV in diastole. In the LVOT, the flow signals take on blue color because they are directed away from the transducer. The small area of red signals completely surrounded by blue represents aliasing owing to the low Nyquist limit of 0.39 m/sec. Red signals (flow toward the transducer) in the RV represent flow moving toward the PA in diastole. During systole (E), the LVO and the aorta move anteriorly, and hence the flow signals take on a red color. Scattered blue signals within the red represent aliasing. Examination from a low parasternal transducer position (F,G,H) shows red diastolic mitral inflow signals (flow toward the transducer), but the systolic signals in the LVO and aortic root are colored blue (flow away from the transducer) due to their posterior orientation in this imaging plane. In some instances, power mode examination (I) may aid in better visualization of the flow signals. Color M-mode examination (J–N), because of its rapid frame rate, is more accurate than color 2D examination in timing flow events in the cardiac cycle.

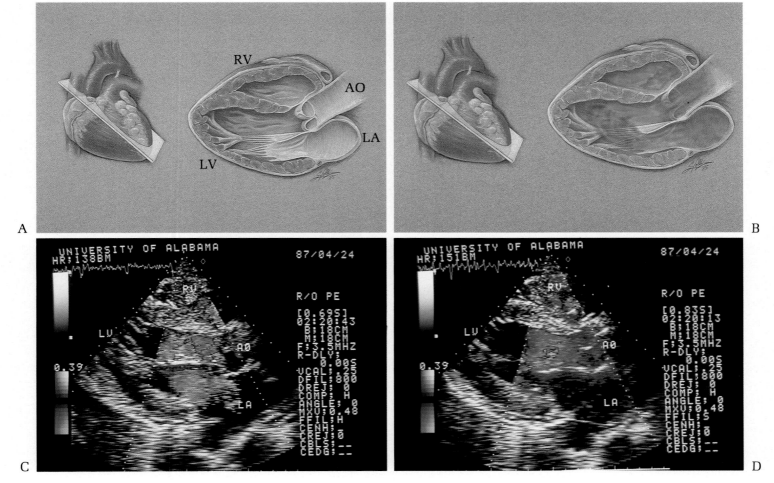

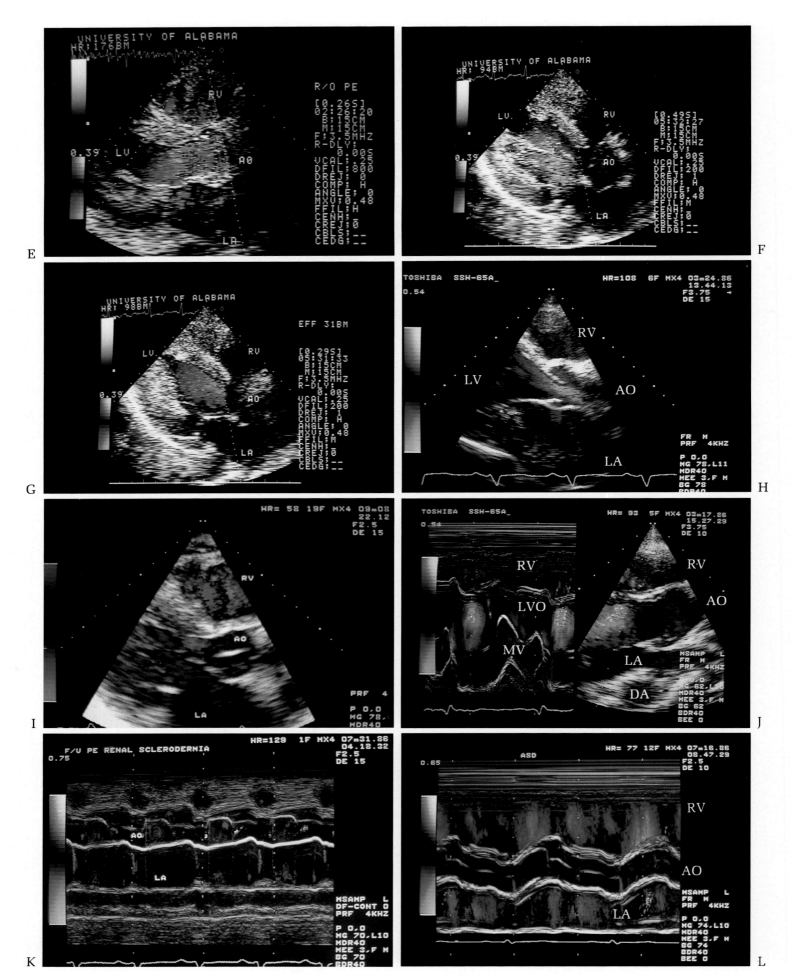

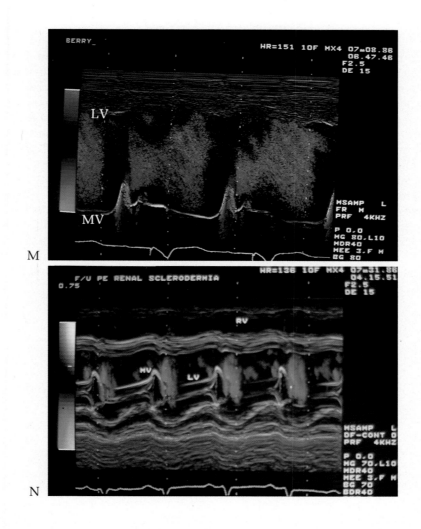

M

N

Figure N-2   **Aortic short axis view.** (A–K) Flow signals (red) are visualized moving from the IVC into the RA and then through the open TV into the RV during diastole. During atrial systole, flow signals move in a retrograde direction into the IVC from the RA (H). Discrete narrow bands of flow signals (PV, F) in the LA (red and blue) in E and F represent pulmonary venous inflow. Their origin helps to identify the openings of the PVs into the LA that are generally not visualized on 2D examination. Color M-mode examination of the IVC in K reveals the presence of flow signals in it throughout the cardiac cycle. The examination of the RVOT (power mode, L) demonstrates anteriorly directed red signals taking up blue color as they move posteriorly toward the PA during systole. Systolic interrogation of the PA by color 2D, M-mode, and pulse Doppler (M–P) reveals posteriorly directed (blue) normal antegrade flow. B = Doppler baseline, SV = position of sample volume, F = flow signals. The red and yellow signals (AL) completely surrounded by blue in O and P represent mild aliasing. Q and R represent color M-mode studies that show retrograde flow in the PA and RVO (red signals) during pulmonary valve closure and later in diastole related to mild PR (arrows), often seen in apparently normal subjects. The systolic reddish-yellow signals completely surrounded by blue in the RVO and PA in Q are due to aliasing.

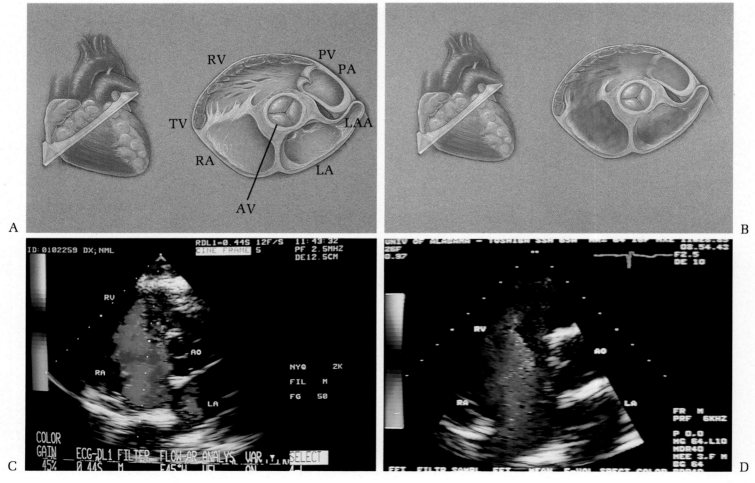

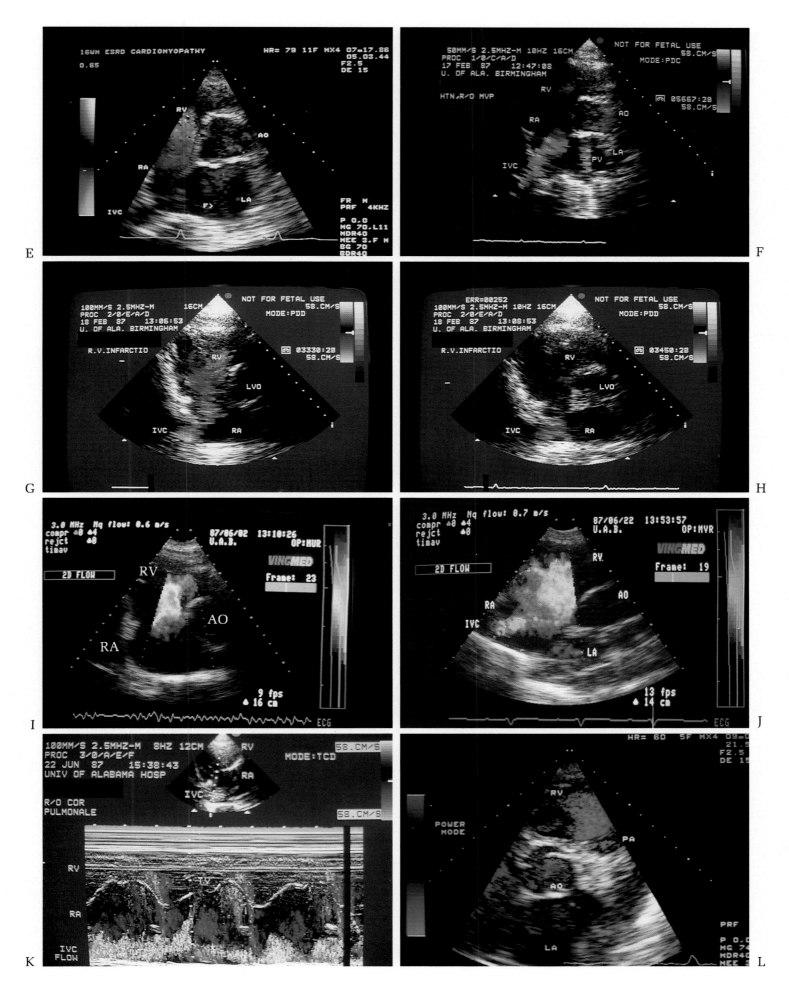

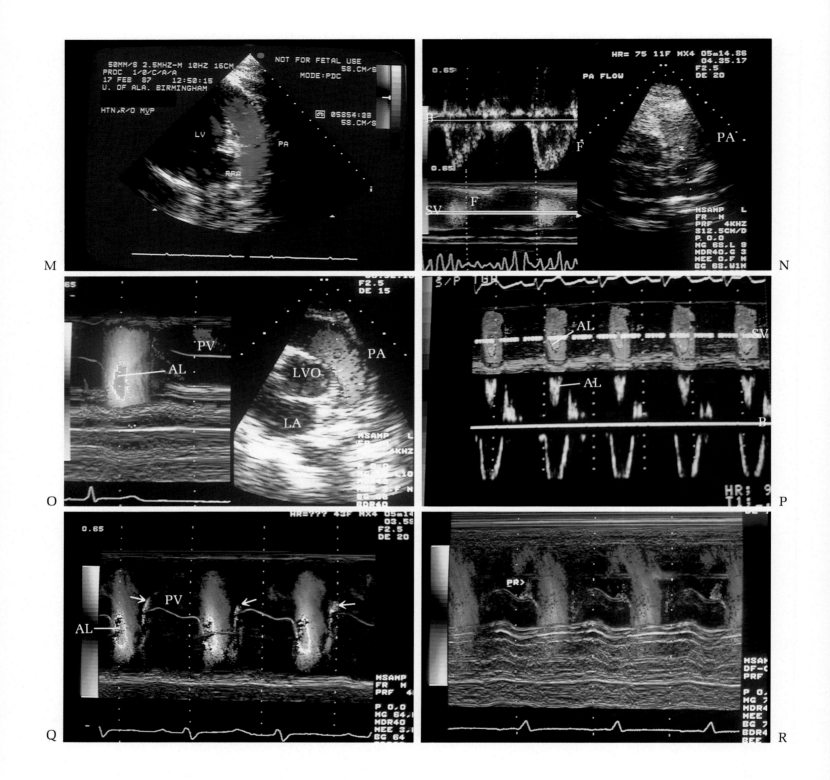

Figure N-3 **Aortic short axis view: Examination of the pulmonary arteries.** (A–G) Color Doppler examination demonstrates posteriorly directed (blue) antegrade flow in the MPA and its proximal RPA and LPA branches.

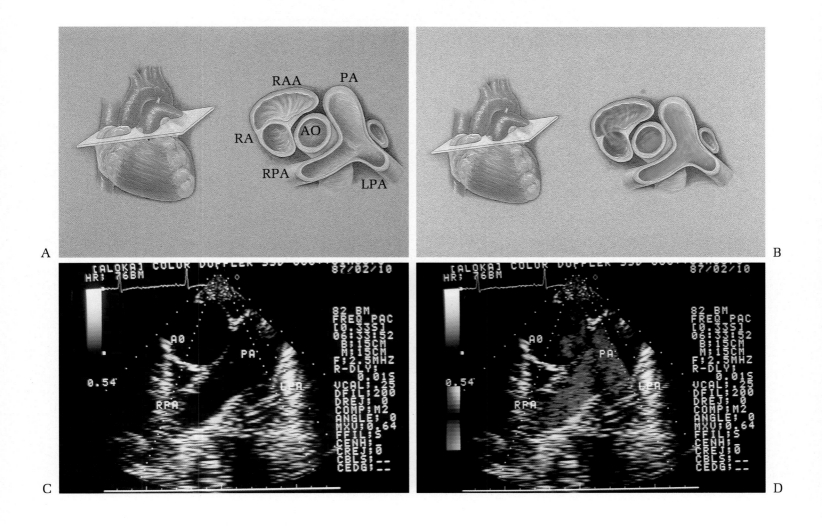

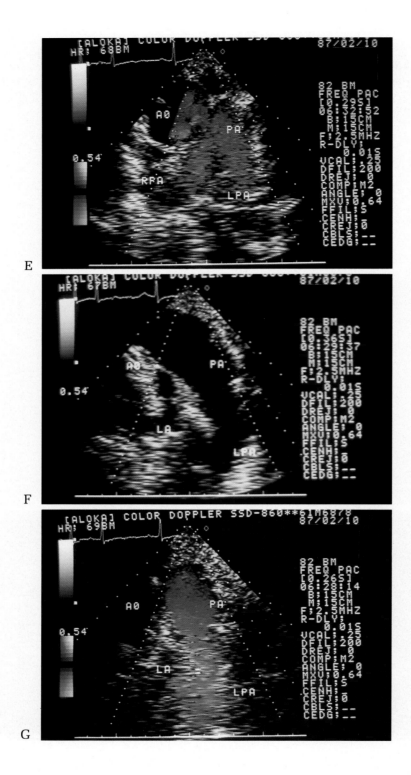

E

F

G

Figure N-4   **Aortic short axis view: Examination of the atrial appendages.** (A–H) The high left parasternal transducer approach is useful in delineating the pointed LAA and the relatively more rounded RAA. Flow signals (red) are visualized moving into the RAA during ventricular systole and moving out of it into the RA during late ventricular diastole (G,H).

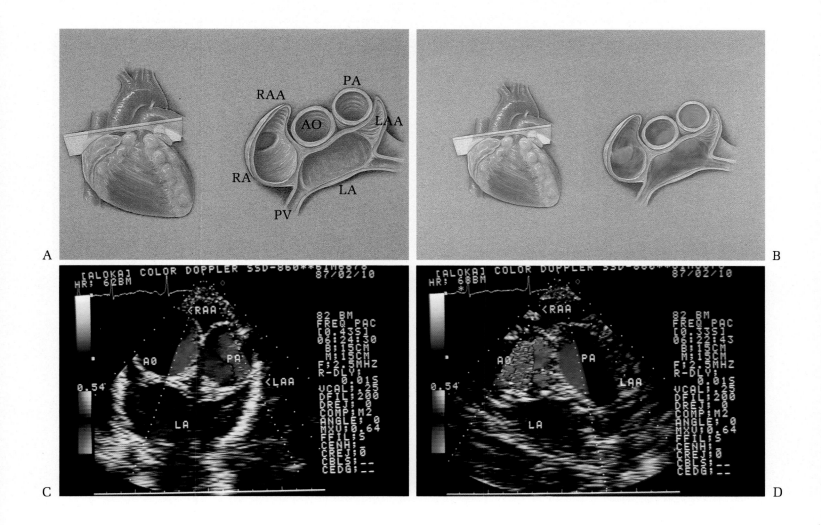

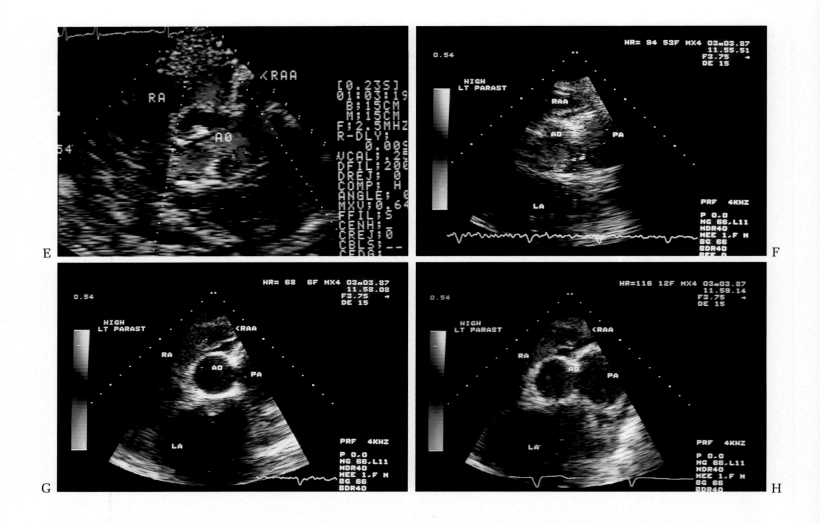

Figure N-5 **Aortic short axis view: Examination of the coronary arteries.** Color Doppler examination (A – F) demonstrates flow signals in the entire LMCA and the proximal LAD and CX branches. Color M-mode (B) and pulse Doppler (C) studies in a 40-year-old man demonstrate late systolic and pandiastolic flows (FL) in the LMCA. B = Doppler baseline. Note the presence of associated mild PR in this patient. Coronary flow patterns may be visualized clearly in some patients in whom the LMCA and its proximal branches are poorly imaged by 2D echocardiography (H,I). The relatively high velocity signals (red in I, blue in A) visualized in the aortic root directly opposite the orifice of the LMCA represent flow acceleration (FA), which may be helpful in searching for the origin of the LMCA during 2D examination. J shows flow signals filling the short LMCA and the proximal LAD branch. Color M-mode examination (K) in a 56-year-old man shows flow signals (red) in the left main coronary artery (LMCA) during diastole. The blue signals visualized in systole represent superimposed pulmonary artery flow. L represents color M-mode examination in another adult, showing flow signals in the LMCA in late systole and early diastole with only minimal superimposition of flow signals (green and yellow) from the adjacent PA in midsystole. The power (amplitude) mode examination (M – P, 51-year-old man) may delineate flow signals in the LMCA (L) and its branches better than regular color Doppler imaging in some patients. The arrow in M points to the LMCA, while the arrow in O denotes the LAD. Q shows flow signals in the proximal RCA, also viewed in the aortic short axis plane in a 40-year-old man.

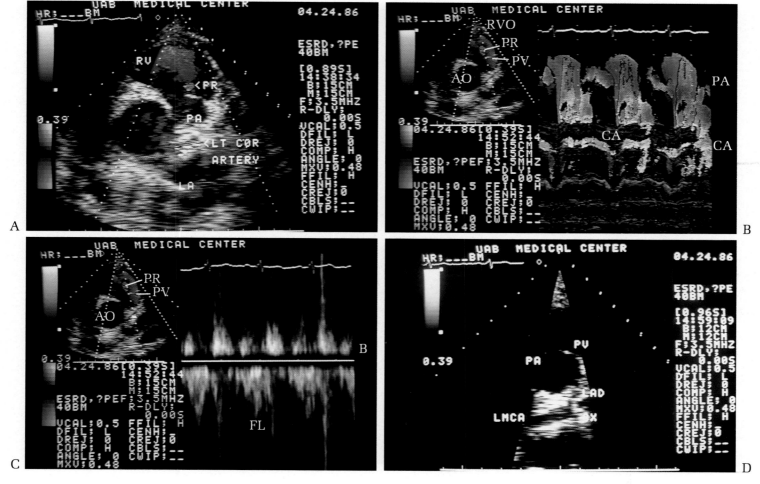

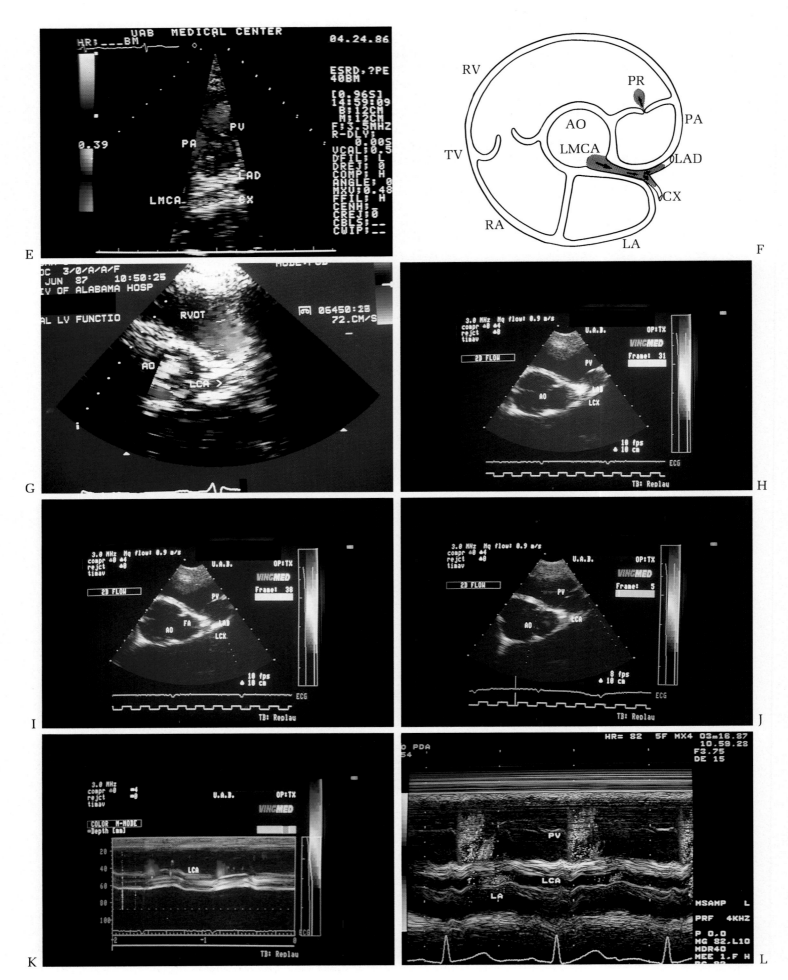

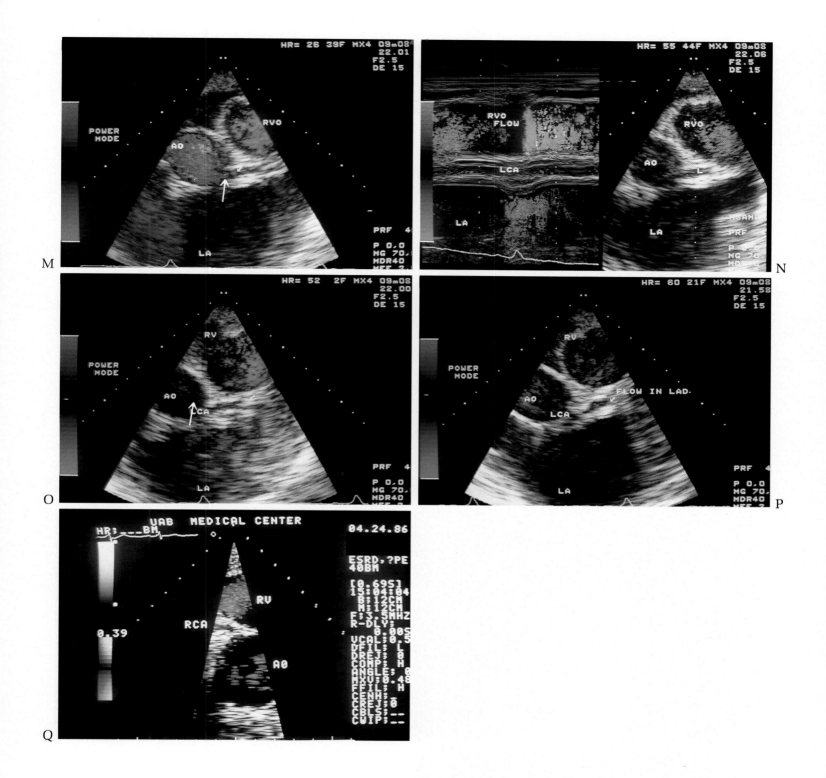

Figure N-6   **Short axis view at the level of the mitral valve.** Color Doppler examination (A,B,C) demonstrates flow signals in the open mitral orifice and in the RV (red). Transducer angulation (RV inflow plane) demonstrates prominent flow signals moving from the coronary sinus (CS) into the RA and RV during diastole (D,E).

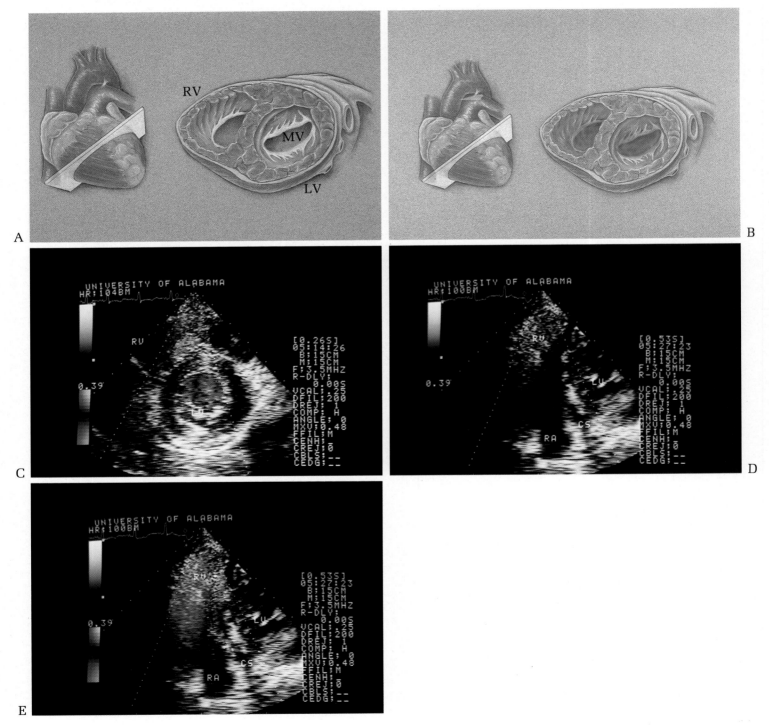

Figure N-7   **Apical 4-chamber plane.** (A–I) During diastole, flow signals (red) are seen moving from the atria through the atrioventricular valves into both ventricles. Because the TV opens slightly earlier than the MV, flow signals tend to appear first in the RV and then in the LV during diastole. This, however, is not often evident during color 2D examination because the frame rates are relatively slow. In E, the bright yellowish-red signals in the LV indicate higher velocities in the left heart, while the dull red signals in the RV are related to lower velocities in the right heart. In G, the blue signals present within the reddish-yellow signals represent aliasing. In H (power mode examination) and I (low reject), the flow signals outline well most of the LV endocardium. During systole (J–M), blue signals in the LV represent flow directed toward the aortic root. In M (color M-mode), the small area of red signals surrounded by blue signals in the LV represents aliasing. In N (late diastole), flow signals (red) are seen moving from the LA through the open MV into the LV and then swirling around toward the LVOT (blue).

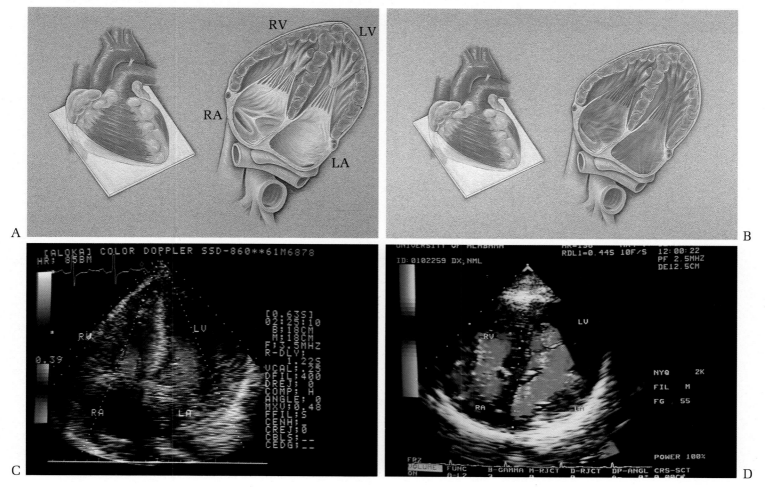

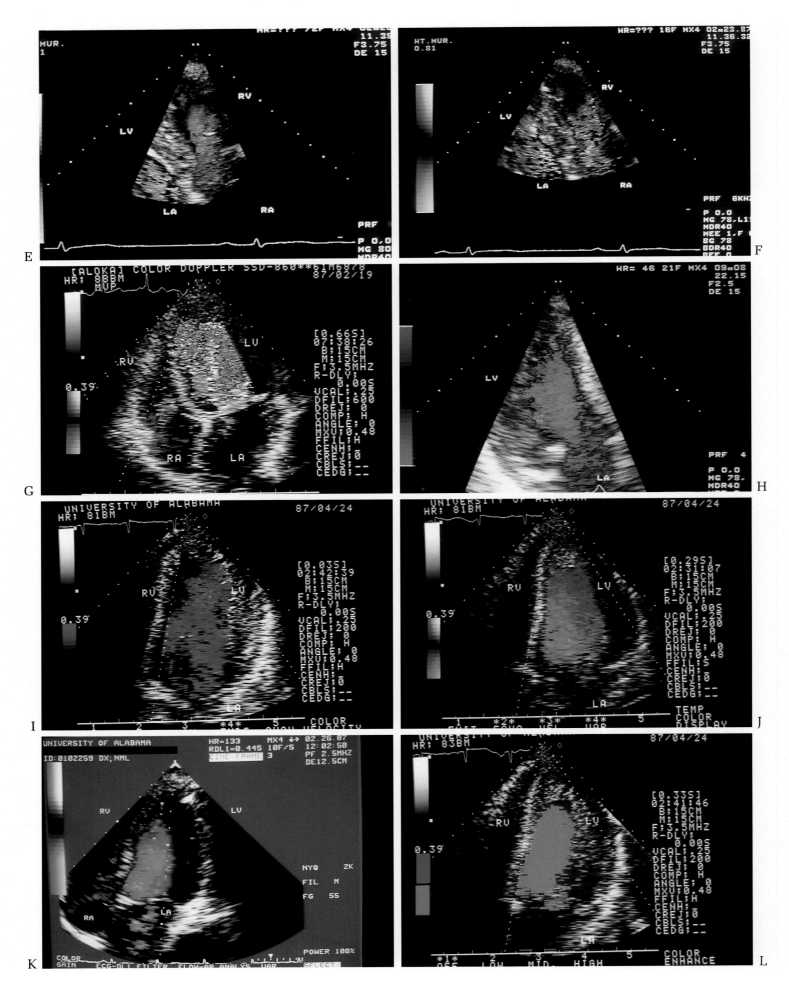

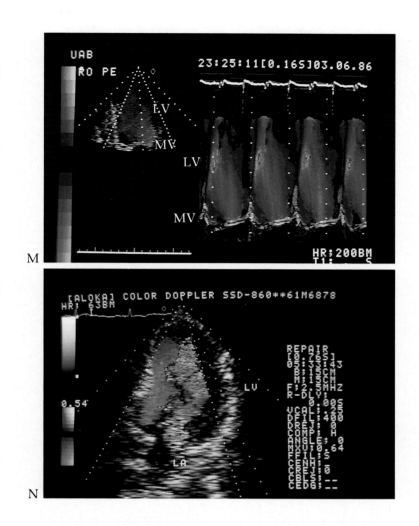

Figure N-8 **Apical 2-chamber view.** In this view (A,B) also, flow signals are seen moving from the LA into the LV (red) and then swirling toward the LVOT (blue). The blue signals within the red signals in the LV are due to aliasing.

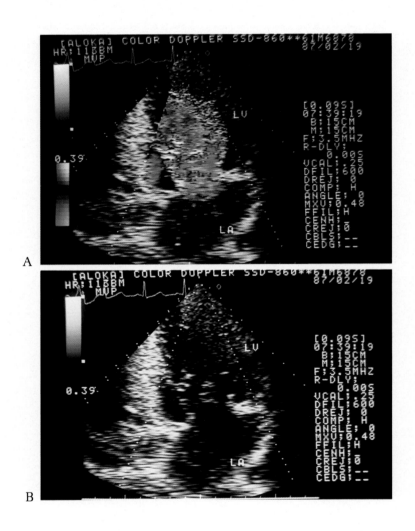

Figure N-9 **Apical long axis view.** (A,B,C) In this view, flow signals are moving from the LA through the open MV into the LV (red) and then are directed toward the aortic root (blue).

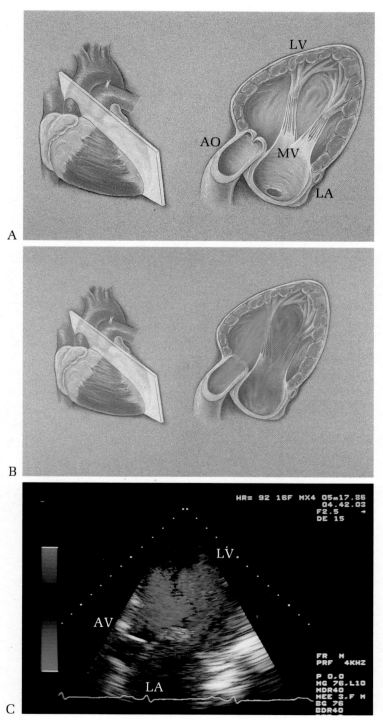

Figure N-10 **Subcostal examination: Inferior vena cava and atrial septum.** Flow signals (blue) are seen moving from the HVs into the IVC (A–E). Here PV = pulmonary vein. Color M-mode examination (F,G,H) demonstrates prominent flow signals in systole (S wave) and diastole (D wave), representing antegrade flow toward the IVC. During atrial systole (G), flow signals (A, red) are seen moving retrogradely and represent flow moving from the RA into the IVC and HVs. Retrograde flow (arrow) in the HVs may also be observed with a premature ventricular contraction (H). In I, the atrial septum (AS) is clearly visualized and the red flow signals in the RA represent flow from the SVC.

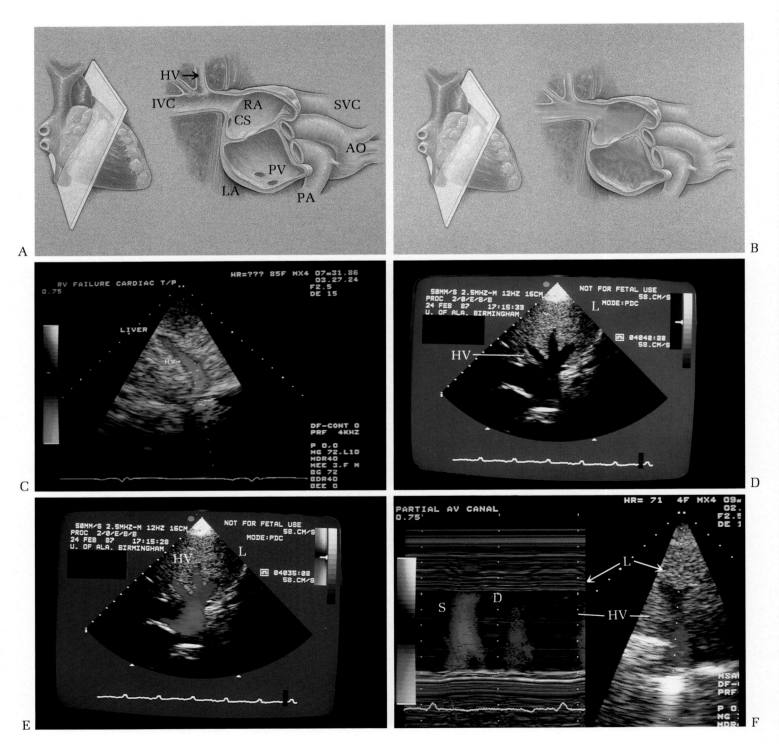

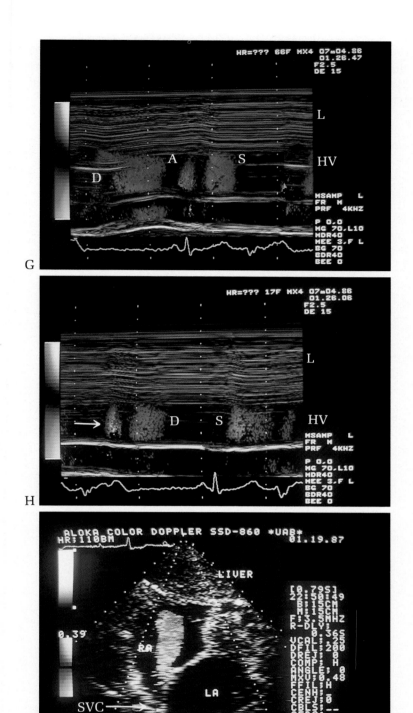

Figure N-11   **Subcostal examination: Examination of the abdominal aorta.** (A,B,C) The abdominal aorta (AA) is visualized to the left of the IVC and prominent flow signals are visualized in its lumen during systole.

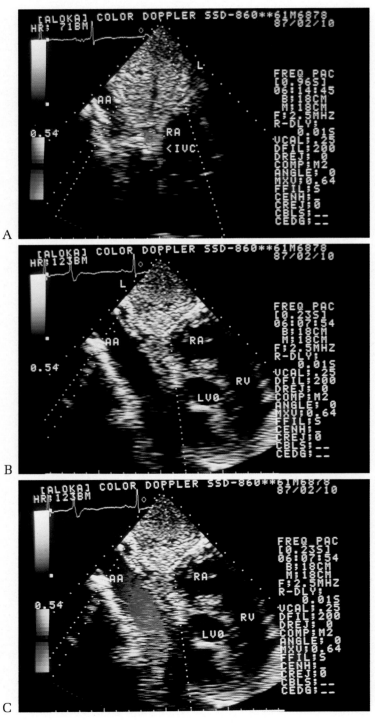

Figure N-12   **Subcostal examination: 4-chamber plane.** (A,B,C) The systolic frame (C) shows prominent flow signals (blue) in the LV moving posteriorly toward the aortic root. Posteriorly directed signals are also seen in the RV.

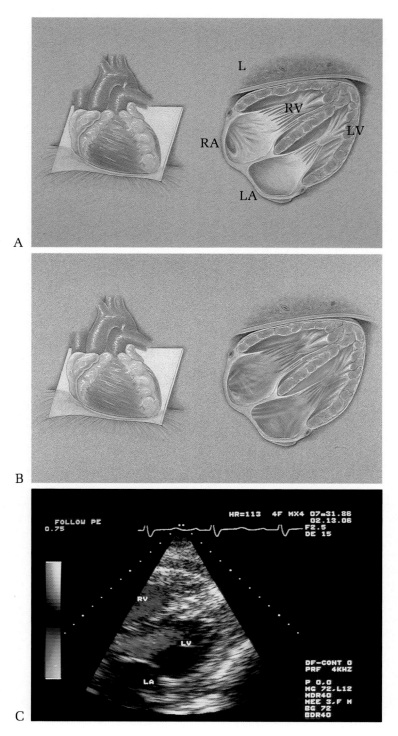

Figure N-13 **Subcostal examination: Long axis plane.** (A,B,C) In this view, the red signals represent mitral inflow and the blue is flow directed toward the aortic root.

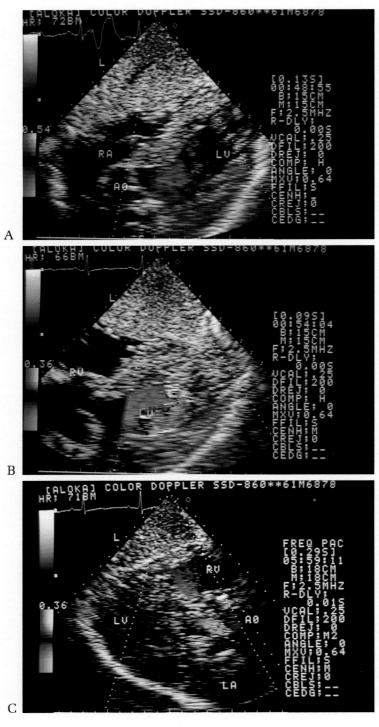

Figure N-14   **Subcostal examination: Short axis plane.** In this view also, flow signals are visualized directed toward (red) and away from (blue) the transducer.

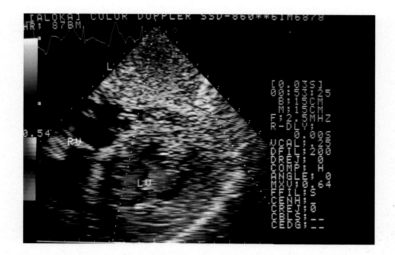

Figure N-15 **Subcostal examination: RV inflow – apical – outflow plane.** (A – H) Flow signals are seen moving from the RA into the RV and then through the PV into the PA. The red signals within the blue in the RVO in F are due to aliasing. In G and H, prominent flow signals are also visualized moving from the SVC into the RA.

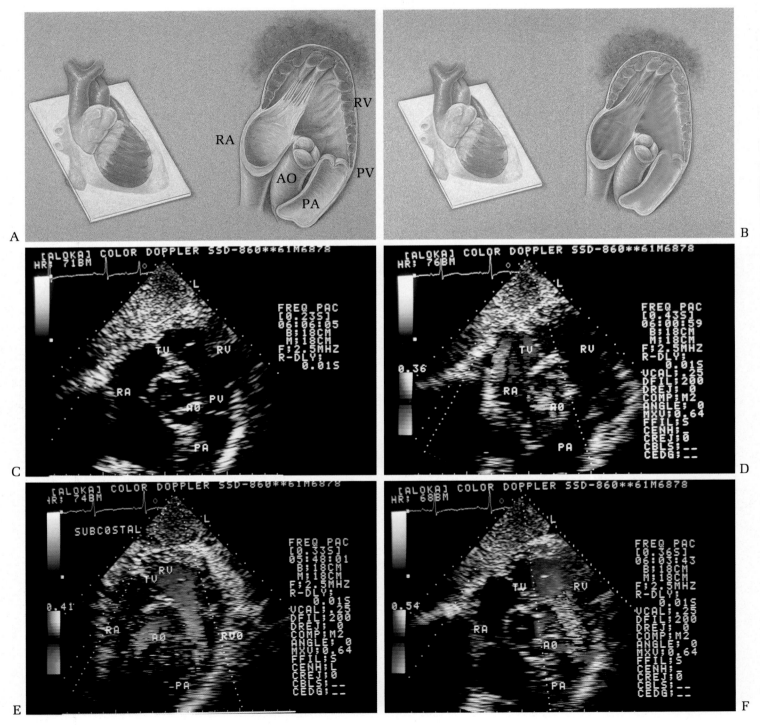

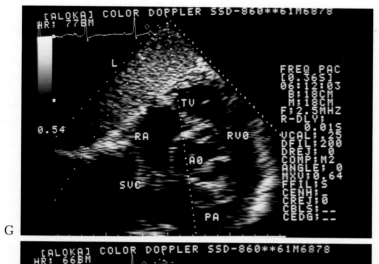

G

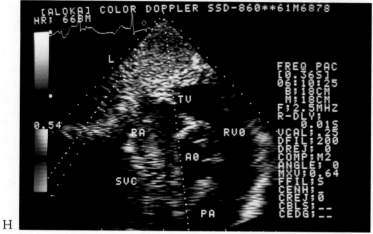

H

Figure N-16 **Suprasternal examination: Long axis plane.** Prominent flow signals are seen moving superiorly into the AA and arch and then directed inferiorly into the DA (A,B). Blue signals within the red in the AA in C represent aliasing. Pulse Doppler and color M-mode examination (D) also show superiorly directed flow in the ascending aorta. Flow signals are seen completely filling the proximal portion of the IA in E. The transducer is slightly angled to the left to demonstrate flow signals in the LPA in F. In this frame (F), red signals in the AA represent superiorly directed flow, while the blue signals in the proximal DA indicate inferiorly directed flow. Scattered blue signals within the red in the AA and red signals within the blue in the proximal DA are due to aliasing (first wrap-around). Virtual nonvisualization of flow signals in the midportion of the aortic arch in G is related to perpendicular orientation of the Doppler ultrasonic beam to the flow direction, resulting in absence of significant Doppler frequency shifts. Blue signals in the IA and red signals inside the blue in the DA represent aliasing. The large black areas seen within the red aliased signals in the proximal DA in H represent velocities close to twice the Nyquist limit. The predominantly blue signals seen inferiorly outside the lateral border of the DA in H and I (arrow) also represent flow signals in another segment of the same vessel, both segments being viewed simultaneously as the DA first courses posteriorly and laterally and then takes up an anatomically medial orientation. Flow patterns in the AA and arch using two different flow maps from the same equipment are shown in J and K. Red aliased signals within the blue in the DA (L) are eliminated (M) by increasing the pulse repetition frequency PRF from 4 KHz to 6 KHz, which raises the Nyquist limit from 0.75 m/sec to 1.13 m/sec. Totally aliased signals (red) in another portion of the DA (arrow, L) are also virtually replaced by blue signals (arrows, M) when the Nyquist limit is raised. Examination of the neck vessels using suprasternal/supraclavicular approaches is aided by color Doppler, which easily detects flow signals even though the vessel is not well visualized by 2D echocardiography. In this example (N), the IA is not well delineated on the 2D image, but pulse Doppler interrogation of the flow signals demonstrates the typical arterial type wave form.

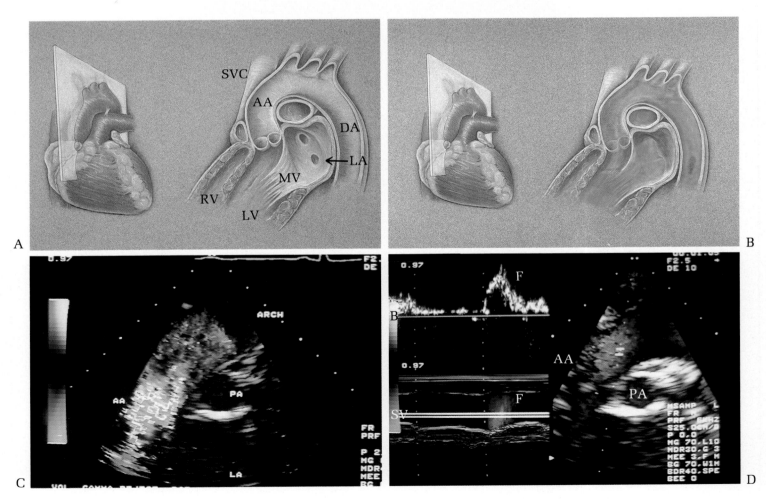

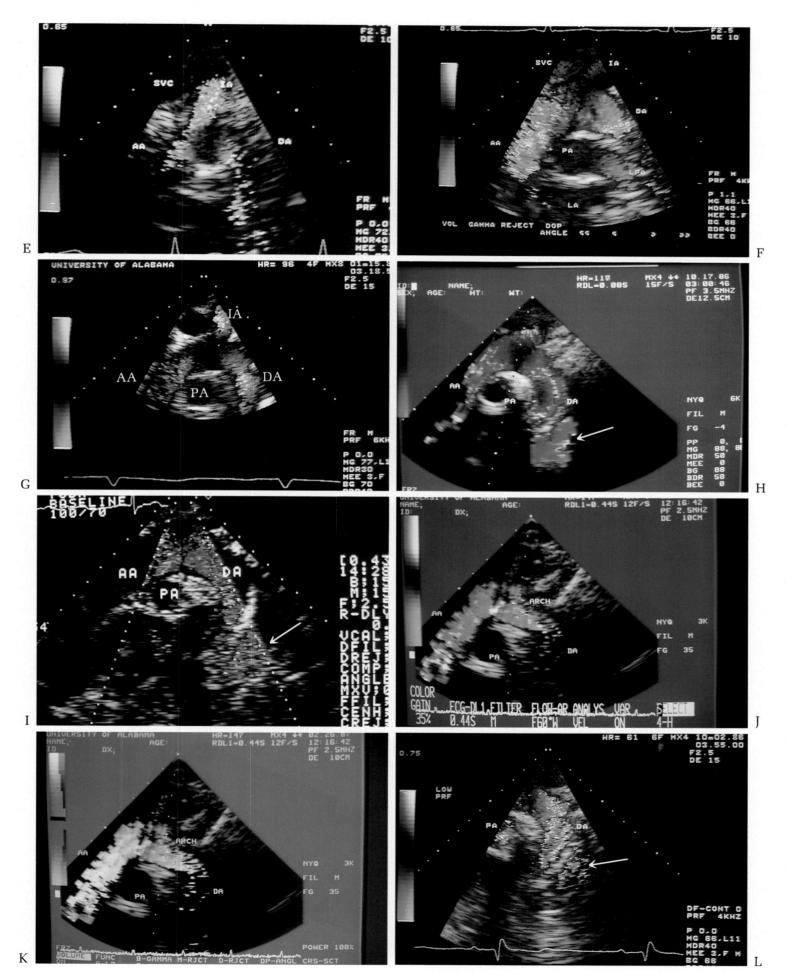

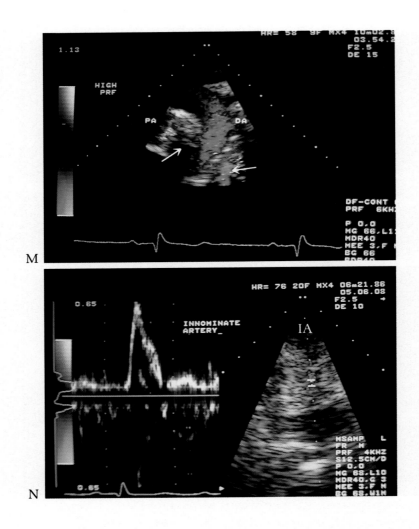

Figure N-17   **Suprasternal examination: Short axis plane.** Flow signals are clearly visualized filling the aortic arch, RPA, and SVC. Pulmonary venous inflow is also visualized in the LA (A,B,C). Careful transducer manipulation in another patient (D) shows flow signals in the MPA and RPA and flow signals moving from the azygos vein into the SVC (E). The mosaic-colored signals visualized in the aortic arch represent turbulence due to aortic stenosis in this patient (D,E). Color 2D and M-mode examination of the SVC (F,G) demonstrate inferiorly directed antegrade flow (S wave and D wave).

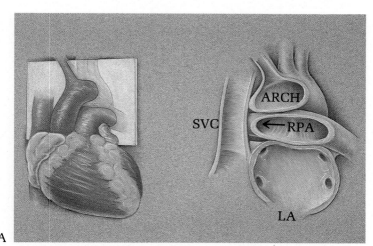

A

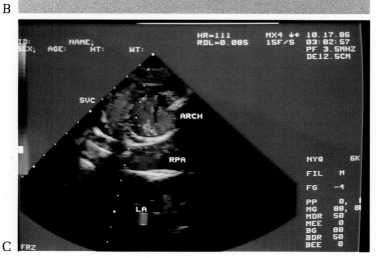

B

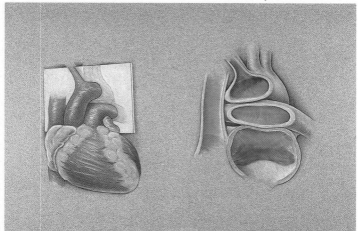

C

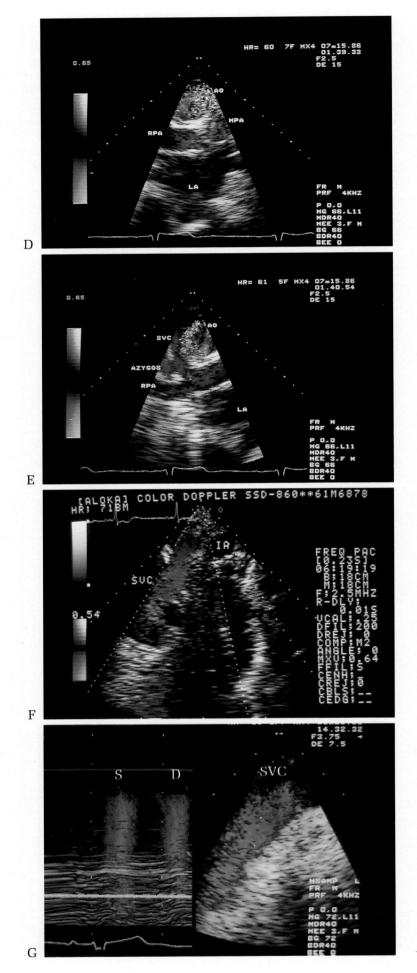

Figure N-18 **Right parasternal examination.** Flow signals are seen moving from the SVC and IVC into the RA and from the PVs into the LA (A,B,C,D,E). CS = coronary sinus; PV = pulmonary vein; EV = eustachian valve, AS = atrial septum. Catheter (C) is clearly visualized in the SVC in F. IVC flow entering the RA through the Eustachian valve EV is clearly shown in G through K. Blue signals in IVC in K represent retrograde flow during atrial systole. Transducer manipulations from the right parasternal approach can also visualize flow signals entering the LA from all the PVs (L,M). PV = pulmonary vein. Two discrete red-yellowish signals represent anteriorly directed flow entering the LA from the left superior and inferior PVs, while the posteriorly directed signals (blue) represent flow from right superior and inferior PVs. Although PV openings are not generally delineated on the 2D images, the sites of origin of the discrete flow signals help to identify their position. Identification of flow jets from all the four PVs excludes the presence of anomalous pulmonary venous connection (L–P). FL = flow. Red signals surrounded by blue in the RA in O are due to aliasing. In Q, R, and S, flow signals are visualized in the DA imaged behind the LA. The blue signals (Q) represent posteriorly directed flow, while the red signals (R,S) indicate anteriorly directed flow in this curved vessel. The mosaic-colored signals in the RA in Q, R, and S are related to turbulence due to TR. In some instances, the LV can also be viewed in this plane in short axis (T) and flow patterns demonstrated in it and in the adjoining chambers. PV = pulmonary valve. In U, the coronary sinus (CS) is visualized and flow signals (red) are seen moving from it into the RA. Superior angulation of the transducer demonstrates flow signals in the AA, aortic arch, and PA (V,W,X). Scattered blue signals in the AA in V and W are due to aliasing. Further leftward angling of the transducer (Y) demonstrates flow signals in the DA and in the LPA. Autopsy specimen (Z) shows a large, fenestrated EV.

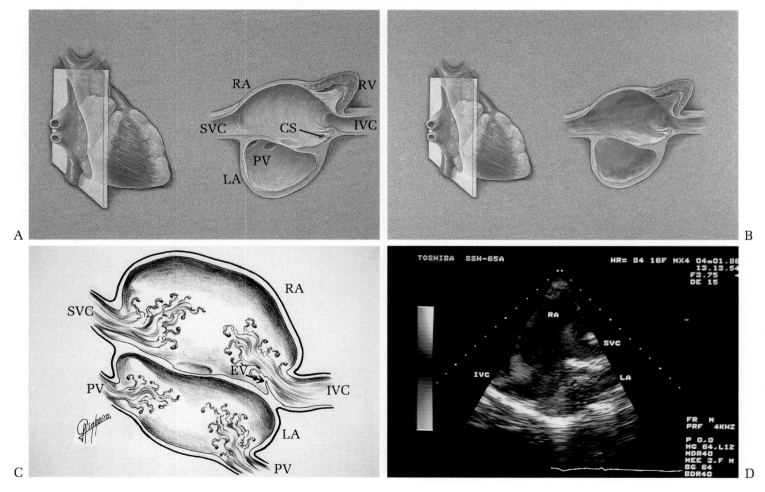

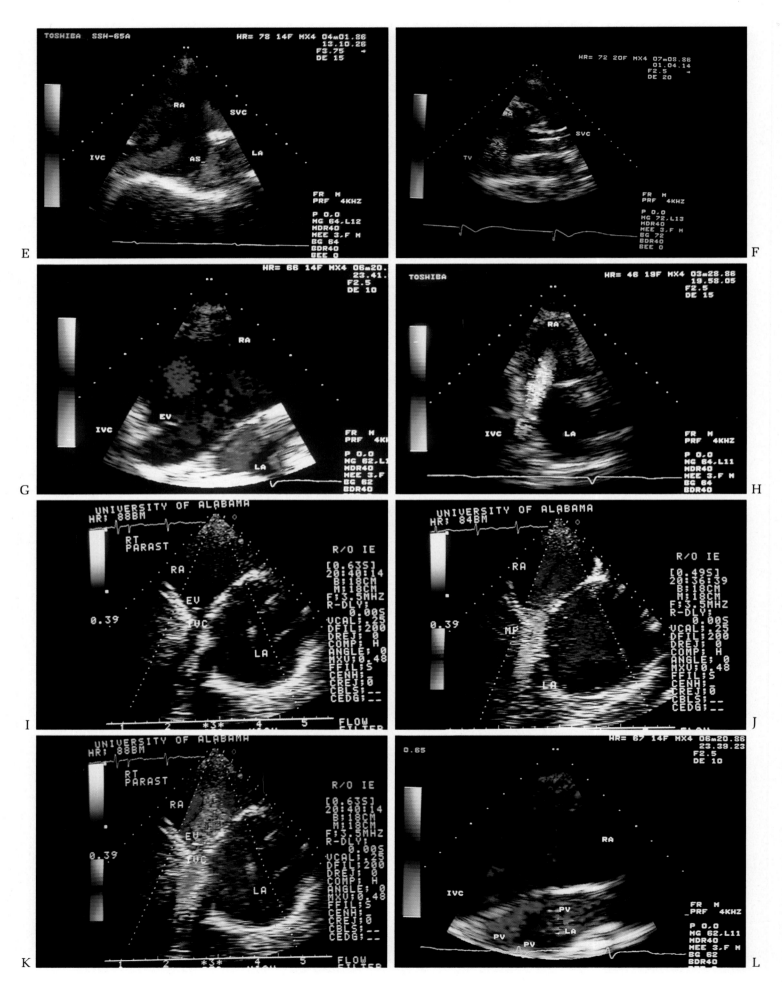

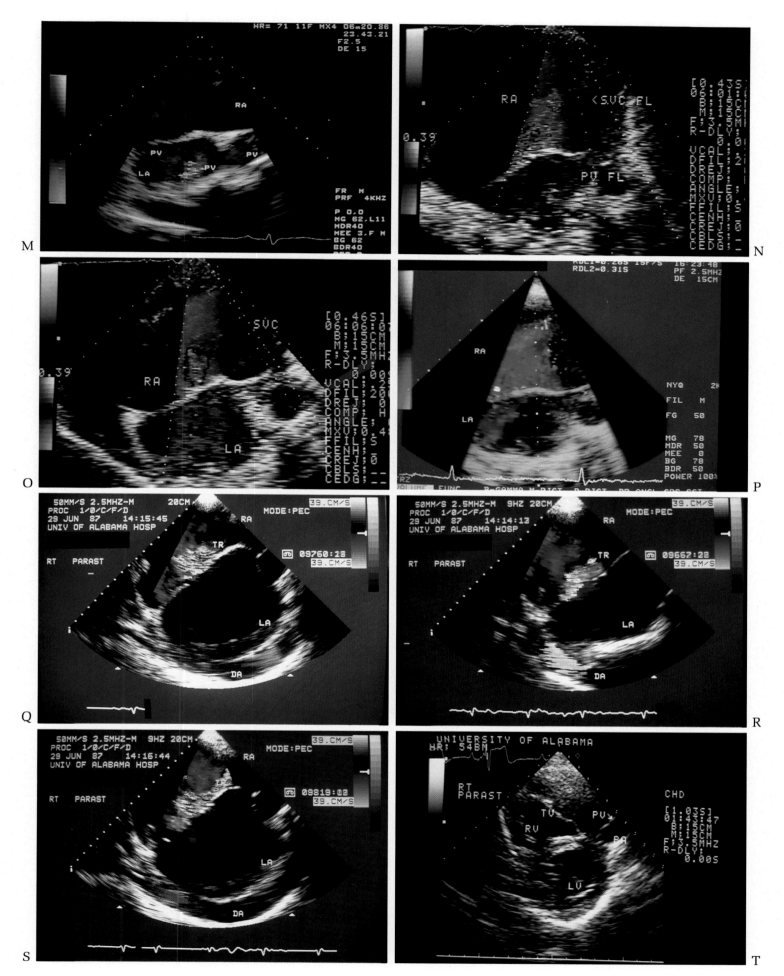

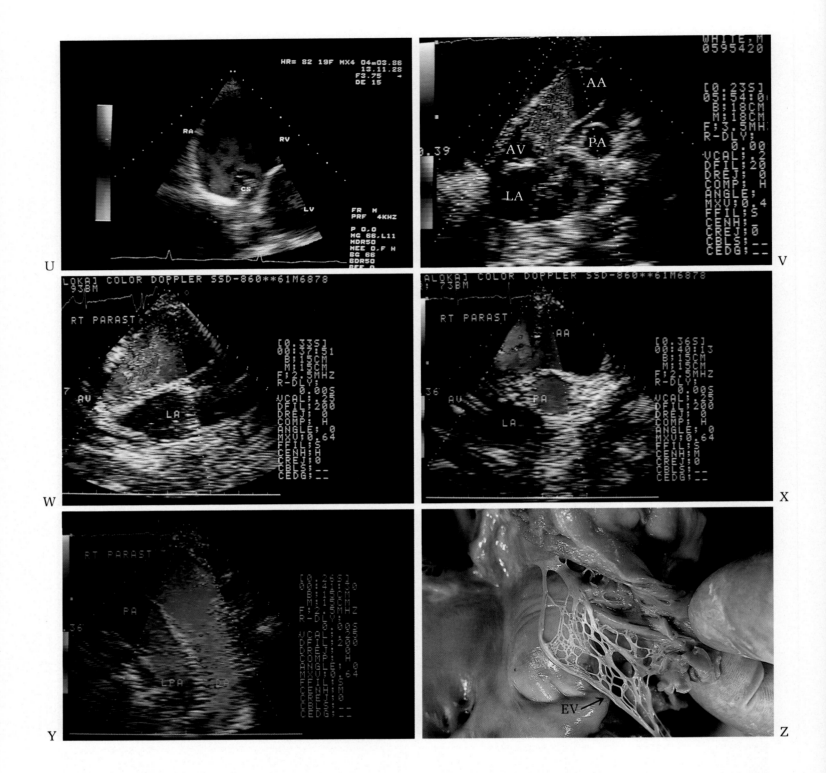

SECTION 2 NORMAL

Figure N-19 **Examination from the back.** In patients with large left or right pleural effusion, thoracic descending aortic aneurysms, or anterior mediastinal masses, the lungs may be displaced, resulting in acoustic access to various cardiac structures and chambers. Prominent flow signals are seen in the LV viewed in short (A) and long axis (B,C) by placing the transducer in a left posterior intercostal space and viewing the heart through the large left pleural effusion (LPL). The DA can also be viewed through the effusion (D).

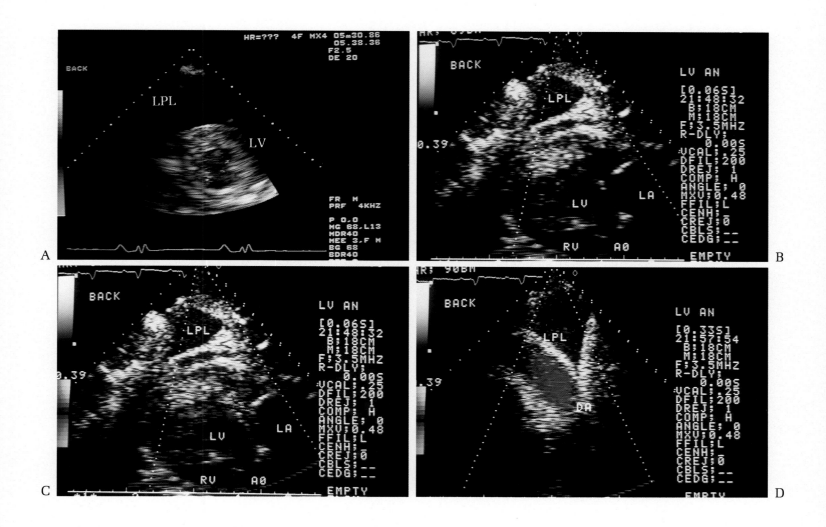

Section 3

MITRAL VALVE

MITRAL VALVE STENOSIS

Color Doppler supplements 2D and pulse Doppler techniques in the assessment of patients with MV stenosis. A narrow band of high-velocity mosaic signals originating from the MV during diastole characterizes MV stenosis in a color Doppler examination. These signals are usually mosaic in color because of turbulence and aliasing. High-velocity signals due to flow acceleration may also be seen on the atrial aspect of the mitral orifice in diastole. Flow acceleration represents a localized area of high-velocity flow located just proximal to a relatively narrow orifice or channel through which flow moves to enter into another chamber. Because it is often observed proximal to a stenotic lesion, it helps to localize the site of stenosis.

The width of the mitral stenotic jet at its origin from the MV reflects its severity. Small width indicates a severe stenotic lesion and larger width indicates a less severe stenotic lesion. It is important to measure this width at the MV level because the stenotic jet tends to widen considerably shortly after its exit from the MV orifice.

Because the mitral stenotic jet usually appears to be directed toward the left ventricular apex, the apical 4-chamber imaging plane provides the best view to place the continuous Doppler cursor line parallel to the flow to obtain the maximum velocity of the mitral stenotic jet. Using the color flow signals as a reference to position this cursor parallel to the flow provides a more reliable estimation of the velocities, and thus a more reliable calculation of the mean pressure gradient and the MV area by using the pressure half-time method than the blind positioning of this cursor across the MV. In our laboratory, calculating the MV area using the pressure half-time method has been shown to correlate better with the MV area obtained using the Gorlin formula during cardiac catheterization in a color-guided

continuous wave Doppler examination rather than in a conventional continuous wave Doppler examination.

In some patients, an eccentric mitral jet may be observed. This jet may be directed anteriorly toward the ventricular septum or posteriorly toward the left ventricular posterior wall. This often happens after balloon valvotomy or surgical mitral commissurotomy. It has also been noted, however, in patients who have not undergone these procedures. In these patients, the use of the parasternal long axis rather than the apical 4-chamber view may be more suitable for the parallel alignment of the Doppler cursor with the stenotic jet.

In some patients, associated aortic and/or tricuspid regurgitation may be present. Differentiating the aortic regurgitant jet from the mitral stenotic jet in patients who have both these lesions is not usually difficult because these jets can be observed originating from their respective valves during diastole. Later during diastole, however, the two jets merge further in the LV, making it difficult to reliably separate the two areas of flow disturbances.

In an occasional patient, the mitral stenotic jet may be seen bifurcating, and sometimes two discrete jets can be observed. One of these jets or one portion of this bifurcating jet may be seen directed anteriorly toward the ventricular septum and the other jet or the other portion is seen directed posteriorly toward the left ventricular posterial wall.

When associated tricuspid regurgitation (TR) is present in a patient with mitral stenosis, the pulmonary artery pressure can be measured by color-guiding the continuous wave Doppler cursor line parallel to tricuspid regurgitant signals to obtain the maximum velocities in the flow. With the Bernoulli equation, the peak systolic pressure gradient across the tricuspid valve (TV) can be calculated, and then assuming a right atrial pressure of 10 mm Hg, the pulmonary artery systolic pressure can be calculated. This allows a reliable assessment of the presence and severity of pulmonary hypertension. Other associated lesions such as an atrial septal defect (ASD), aortic regurgitation, aortic stenosis, and pulmonary regurgitation can also be evaluated and delineated by color Doppler.

Color Doppler is useful in assessing the effect of balloon valvuloplasty on mitral stenosis. In our experience, color Doppler shows the mitral stenotic jet widening at the level of the MV following successful performance of this catheter procedure in many of the patients with this stenotic lesion. This reflects an increase in the MV area. Color Doppler also shows a decrease in the amount of turbulence and aliasing occurring in the LV, and any increase in the MV area using the pressure half-time method and decrease in the mean pressure gradients can be reliably estimated by color-guided continuous wave Doppler. Any change in the pre-existing mitral regurgitation (MR) or the development of new MR following this procedure can also be assessed by color Doppler.

MITRAL REGURGITATION

Pulsed Doppler provides only a limited amount of information on the severity of MR. For example, it often erroneously indicates the presence of severe MR in patients with systemic hypertension. The severity of MV regurgitation is classified according to the maximum width of the mitral regurgitant jet and the distance it extends into the LA. This width and length of the jet depend significantly on the pressure gradient occurring across the MV during systole. In patients with systemic hypertension, the pressure gradient across the MV is high and may cause the regurgitant jet to extend almost to the back wall of the LA even when severe mitral valve regurgitation is not present. In addition, severe MR may be underestimated by pulsed Doppler if the regurgitant jet is eccentrically directed toward the atrial septum or toward the left atrial posterior wall in the apical 4-chamber view, because this may result in absence of high-velocity aliased signals near the back wall of the LA. In general, we have found that the distance to which the mitral regurgitant jet extends into the LA does not correlate well with the severity of the regurgitation. Pulsed Doppler is also tedious and time-consuming, especially when an attempt is made to map out the area of disturbed flow in multiple planes. Color Doppler, by providing multiple sample volumes almost simultaneously in the LA, eliminates the time-consuming mapping of the mitral regurgitant jet in any given plane.

MV regurgitation is indicated by color Doppler displaying systolic retrograde flow signals in the LA, which originate from the MV. These signals are often mosaic in color because of the presence of high-velocity turbulent flow, but in some cases, the mosaic color is not seen because either the ultrasonic beam is not oriented parallel to the flow in some of the available imaging planes,

or mean velocities rather than peak velocities are displayed by color Doppler.

A localized area of flow acceleration may be seen on the ventricular side of the MV. The site of this flow acceleration is usually located exactly opposite the site of the mitral defect, allowing identification of the site of the anatomical defect in the MV. The site of the defect can also be found by color Doppler displaying the flow patterns moving through the MV. For example, a congenital "hole" or a defect due to endocarditis may be clearly outlined by color flow signals moving through it into the LA. In one patient with one of these defects, we have observed two separate jets of MR moving through the hole and the area of coaptation of the mitral leaflets. 2D echocardiography cannot be used in this determination because it may not be possible to differentiate the anatomical defect or the small area of discontinuity in the anterior mitral leaflet from a normally occurring "echo dropout."

The severity of MR is estimated by noting the portion of the LA occupied by the regurgitant signals. This is expressed in terms of a ratio of the maximum area of regurgitant flow to the area of the left atrial cavity measured in the same frame. The maximum regurgitant area is determined from the areas planimetered in three orthogonal imaging planes: the long axis, short axis, and apical 4-chamber plane. In planimetering this area, both the mosaic signals resulting from the disturbed flow and the laminar flow signals moving in a phasic manner with the disturbed flow are used, because the systolic laminar flow signals usually seen at the distal end of mosaic signals represent mitral regurgitant flow with velocities lower than the Nyquist limit. These low-velocity signals can also result from the nonperpendicular orientation of the ultrasonic beam to the direction of the high-velocity regurgitant flow. Other left atrial flow signals which do not move in a phasic manner with the disturbed flow, however, are not included in the area estimation because these signals, in all likelihood, represent pulmonary venous flow. In general, if the regurgitant jet occupies less than 20% of the left atrial cavity, the MV regurgitation present corresponds to the mild or grade 1/3 regurgitation determined by angiocardiography using Nagle's criteria. When the jet occupies between 20 and 40% or more than 40% of the LA, the MV regurgitation corresponds respectively to the moderate or grade 2/3 or severe or grade 3/3 regurgitation classification used by angiocardiography.

Although MR may be present throughout systole, the maximum area of the MR is measured at only one specific instant in time. This area, however, needs to be determined from areas measured during the entire period during which the MR occurs. This would be tedious, time-consuming, and not always reliable, because the size of the measured areas depends on the interrogation angle between the Doppler ultrasonic beam and the flow direction, which varies with the movement of the heart. In general, we have found that the accuracy of the MR assessment does not improve by making area measurements throughout the cardiac cycle. In addition, to obtain the maximum regurgitant jet area, the transducer also must be angled in various directions, because minimal transducer angulations can produce significant changes in the area size.

When a mitral regurgitant jet is narrow at its origin from the MV, the presence of a small defect in the valve is usually indicated. In many patients, however, MV regurgitation results from left ventricular dysfunction or dilatation rather than from an anatomic defect in the MV. This can cause the regurgitant jet to appear wide at its origin from the valve. In patients with huge left atria, the full extent of the MV regurgitation may not be correctly assessed, especially if the acoustic window is small and, thus, a complete interrogation of the LA is impossible. In addition, the severity of MR in patients with very low cardiac outputs may be underestimated because the resultant lower pressure gradient across the MV causes the regurgitant jet to be less turbulent and to become smaller in size (Fig. 3-1).

The severity of MR may not always be correctly assessed using color Doppler because the area of reversed flow signals rather than the actual amount of blood flowing back through the mitral orifice during systole is obtained. It also may not be correctly assessed because the area of systolic turbulence produced by MR is larger than the actual size of the mitral regurgitant jet. The

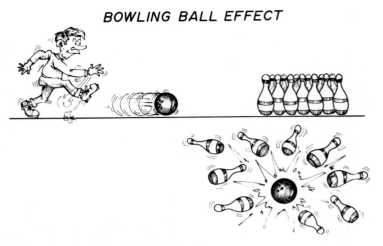

BOWLING BALL EFFECT

Figure 3-2 "Bowling ball effect." The severity of the regurgitant lesion can be overestimated because moving flow from the regurgitant jet impacts on stationary blood cells already present in the LA and thus causes them to move and to show a Doppler shift. This "bowling ball" effect increases the area of turbulence and the color Doppler displays a larger area of turbulence. The area of turbulence is also significantly increased because of entrainment. This phenomenon occurs when the jet moves into the chamber, pulling or "sucking" stationary red blood cells into its flow.

additional area of turbulence results from the "bowling ball" effect or the moving flow from the regurgitant jet impacting on stationary blood cells already present in the LA and causing them to move and to show a Doppler shift (Fig. 3-2) and from entrainment that occurs when the jet moves into the chamber, pulling or "sucking" stationary red blood cells into its flow. Vegetations on the MV, producing considerable dispersion of the mitral regurgitant jet, and heavy fibrosis or calcification in a vegetation attenuating the ultrasonic beam also cause poor visualization of MV regurgitation and hence underestimation of its severity. Using the right parasternal imaging plane, however, this regurgitation may be well visualized in the LA because the LA can be interrogated without the ultrasonic beam having to pass through the vegetation or a calcified MV. Posterior MV leaflet prolapse often causes the mitral regurgitant jet to be directed anteriorly toward the aortic root rather than superiorly so that the flow signals seen using the long axis imaging plane are red rather than the usual blue or the blue and mosaic colors resulting from the normal posterior direction. Significant underestimation of severity of the MV regurgitation occurs if these red signals are considered to be associated with the pulmonary venous inflow rather than the MV regurgitation.

We have found the inter-observer variability in the measurement of the maximum regurgitation area and, thus, in the estimation of the severity of the MV regurgitation to be fairly low. Intermachine variability often exists, however, because of the different capabilities of the available color Doppler systems to detect the low-velocity flows. This intermachine variability is, in our experience so far, not significant enough to change the grading of MR in most patients. Therefore, the severity

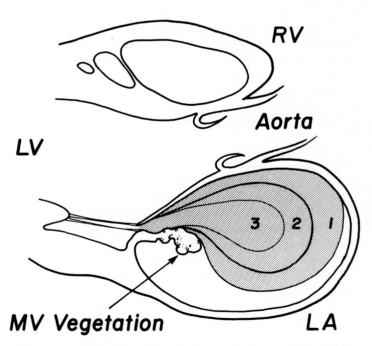

Figure 3-1 Effect of cardiac output on mitral regurgitation. This schematic of a parasternal long axis view shows severe MR resulting from a flail posterior leaflet and a large vegetation on the valve. Even though the MR is severe, a low cardiac output may cause its severity to be underestimated. This is due to the fact that the lower pressure gradient across the MV resulting from the low cardiac output causes the regurgitant jet to be less turbulent and much smaller in size. In general, for normal cardiac outputs, the presence of severe MR is indicated when a large area of reversed flow signals is displayed (1). As shown by this figure, this area decreases as the cardiac output decreases (2), and when the cardiac output is very low, the area of flow signals decreases markedly (3).

of the MV regurgitation present can be reliably assessed with any of the commercially available color Doppler systems.

To overcome some of the intermachine variability, the settings need to be adjusted for each system to provide the same optimal flow information. For example, the gain setting needs to be adjusted and standardized for a reliable estimation of the severity of MV regurgitation. As the gain is lowered, the flow signals begin to disappear and as it is increased, static or white noise begins to appear. To calculate the maximum area of disturbed flow due to MV regurgitation, the gain needs to be set so that the white noise just begins to appear. Another example is the color threshold setting or, in other words, the control of the strength of the 2D imaging signals versus the color flow signals on a color Doppler system. This setting determines whether or not the low-velocity flows are detected. When the color threshold is "high" or "on," depending on the system, the 2D imaging signals are stronger, causing the presence of ghosting artifacts, and thus the loss of the low-velocity flow signals, resulting in erroneous calculation of the area of disturbed flow. If the thresholding is "off" or "low," however, the color flow signals are stronger than the 2D imaging signals and the low-velocity flow signals are observed. A final example is the use of the power or amplitude mode, available on only some color Doppler systems. We have been investigating the use of this mode in providing a better quantitative estimation of MV regurgitation, because it is expected to be independent of the Doppler interrogation angle and gives flow information about the concentration of the blood cells in the left atrial cavity. When this mode is on, however, the MR signals may be hard to distinguish from the pulmonary venous inflow signals. The amplitude mode also depends greatly on the gain setting, which may be a significant disadvantage. Therefore, using both the amplitude and velocity modes may provide the most reliable information about the severity of MR.

The color Doppler assessment of MR may not always correlate well with angiography. Angiography, however, is not an ideal "gold standard," because it is highly subjective, and angiographic evaluation of MR depends on variables such as the enlargement of the LA and the amount of radio-opaque contrast material injected. It also depends on the position of the catheter through which the radio-opaque dye is injected. For example, when the catheter is positioned too close to the mitral leaflets, artificial MV regurgitation will be produced. The calculation of regurgitant jet fractions by cardiac catheterization is also not ideal because both the Fick and thermo-dilution techniques used for the measurement of cardiac output show considerable variability. A small error in the estimation of the angiographic total left ventricular stroke volume and the effective stroke volume across the AV can cause a disproportionately large error in the calculation of the regurgitant volumes and fractions. In addition, the assumption made in these calculations that the LV has a standard geometric configuration may not be valid.

Color Doppler is considered better than angiocardiography in assessing the changes in the severity of MR because MR is a dynamic event that depends on the pressure gradient between the ventricle and the atrium and the type of activity the patient is engaged in. Angiography cannot observe this dynamic change because when it is performed, the patient is either sedated or premedicated. Thus, the severity is assessed at only one point in time and, being invasive, the procedure cannot be done repeatedly. Color Doppler, however, is completely noninvasive, and may be performed whenever necessary under various clinical conditions to evaluate the presence and severity of MV regurgitation.

Although the presence of a small amount of MV regurgitation can be easily detected by pulsed Doppler and continuous wave Doppler, it may not be easily detected by color Doppler, and thus multiple 2D imaging planes may be needed to detect its presence. Imaging in multiple planes must be done to obtain a complete picture of the mitral regurgitant jet because this jet has three dimensions, and at any given time only two dimensions of the jet are shown in any given plane. When the presence of MR is questionable by color Doppler due to the difficulty in differentiating a small jet of MR from a ghosting artifact caused by MV motion, the use of the hand-grip maneuver may be helpful. With this maneuver, the blood pressure and the afterload increase, causing the pressure gradient across the MV and the area of disturbed flow in the left atrial cavity to increase during systole. This allows the mitral regurgitant flow signals to be differentiated from the ghosting artifact.

MR may occur in some patients only during exercise and, in some patients studied by us, this appeared to be a good indicator of ischemic heart disease, especially three-vessel disease. The exact cause of the development of MR during exercise is not clear, but it is probably related to ischemic left ventricular dysfunction or papillary muscle dysfunction produced by ischemia, which, in turn, is induced by exercise.

Color Doppler evaluation of MR has also been found useful in patients with cardiac transplantation who develop acute rejection with myocyte necrosis seen on endomyocardial biopsy. In these instances, because of left ventricular dysfunction, MR may develop or increase significantly in severity, indicating acute rejection. This MR disappears or decreases considerably when the acute rejection is alleviated after chemotherapy. When MR does not develop or increase in severity, the acute rejection process is absent in the cardiac transplant patient. A color Doppler examination may thus reduce the need for multiple endocardial biopsies, which presently are routinely performed in the follow-up of these patients.

Color Doppler is also useful in the assessment of diastolic MV regurgitation and associated lesions such as aortic, tricuspid, and pulmonary regurgitation. For example, color Doppler clearly delineates diastolic MV regurgitation by displaying flow signals moving through a partially closed MV into the LA. This occurs in some patients with severe aortic regurgitation (AR) which results from the left ventricular end diastolic pressure being higher than the left atrial pressure during late diastole. Diastolic MR may also be observed when the pulmonary regurgitation (PR) interval is prolonged, as may occur in first-degree or complete atrio-ventricular block.

For timing events in the cardiac cycle and also timing the onset and duration of MV regurgitation, a color M-mode examination is better than a 2D examination because its faster frame rate prevents overlapping of flows from occurring at adjacent but different times in the cardiac cycle. Most MV regurgitations, even mild, are pansystolic even though the murmurs are not audible on clinical examination throughout the duration of systole. In some patients with MV prolapse, color M-mode clearly shows MR occurring only during middle to late systole and, as mentioned previously, patients with first-degree atrioventricular block or severe AR may show diastolic MR.

REFERENCES

Mitral Valve Stenosis

1. Hatle, L., Bjorn, A., and Tromdale, A.: Noninvasive assessment of atrioventricular pressure half-time by Doppler ultrasound. Circulation 60:1096, 1979.
2. Switzer, D.F., and Nanda, N.C.,: Limitations of pulsed and continuous-wave Doppler echocardiography (Editorial). Echocardiography: A Review of Cardiovascular Ultrasound 2:207, 1985.
3. Skelton, T.N., and Kisslo, J.: Real-time Doppler color flow mapping in stenotic valvular lesions. Echocardiography: A Review of Cardiovascular Ultrasound 2:523, 1985.
4. Khandheria, B.K., and Tajik, A.J., Relder, G.S., Callahan, M.H., Nishimura, R.A., Miller, F.A., and Seward, J.B.: Doppler color flow imaging: A new technique for visualization and characterization of the blood flow jet in mitral stenosis. Mayo Clin. Proc. 61:623, 1986.
5. Kan, M.N., Goyal, R.G., Helmcke, F., and Hsiung, M.C.: Color Doppler assessment of severity of mitral stenosis (Abstract). Circulation 74 (Suppl. II) II-145, 1986.
6. Nanda, N.C.: Color Doppler flow mapping of stenotic and regurgitant natural heart valves. 39th Annual Conference on Engineering in Medicine and Biology, Baltimore, September 13–16, 1986.
7. Villa Costa, I., Aggarwal, K.K., Bulle, T., Dean, L., Baxley, W., and Nanda, N.C.: Color Doppler flow imaging in balloon valvotomy (Abstract). Circulation 72 (Suppl. IV) IV-1987.

Mitral Regurgitation

1. Abbasi, A.S., Allen, M.W., DeCristofaro, D., and Ungar, I.: Detection and estimation of the degree of mitral regurgitation by range gated pulsed Doppler echocardiography. Circulation 61:43, 1980.
2. Chandraratna, P.A.N., Mirago, E.S., and Wade, N.: Demonstration of regurgitant stream shape and direction in mitral and tricuspid regurgitation by two-dimensional Doppler color flow mappng. J. Am. Coll. Cardiol. 5:454, 1985.
3. Switzer, D.F., and Nanda, N.C.: Color Doppler evaluation of valvular regurgitation. Echocardiography: A Review of Cardiovascular Ultrasound 2:533, 1985.
4. Saenz, C.B., Deumite, N.J., Roitman, D.I., Moos, S., Nanda, N.C., and Soto, B.: Limitations of color Doppler in quantitative assessment of mitral regurgitation (Abstract). Circulation 72 (Suppl. III):III-99, 1985.
5. Miyatake, K., Izumi, S., Okamoto, M., Kinoshita, N., Asonuma, H., Nakagawa, H., Yamamoto, K., Takamiya, M., Sakakibara, H., and Numura, Y.: Semiquantitative grading of severity of mitral regurgitation by real-time two-dimensional Doppler flow imaging technique. J. Am. Coll. Cardiol. 7:82, 1986.
6. Konstadt, S., Thys, D., Mindich, B., Kaplan, J., and Goldman, M.E.: Validation of quantitative intraoperative transesophageal echocardiography. Anesthesiology 65:418, 1986.
7. Hsiung, M.C., Nanda, N.C., Kirklin, J.K., Bittner, V., and Smith, S.: Usefulness of color Doppler in the early detection of cardiac allograft rejection (Abstract). Circulation 74 (Suppl. IV):IV-180, 1986.
8. Hsiung, M.C., Zachariah, Z.P., Perry, G., and Nanda, N.C.: Color Doppler evaluation of mitral regurgitation in pacemaker patients before and during exercise (Abstract). Clin. Res.: 34:308A, 1986.
9. Zachariah, Z.P., Hsiung, M.C., Nanda, N.C., Roitman, D.I., and Storey, O.: Color Doppler assessment of mitral and tricuspid regurgitation induced by supine exercise in ischemic heart disease (Abstract). South. M. J. 79:7, 1986.
10. Saenz, C.B., Roitman, D., Deumite, J.N., and Nanda, N.C.: Assessment of mitral regurgitation with color Doppler during isometric exercise (Abstract). South. Med. J. 79:6, 1986.
11. Goldman, M.E., Fuster, V., Guarino, T., and Mindich, B.P.: Intraoperative echocardiography for the evaluation of valvular regurgitation: Experience in 263 patients (Abstract). Circulation 74 (Suppl. I.):I-143, 1986.
12. Czer, L.S., Maurer, G., DeRobertis, M., Bolger, A.F., Kass, R.M., Lee, M.E., Blanche, C., Chaux, A., and Matloff, J.M.: Intraoperative evaluation of mitral regurgitation: Superiority of Doppler color flow mapping (Abstract). Circulation 74 (Suppl. II)II:394, 1986.
13. Helmcke, F., Nanda, N.C., Hsiung, M.C., Soto, B., Adey, C.K., Goyal, R.G., and Gatewood, R.P.: Color Doppler assessment of mitral regurgitation with orthogonal planes. Circulation 75:175, 1987.
14. Zachariah, Z.P., Hsiung, M.C., Nanda, N.C., Kan, M.N., and Gatewood, R.P. Jr.: Color Doppler assessment of mitral regurgitation induced by supine exercise in ischemic heart disease. Am. J. Cardiol. 59:1266, 1987.
15. Wong, M., Matsumura, M., Suzuki, K., and Omoto, R.: Technical and biologic sources of variability in the mapping of aortic, mitral and tricuspid color flow jets. Am. J. Cardiol. 60:847, 1987.
16. Otsuji, Y., Tei, C., Kisanuki, A., Natsugoe, K., and Kawazoe, Y.: Color Doppler echocardiographic assessment of the change in the mitral regurgitant volume. Am. Heart J. 114:349, 1987.
17. Perry, G.J., and Nanda, N.C.: Recent advances in color Doppler evaluation of valvular regurgitation. Echocardiography: A Review of Cardiovascular Imaging 4:503, 1987.
18. Cooper, J., Kapur, K.K., Fan, P.H., and Nanda, N.C.: Conventional and color Doppler assessment of mitral regurgitation in mitral valve prolapse (Abstract). Clin. Res. 35:270A, 1987.

SECTION 3   MITRAL VALVE

In this section, various lesions affecting the MV are illustrated.

Figure MV-1   **Mitral stenosis.** (A) Autopsy specimen shows a markedly thickened MV with calcification and fibrosis, characteristic of rheumatic involvement. (B) The same MV is viewed in cross section from the atrial aspect. Note the narrowed orifice and heavy fibrosis and calcification. (C) Another autopsy specimen shows heavily calcified and fibrotic mitral leaflets, commissural fusion, markedly narrowed orifice, and a large LA. (D) Another autopsy specimen shows a narrow, irregular slit-like mitral orifice and heavily calcified leaflets. (E) Another autopsy specimen shows a slit-like mitral orifice and a huge LA.

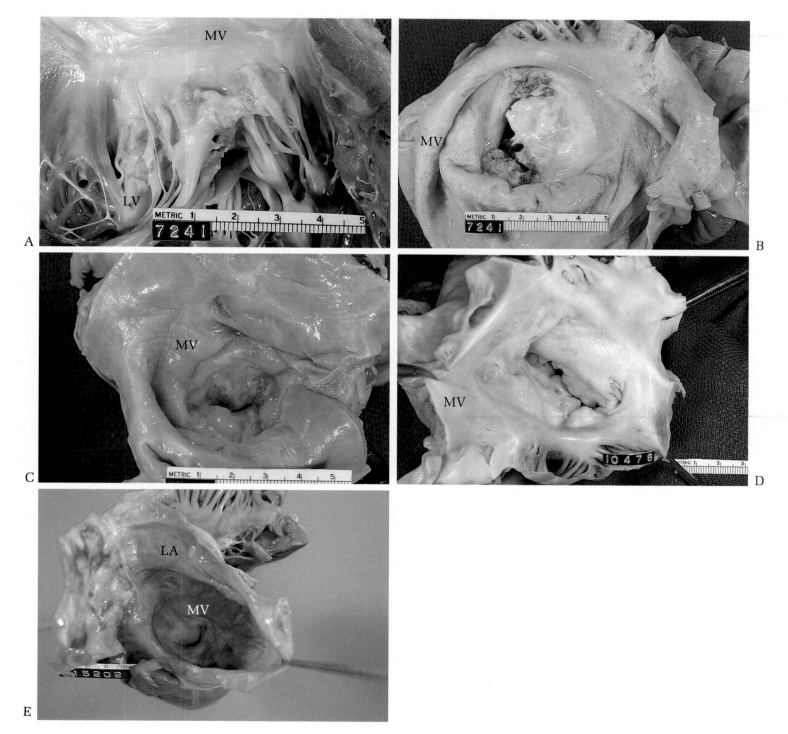

SECTION 3   MITRAL VALVE

Figure MV-2   **Mitral stenosis.** Autopsy specimen shows thickened and fused chordae tendineae (arrow) in a patient with rheumatic MV stenosis.

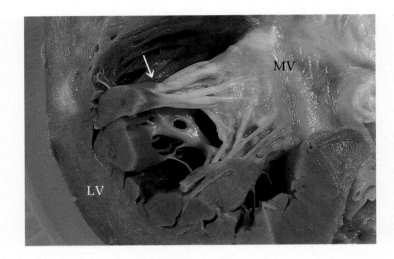

SECTION 3 MITRAL VALVE

Figure MV-3 **Mitral stenosis.** (A) 2D echocardiogram shows the narrow mitral orifice area 1.5 cm²) in short axis plane. (B) Apical 4-chamber view obtained from the same patient shows restricted opening of the mitral leaflets. Color flow examination (C) in the apical 4-chamber view shows a narrow band of flow signals (arrow) originating from the MV in diastole, characteristic of MS. Blue signals within the red are due to aliasing. The red flow signals seen on the atrial aspect of the mitral orifice represent flow acceleration (FA), often noted proximal to a stenotic lesion. FA represents a localized increase in the velocity, produced by flow moving from a high-pressure chamber into a low-pressure chamber through a small opening (a sort of "suction effect") and helps to localize the site of stenosis. Nonvisualization of flow signals in the remainder of the LA is related to the presence of low-flow velocities below the instrument threshold setting.

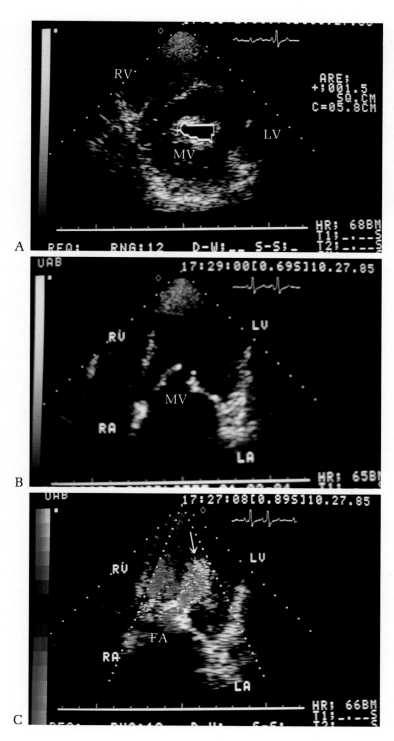

SECTION 3 MITRAL VALVE

Figure MV-4 **Mitral stenosis.** (A) Apical 4-chamber view in an adult shows a mosaic pattern of colors emerging from the narrowed mitral orifice resulting from turbulence, aliasing, and high flow velocities. Flow acceleration is seen as a localized area of red signals on the atrial aspect of the mitral orifice (arrow). B and C are schematics.

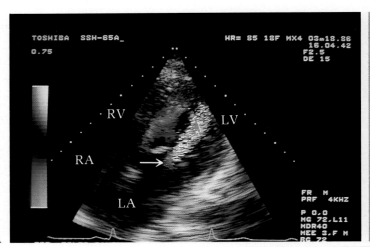

A

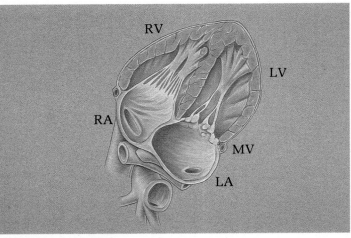

B

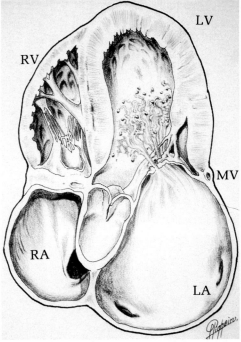

C

SECTION 3   MITRAL VALVE

Figure MV-5   **Mitral stenosis: Status postcommissurotomy.** Apical 4-chamber view (right) in a 44-year-old woman shows a wide flow jet originating from the mitral orifice in diastole, indicating alleviation of obstruction. The pulse Doppler velocity waveform (left) shows a rapid diastolic closing slope, also suggesting relief of MS. The systolic signals below the Doppler baseline represent MR in this patient.

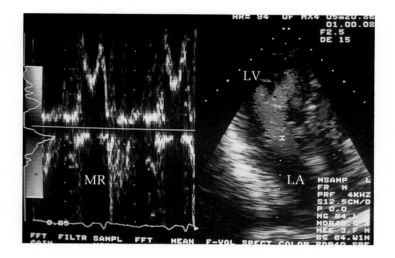

SECTION 3   MITRAL VALVE

Figure MV-6   **Mitral stenosis.** Continuous wave Doppler cursor line is placed parallel to the MS signals in the apical 4-chamber view to obtain the maximal velocity of the MS jet. This facilitates reliable calculation of the mean pressure gradient and the MV area using the pressure half-time method. The MV area was calculated as 0.8 cm^2 in this patient.

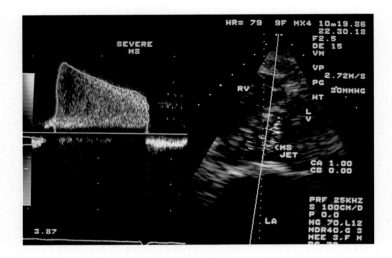

Figure MV-7 **Mitral stenosis: Color M-mode examination.** Color M line cursor is placed through the MS jet obtained in the apical 4-chamber to obtain color flow patterns in this patient. Note the mosaic pattern of colors recorded in front of the mitral leaflets in diastole, characteristic of MS.

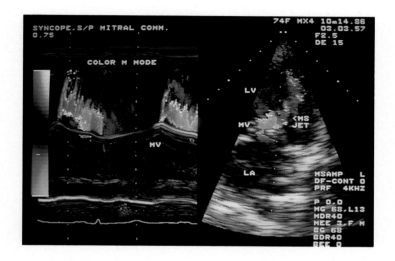

Figure MV-8   **Mitral stenosis.** (A) Apical 4-chamber view shows 2 discrete jets (J1 and J2) originating from the MV in diastole in this patient with MS. (B) Schematic shows two discrete jets of MS and a large LA.

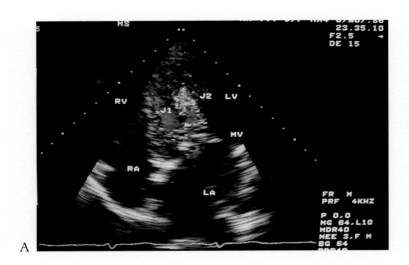

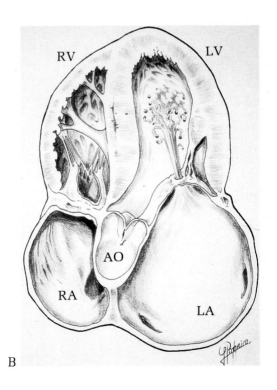

Figure MV-9 **Mitral stenosis associated with aortic regurgitation.** (A) In diastole, a thin band of red signals is seen originating from the AV indicative of AR and a wider MS jet originates from the mitral leaflets. The blue flow signals in the mitral jet contained within the red signals are due to aliasing. The red signals on the atrial aspect of the mitral orifice represent flow acceleration (arrow). (B) Expanded view shows flow signals due to AR and MS in the same patient. (C,D) Schematic shows two discrete jets originating from the MV and AV in diastole (arrows). Note that the AR signals merge with the MS flow signals downstream in the LV, making it difficult to reliably separate the areas of flow disturbance originating from the two valves. (E) Low parasternal long axis view in a 59-year-old man shows merging of MS and AR jets in the LV. ACC=flow acceleration; AI=aortic regurgitation.

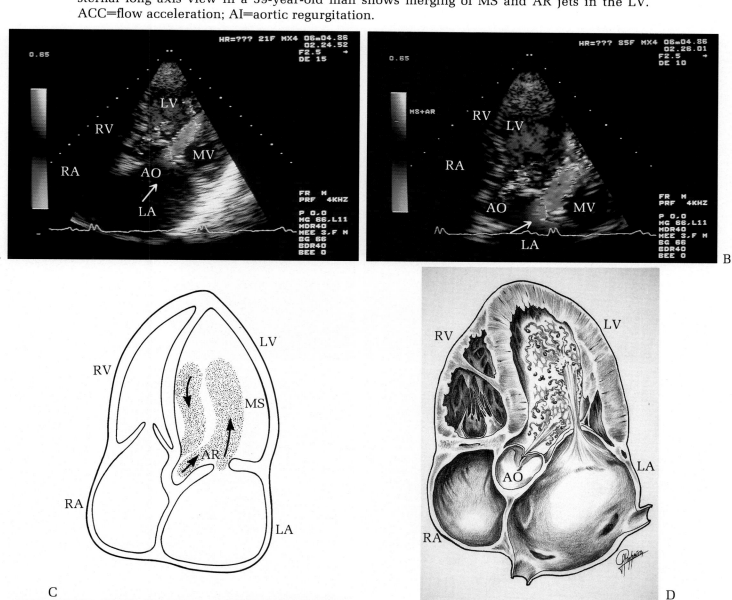

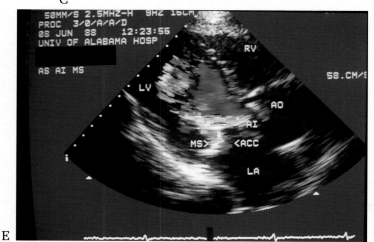

SECTION 3 MITRAL VALVE

Figure MV-10   **Mitral stenosis.** (A) Apical 4-chamber view in another adult with MS shows blue signals and a mosaic pattern of colors due to aliasing and disturbed flow taken at a pulse repetition frequency (PRF) of 4 KHz. The Nyquist limit is 0.75 m/sec. (B) The PRF in the same patient has been increased to 6 KHz, eliminating aliasing so that the MS jet is now predominantly red in color. The high PRF increases the Nyquist limit to 1.13 m/sec so that higher velocities can be resolved by the system without aliasing. (C) Here the color baseline has been modified (arrows), increasing the Nyquist limit and eliminating the red color so that all flow signals originating from the MV appear blue. (D) Here the baseline has been moved in the opposite direction, causing the mitral flow signals to take up red color.

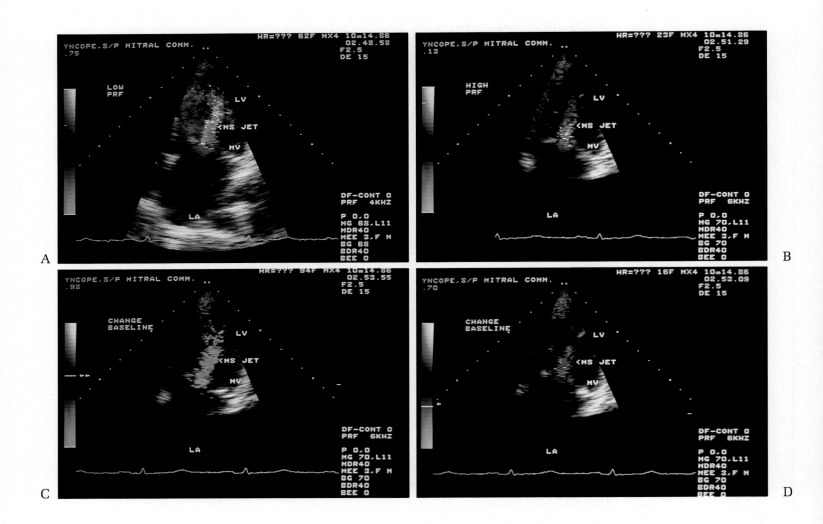

SECTION 3   MITRAL VALVE

Figure MV-11   **Mitral stenosis.** (A,B) Schematics show thickened and calcified mitral leaflets viewed in the long axis plane in diastole (A) and systole (B). (C) 2D long axis view shows a narrow band of mosaic-colored signals originating from the mitral leaflets in diastole in the long axis view, typical of MS. The red signals on the atrial aspect of the narrowed mitral orifice represent flow acceleration (ACC). The LA is markedly enlarged. (D,E) Long axis views in two other patients with MS also show a narrow band of diastolic mosaic-colored signals moving through the mitral orifice into the LV. The red signals on the atrial aspect of the MV represent flow acceleration (ACC).

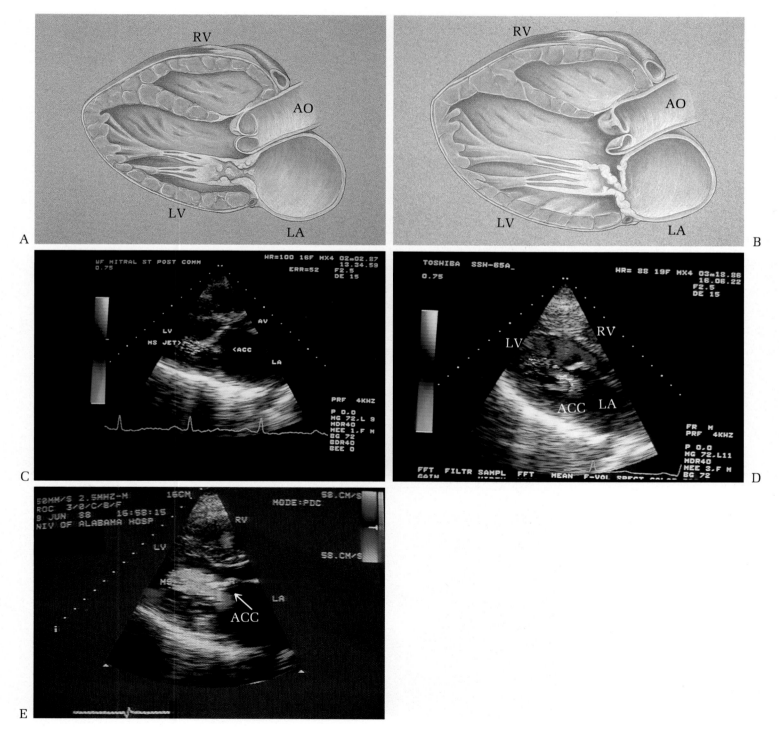

SECTION 3   MITRAL VALVE

Figure MV-12   **Mitral stenosis.** (A) Long axis view shows the MS jet bifurcating; one portion is directed anteriorly toward the VS (red) and the other is directed toward the left ventricular posterior wall (blue). The arrow points to flow acceleration. (B,C) Long axis views (using two different flow maps) in another patient also show bifurcation of the MS jet, one directed toward the VS, the other toward the LV posterior wall. A=flow acceleration.

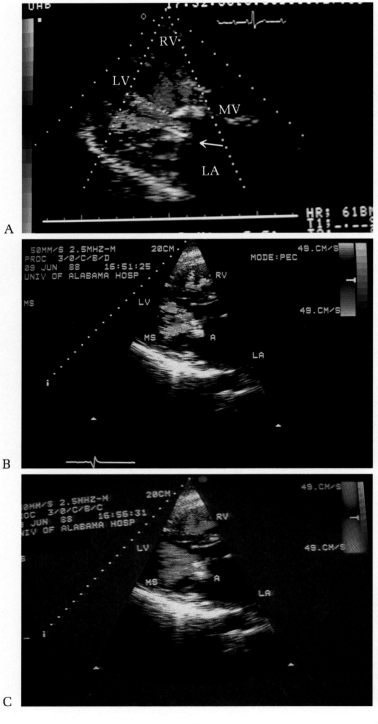

SECTION 3   MITRAL VALVE

Figure MV-13   **Mitral stenosis.** The long axis view in a 21-year-old woman shows MS jet signals (yellow) directed anteriorly toward the VS. Note that the flow signals remain narrow throughout and do not widen.

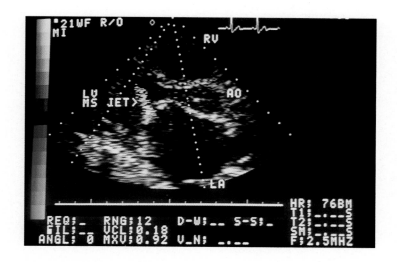

SECTION 3 MITRAL VALVE

Figure MV-14 **Mitral stenosis.** Red and blue signals within and outside the narrowed mitral orifice in diastole represent the high-velocity mitral inflow viewed in short axis.

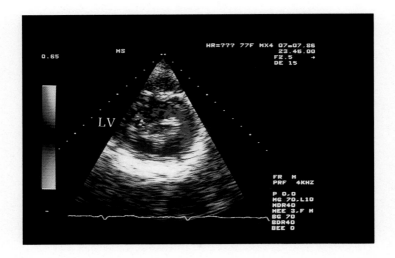

SECTION 3   MITRAL VALVE

Figure MV-15   **Mitral stenosis: Balloon valvotomy.** Baseline long (A) and short axis (B) views in a 50-year-old woman show a narrow mosaic-colored MS jet and a MV orifice area of 1.0 cm² by computerized planimetry. There is no evidence of MR. Following successful balloon valvotomy, the MS jet, also viewed in the long axis plane, shows considerable widening with no significant aliasing or turbulence (C) and the MV area increased to 2.5 cm² (D). E shows a small area of blue signals in the LA during systole, indicating mild MR, which developed after balloon valvotomy. This patient also has associated moderate AR (A,C).

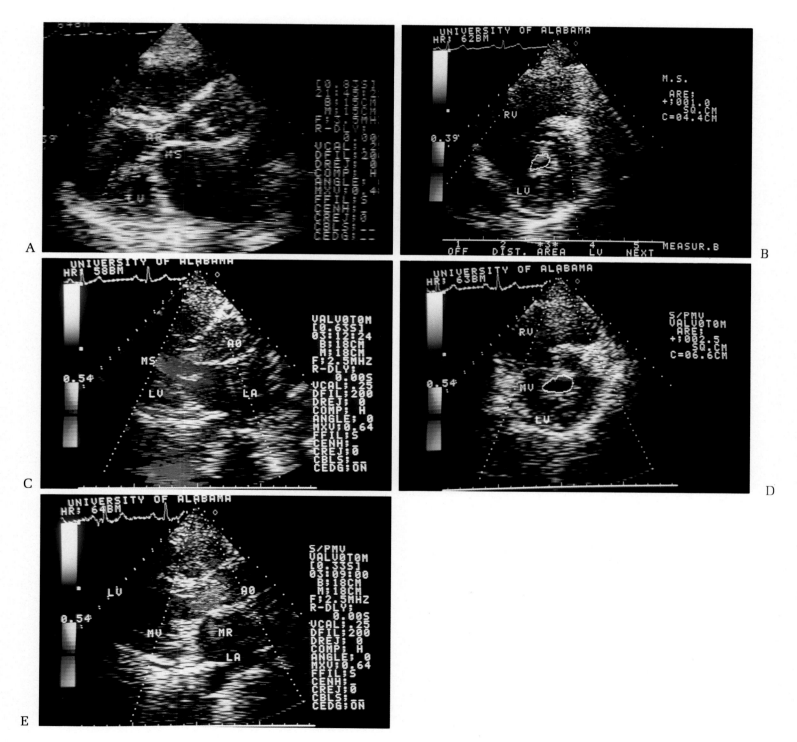

SECTION 3 MITRAL VALVE

Figure MV-16 **Mitral stenosis: Measurement of pulmonary artery pressure.** Patient, a 27-year-old woman, has developed MV restenosis following successful commissurotomy in 1979, and her MV area, shown by echocardiography and Doppler pressure half-time method, is 0.5 cm². Because she also has associated TR, shown by color Doppler, the continuous-wave Doppler cursor line is placed parallel to the TR signals to obtain a peak velocity of 5.25 m/sec. This translates into a peak systolic pressure gradient of 110 mm Hg across the TV using the Bernoulli equation. Assuming a right atrial pressure of 10 mm Hg, the PA systolic pressure is calculated as 120 mm Hg (systemic level pulmonary hypertension). The patient underwent balloon valvotomy with an increase in the MV area to 2.0 cm²; new developments were moderate MR and reduction in PA pressure to 60 mm Hg.

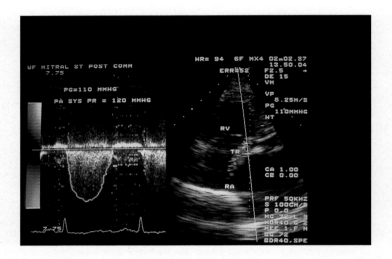

SECTION 3 MITRAL VALVE

Figure MV-17 **Mitral stenosis associated with tricuspid valve stenosis.** Low parasternal 4-chamber view shows a very narrow band of mosaic-colored flow signals originating from the TV in diastole, suggesting the presence of severe TS. Note the considerable widening of the TS jet further downstream in the RV. Mosaic-colored signals in the LV in diastole represent disturbed flow due to MS.

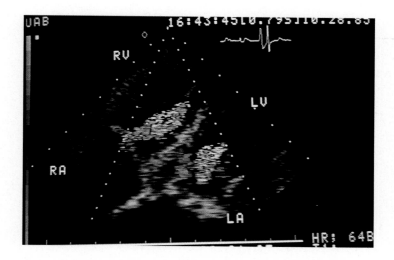

SECTION 3   MITRAL VALVE

Figure MV-18   **Mitral stenosis with mitral regurgitation.** Autopsy specimen shows thickened mitral leaflets, fixed in the partially open position, indicating a severely incompetent and stenotic MV.

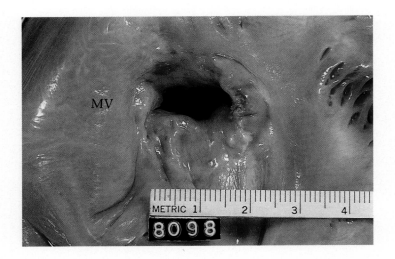

SECTION 3   MITRAL VALVE

Figure MV-19   **Mitral regurgitation.** (A) Parasternal long axis view in an 18-year-old woman shows mosaic-colored MR signals originating from the posterior portion of the MV and directed into the LA along its posterior wall. FA (flow acceleration) represents a localized area of increased velocity on the ventricular side of the mitral leaflets and exactly opposite the origin of the MR jet. (B) Color M-mode recording in this patient shows mosaic-colored signals persisting throughout systole, indicating pansystolic MR. Color M-mode is more reliable than color 2D imaging for timing flow events.

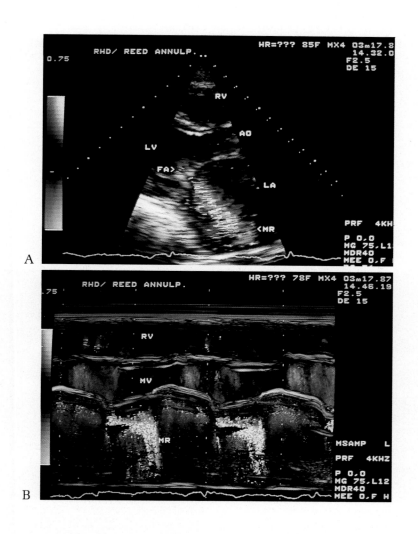

Figure MV-20   Mitral regurgitation. (A) Long axis view in another patient with lupus erythematosus shows mosaic-colored systolic signals due to MR originating from the MV and moving posteriorly into the LA. The red signals next to the mosaic signals represent regurgitant signals which have swirled around, or prominent pulmonary venous flow. (B) Minimal angulation of the transducer causes a much larger area of the LA to be filled with mosaic-colored signals. Also, the red signals appear to be continuous with the mosaic and blue signals, suggesting that they are part of the MR jet and not pulmonary venous flow. Note that MR now appears to be more severe than in A, underlining the importance of angling the transducer in various directions to obtain the maximal area of the flow disturbance, which can then be used to evaluate the severity of MR. (C) The mosaic pattern is more dramatically visualized in the LVO-pulmonic plane, which also demonstrates normal systolic flow signals in the MPA. (D) Short axis view taken at the level of the high LVO also shows mosaic-colored signals occupying a large portion of the LA in this patient, indicative of severe MR. (E) The two ECG gated frames in this patient show MR signals moving through the MV into the LA during the isovolumic contraction period of the LV (left, both AV and MV are closed) and more extensive filling of the LA later in systole (right, AV is fully open). (F,G) Color M-mode studies in this patient demonstrate mosaic-colored signals throughout systole, signifying pansystolic regurgitation.

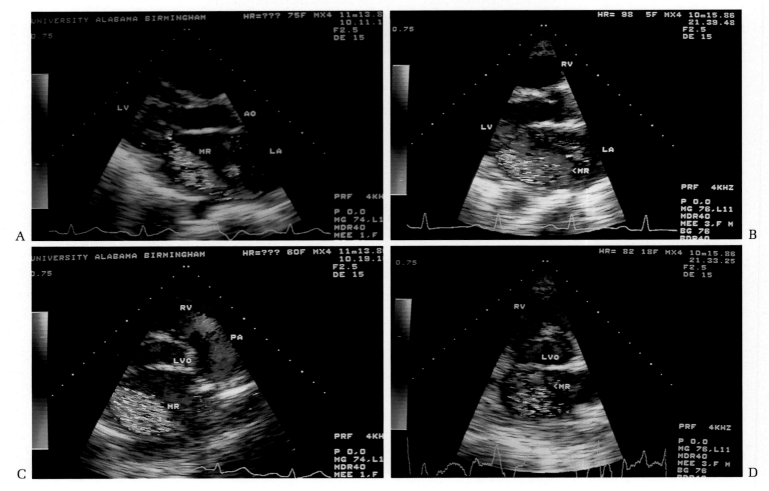

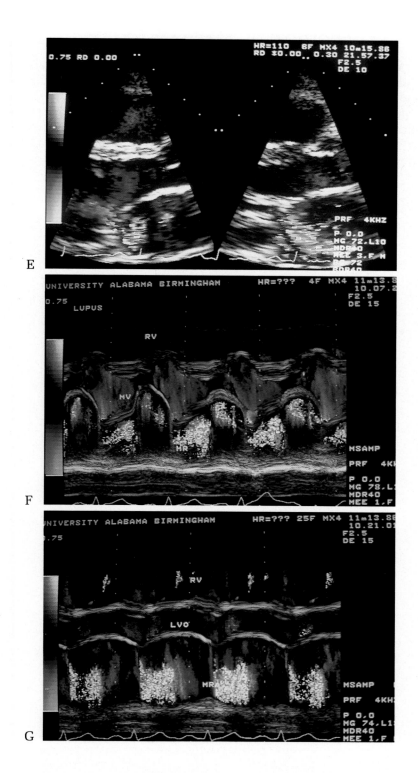

SECTION 3 MITRAL VALVE

Figure MV-21 **Mitral regurgitation.** In this patient, the long axis view initially shows mosaic-colored signals of MR filling approximately 40% of the LA (A), but minimal angulation of the transducer demonstrates the presence of more severe MR with the flow signals practically occupying the whole LA (B). The red signals represent anteriorly directed flow due to a "swirling" effect resulting from deflection of the jet by the atrial wall. Presence of swirling is a good indicator of severe regurgitation. The aortic short axis view (C) also shows mosaic-colored signals filling most of the LA.

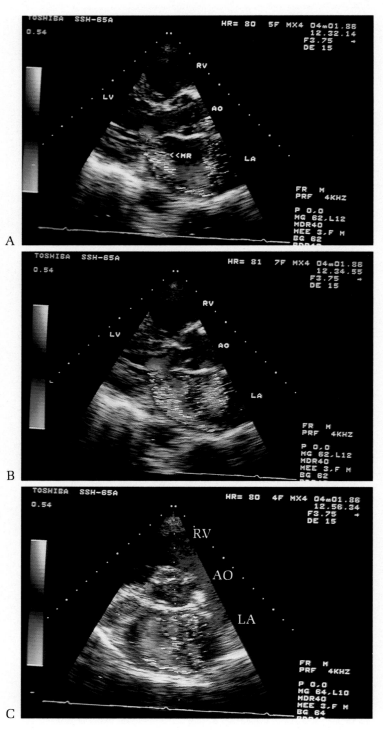

SECTION 3   MITRAL VALVE

Figure MV-22   **Severe mitral regurgitation.** (A) Long axis view. The mosaic-colored signals moving through the MV and filling virtually the entire LA during systole indicate the presence of severe MR in a 50-year-old man. The blue signals in the LVOT represent relatively low-velocity normal flow directed into the aorta. (B) Examination of same patient with different commercially available equipment also shows the presence of severe MR. Although the pattern of colors is different, the area of disturbed flow is essentially similar. The short axis view (C) also shows mosaic-colored regurgitant signals in the LA.

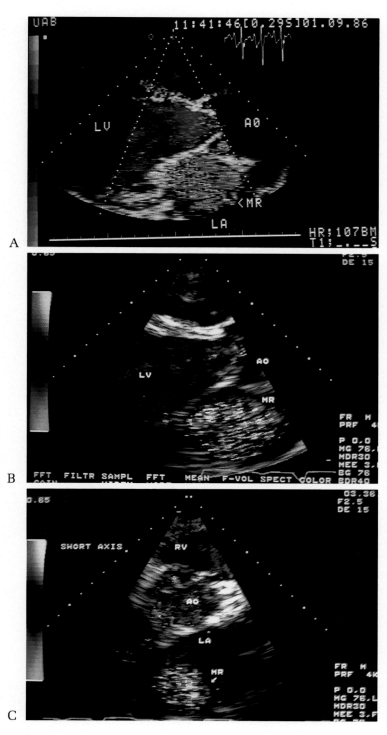

SECTION 3 MITRAL VALVE

Figure MV-23 **Mitral regurgitation.** Long axis view shows bluish-green systolic signals in the LA originating from the MV, indicating MR. Similarly colored signals are also seen moving through the AV and indicate normal flow moving from the LV into the aortic root. Notice that in this patient, no aliasing is seen in the LA and the mosaic pattern of colors is absent, probably because the nonparallel orientation of the Doppler ultrasonic beam to the regurgitant flow direction is such that only the low-velocity vectorial components of the high-velocity jet are recorded. Also, the color Doppler signals represent mean rather than peak velocities.

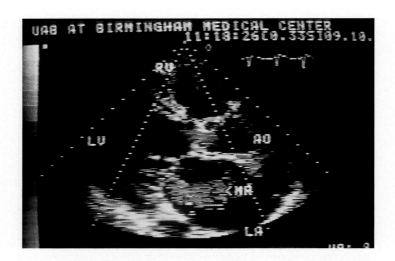

SECTION 3 MITRAL VALVE

Figure MV-24 **Mitral regurgitation viewed in three orthogonal planes.** The mosaic-colored signals due to MR are demonstrated in the parasternal long axis view (A), short axis view (B), and apical 4-chamber view (C). This provides an estimate of the shape and extent of the flow disturbance produced by MR in three dimensions.

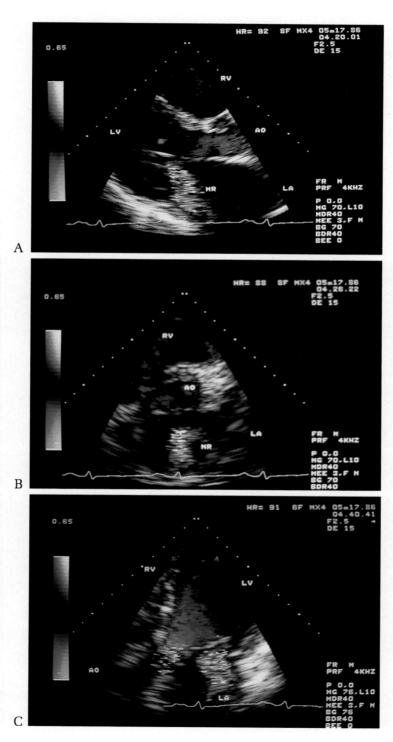

SECTION 3   MITRAL VALVE

Figure MV-25   Mitral regurgitation: Color Doppler assessment of severity. (A) Long axis view shows the maximum area of MR signals measured by planimetry. (B) In the frame where the maximal MR signals are detected, the LA area is also measured by planimetry. (C) Then the maximum area of the MR is recorded in the aortic or high left ventricular short axis view. (D) The left atrial area is next planimetered in the same plane. (E,F) Finally, the maximal area of the flow disturbance produced by MR is obtained in the apical 4-chamber view and its area measured by planimetry. The left atrial area is also measured by planimetry in the same frame (not shown). The percentage ratios of the maximal flow disturbance produced by MR (RJA) to the left atrial area (LAA) is calculated in all three orthogonal planes and the maximum ratio is taken. If this ratio < 20%, MR is considered mild (angiographic grade 1/3); if it is between 20 and 40%, MR is moderate in severity (angiographic grade 2/3); and a percentage ratio > 40% indicates the presence of severe MR (grade 3/3 angiographic regurgitation using Nagle's criteria). (G) Schematic shows the measurement technique.

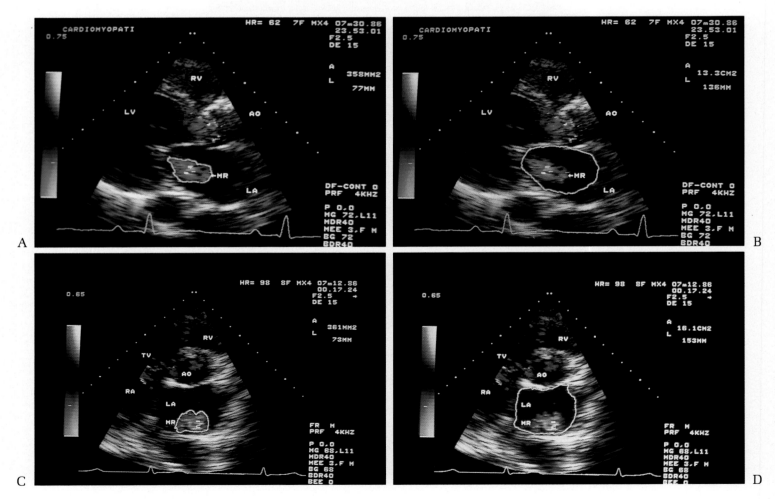

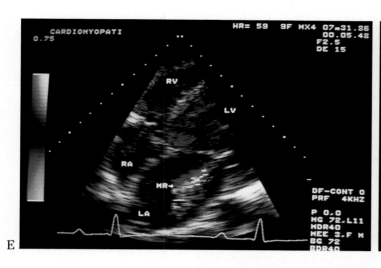

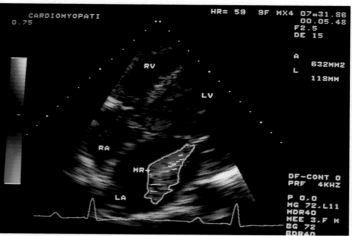

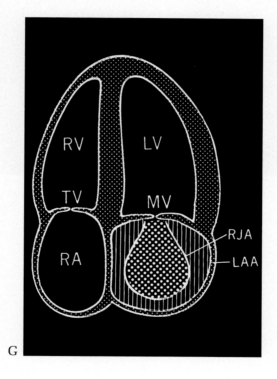

77

SECTION 3 MITRAL VALVE

Figure MV-26 **Mitral regurgitation.** In this long axis view, systolic mosaic-colored signals representing high velocity and turbulence due to MR are noted in the LA immediately below the mitral orifice. Further upstream, however, only blue signals are visualized in the LA because the jet velocity has decreased to below the Nyquist limit of 0.75 m/sec and flow disturbance is minimal. For assessing the severity of MR, these low-velocity blue signals should also be included in the MR area measurement. These signals can be differentiated from pulmonary venous flow because they occur in continuity with the mosaic pattern of regurgitant signals and move with it in the cardiac cycle. The severity of MR will be considerably underestimated if the lower-velocity regurgitant signals are ignored.

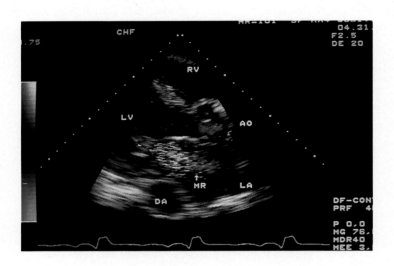

SECTION 3   MITRAL VALVE

Figure MV-27   **Mitral regurgitation: Assessment of severity.** In a 25-year-old woman, MR presents as predominantly red flow signals in the LA during systole in the apical 4-chamber view. This unusual pattern is caused by aliasing and direction of portions of the regurgitant jet toward the transducer. For assessing MR severity, such unusual signals must be taken into account. Their origin from the MV and their occurrence during systole and not diastole help to identify them as MR signals. The red signals on the ventricular aspect of the thickened MV represent aliased flow acceleration.

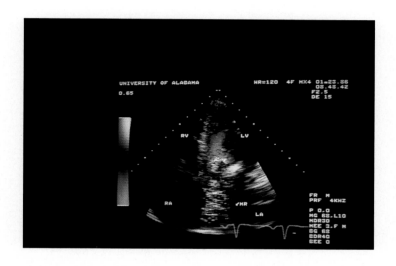

SECTION 3   MITRAL VALVE

Figure MV-28   **Severe mitral regurgitation with swirling.** (A) Apical 4-chamber view during systole demonstrates mosaic-colored signals originating from the thickened MV and directed into the LA. The red signals seen in continuity with mosaic signals are due to swirling of the regurgitant flow in the huge LA. Absence of aliasing in the inferiorly directed regurgitant flow (red) reflects loss of kinetic energy and decreased velocity below the Nyquist limit. (Reproduced with permission from Switzer and Nanda, Doppler color flow mapping. Ultrasound Med. Biol. 11:403–416, 1985). (B) Schematic illustrates the swirling effect in the LA.

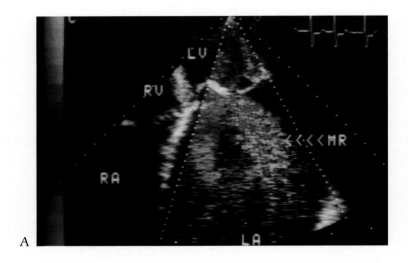

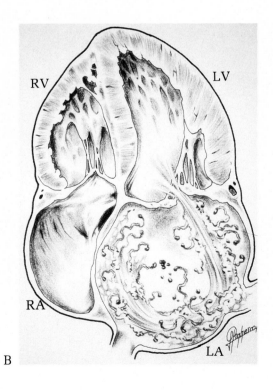

SECTION 3 MITRAL VALVE

Figure MV-29 **Mitral regurgitation with swirling.** (A,B,C) Considerable MR producing swirling in normal or mildly enlarged LA is shown in 3 patients using 3 different commercially available color Doppler systems.

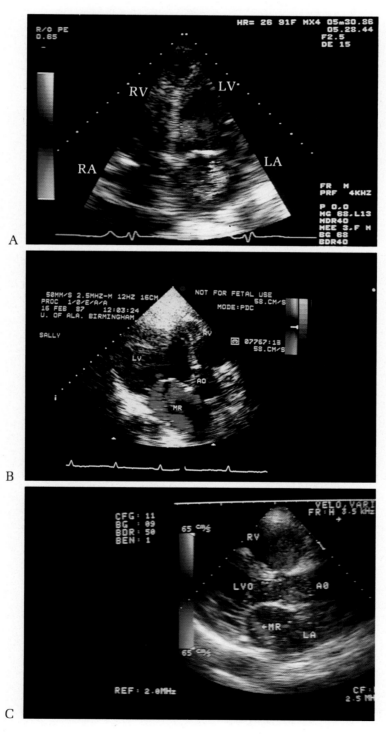

SECTION 3 MITRAL VALVE

Figure MV-30 **Mitral regurgitation.** (A) Schematic explains why, in some patients, MR signals may not appear to originate from the closed MV viewed in long axis. (B) Long axis view in a patient with MR shows mosaic-colored signals in the LA which do not appear to originate from the MV. (C) Minimal transducer angulation in the same patient shows MR signals originating from the MV (right), and color M-mode recording (left) demonstrates pansystolic MR.

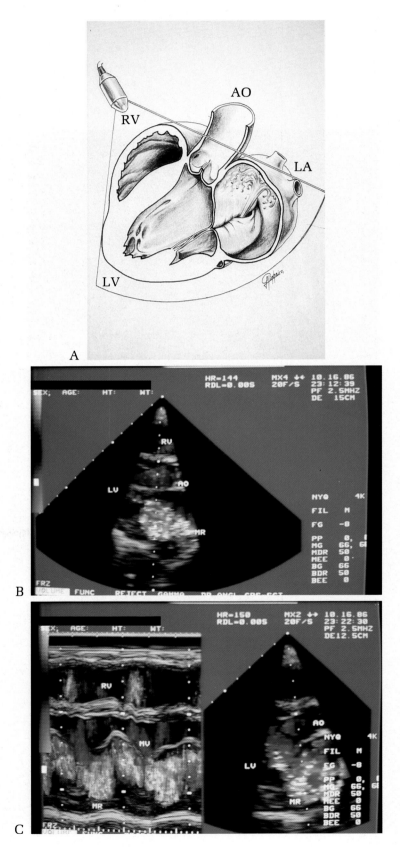

SECTION 3 MITRAL VALVE

Figure MV-31 **Mitral regurgitation.** (A) Apical 4-chamber view shows 2 discrete jets of MR (J1 J2) in a patient with ischemic heart disease. (B) Long axis view shows 2 discrete jets of MR in another patient who has had aortic aneurysm repair and AV replacement. MR in this patient may be secondary to LV enlargement.

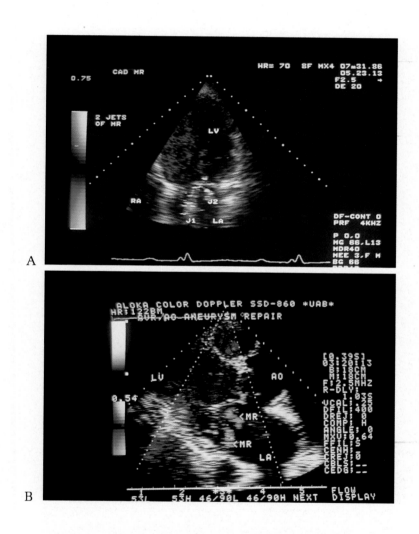

SECTION 3 MITRAL VALVE

Figure MV-32   **Mitral regurgitation.** (A) Aortic short axis view shows MR jet signals in the LA located somewhat posteriorly. Associated TR is also noted. (Reproduced with permission from Switzer and Nanda, Doppler color flow mapping. Ultrasound Med. Biol. *11*:403–416, 1985). (B) Short axis view in another patient shows MR flow signals located adjacent to the posterior wall of LA. Care should be taken not to confuse these signals with normal pulmonary venous flow. (C) Color M-mode recording shows posterior location of MR flow signals in another patient.

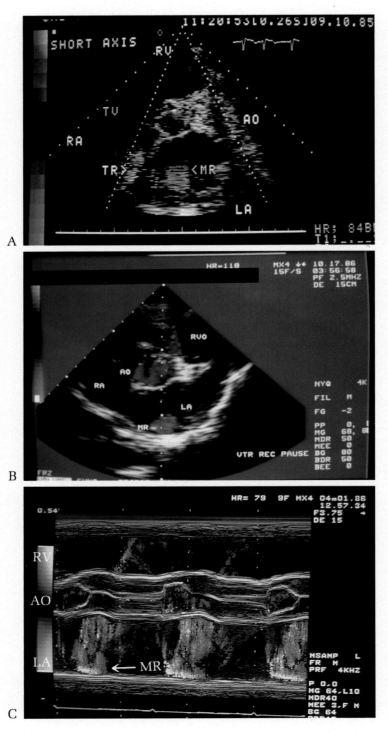

Figure MV-33   **Mitral regurgitation: Hand grip maneuver.** In an apical 4-chamber view (A), a tiny bluish-green area is seen on the atrial aspect of the MV during systole, consistent with minimal MR versus "ghosting" artifact due to rapid MV motion. In such a patient, a hand-grip maneuver accentuates the degree of MR by increasing the pressure gradient across the MV (increase in LV pressure and afterload) and helps to delineate the true nature of color signals. In this particular patient (B), hand grip (HG) increases the area of MR flow signals and also demonstrates the presence of a second MR jet. (Reproduced with permission from Switzer and Nanda, Doppler color flow mapping. Ultrasound Med. Biol. *11*:403–416, 1985). (C) Schematic.

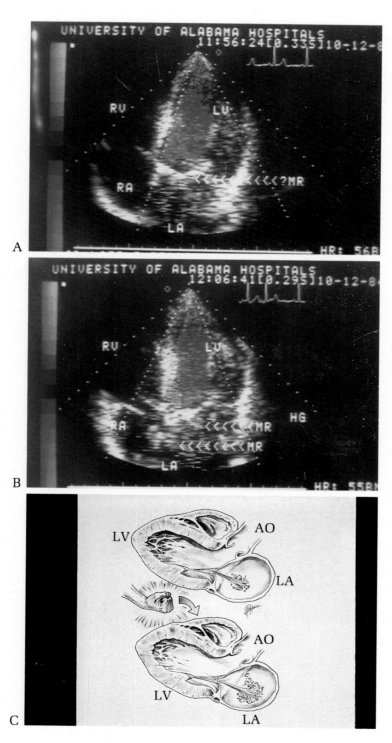

Figure MV-34 **Mitral regurgitation: Right parasternal examination.** (A) Schematic illustrates an enlarged LA viewed from the right parasternal approach. PV=pulmonary vein; CS=coronary sinus. (B,C) Right parasternal studies using two different color Doppler systems show blue, yellow, and mosaic-colored MR signals in the LA of a 50-year-old man with a flail MV. Note bulging of the atrial septum, (AS) into the RA. (D,E,F) Right parasternal examination in a 22-year-old woman with lupus erythematosus shows predominantly blue (D), red (E), and both blue and red (F) MR signals in the LA, depending on transducer angulation. (G) In a patient with congestive cardiomyopathy, the transducer has been angled to show a large portion of the RA and a relatively small portion of the LA which is completely filled with mosaic-colored signals due to MR.

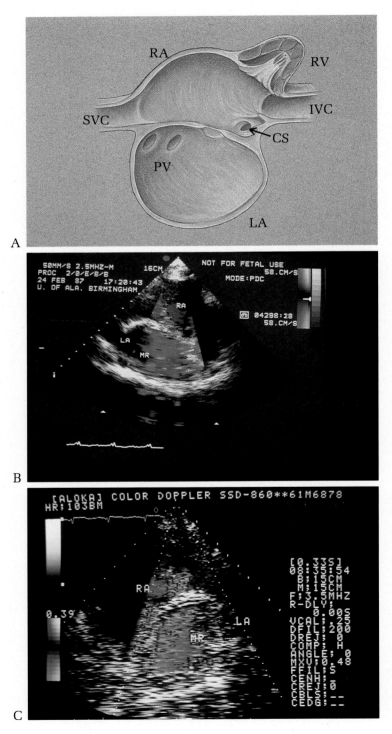

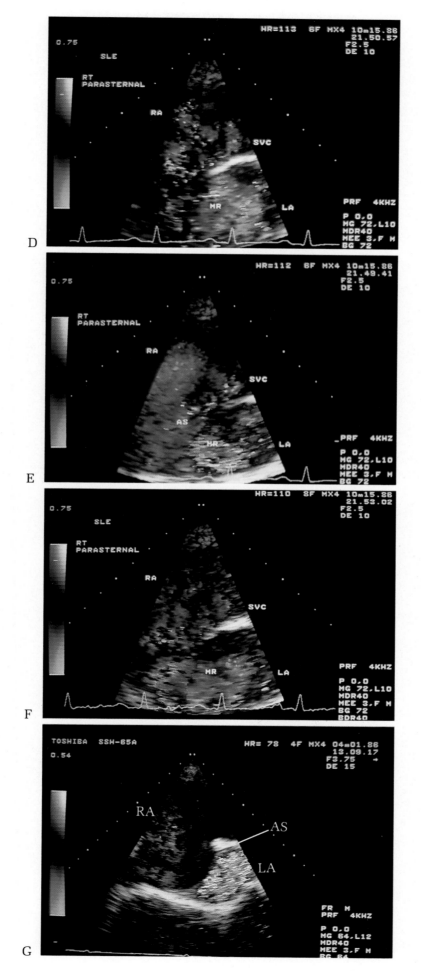

SECTION 3 MITRAL VALVE

Figure MV-35 **Mitral regurgitation: Examination from the left axilla.** In an adult female with rheumatic MV disease and angiographically documented severe MR, color Doppler failed to show any MR signals in the huge LA in any of the parasternal (both left and right), apical, suprasternal, or subcostal views. Examination from the left axilla, however, reveals a larger extent of the LA and shows multiple systolic flow signals (red) consistent with significant MR.

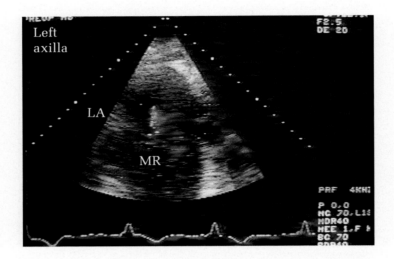

SECTION 3 MITRAL VALVE

Figure MV-36   **Mitral valve prolapse.** (A,B) Autopsy specimens show folding and redundancy of both mitral leaflets in a patient with myxomatous degeneration of the MV. C shows nodular thickening of the mitral leaflets and D and E demonstrate redundancy of the chordae and hooding of the mitral leaflets.

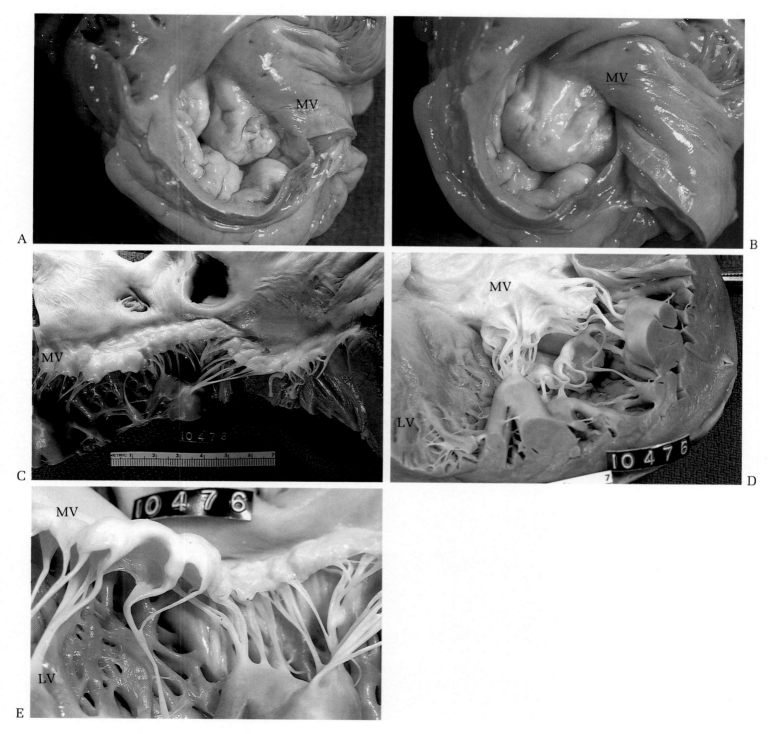

SECTION 3 MITRAL VALVE

Figure MV-37 **Mitral valve prolapse.** (A) Long axis view shows prolapse of the anterior mitral leaflet (MVP) in a young woman. (B) Color M-mode from the same patient shows green and yellow signals in late systole coinciding with posterior displacement of the MV, indicating late systolic MR. (C) Color M-mode recording in an elderly woman with MV prolapse shows mosaic-colored signals of MR (arrow) in middle to late systole.

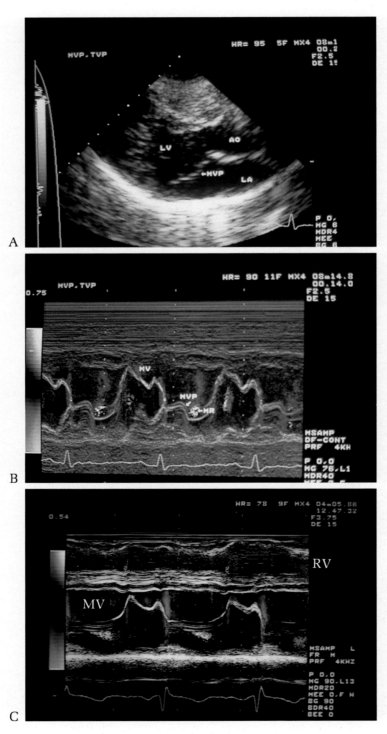

SECTION 3   MITRAL VALVE

Figure MV-38   **Mitral valve prolapse.** Long axis view in a patient with MV prolapse shows a long, thin jet of late systolic MR.

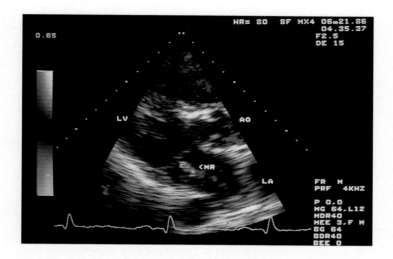

SECTION 3 MITRAL VALVE

Figure MV-39 **Posterior mitral leaflet prolapse.** Apical 4-chamber view (A) in a 73-year-old man with prolapse involving mainly the posterior leaflet. The mosaic-colored regurgitant signals are small and directed anteriorly toward the AS. Minimal transducer angulation demonstrates more severe MR (B). Long axis view (C) shows posterior mitral leaflet prolapse and MR signals directed anteriorly toward the aorta. The blue and red signals on the ventricular aspect of the mitral leaflets in B and C represent aliased flow acceleration (ACC).

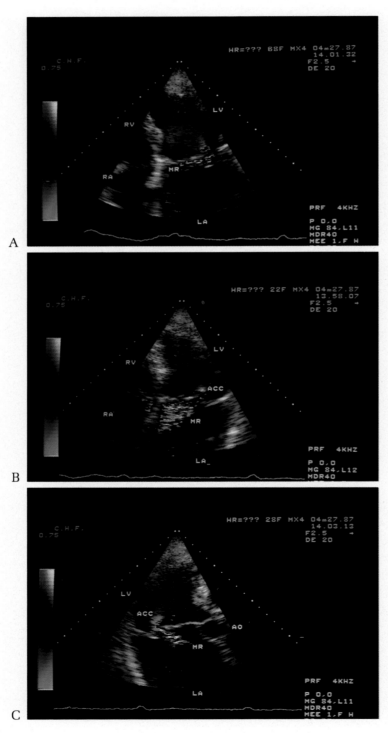

SECTION 3   MITRAL VALVE

Figure MV-40   **Mitral valve prolapse.** (A,B) In a 64-year-old man with MV prolapse, minimal MR is represented by a few yellow and green flow signals that lie in close contact with the anterior leaflet, viewed in low parasternal long axis plane. Apical 4-chamber view (C) delineates the MR signals more clearly, although most of them are still in close contact with the MV. In this patient, the hand-grip maneuver did not increase the flow disturbance.

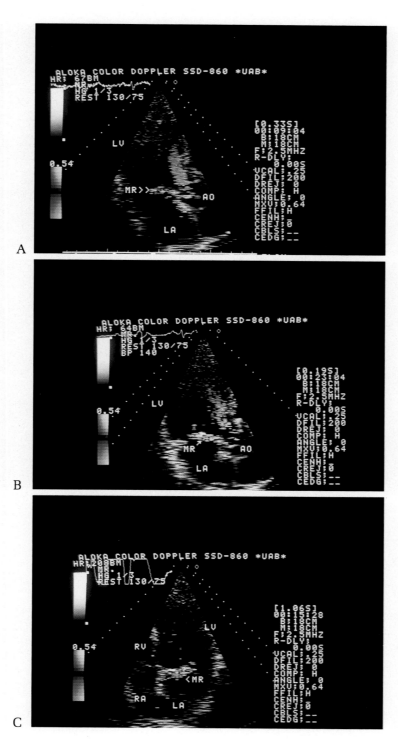

SECTION 3   MITRAL VALVE

Figure MV-41.   **Mitral valve prolapse.** (A, B) Apical views in a 67-year-old woman show prominent prolapse (arrow) of the posterior leaflet into the LA and MR signals moving from the LV into the LA through the separation between the two leaflets. Initially, MR flow signals are predominantly bluish in color, reflecting flow away from the transducer, but they later take on a reddish-yellow appearance due to aliasing and anterior direction of flow (toward the transducer). This finding is commonly seen with posterior mitral leaflet prolapse, which results in the MR jet being directed antero-superiorly. Clinically, the systolic murmur in these patients frequently radiates to the aortic area. Aortic short axis view (C) in the same patient shows mosaic-colored MR flow signals in close proximity to the aortic root. D represents a long axis view in a 49-year-old man with prominent posterior mitral leaflet prolapse, showing the MR jet directed predominantly along the anterior MV leaflet (greenish-yellow signals). FA=flow acceleration. The schematic (E) illustrates anterior and superior direction of the MR jet due to posterior mitral leaflet prolapse.

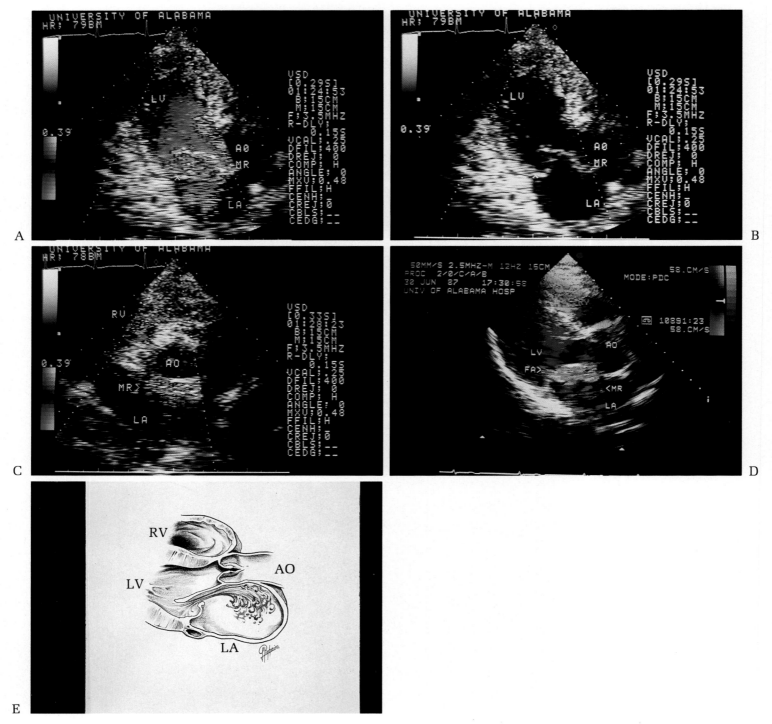

SECTION 3 MITRAL VALVE

Figure MV-42 **Late systolic mitral regurgitation without mitral valve prolapse.** Long axis view in a 74-year-old woman with systemic hypertension and concentric LV hypertrophy shows late systolic flow signals in LA due to MR. The small width of the MR jet at its origin indicates a small defect (either structural or functional) in the MV. The relatively large total area of flow signals, however, suggests more severe MR, probably related to increased pressure gradient across the MV due to systemic hypertension. Because MR in this patient occurred in late systole, it is more likely to be secondary to papillary muscle dysfunction associated with systemic hypertension than due to localized thickening of the MV seen on 2D examination. There was no evidence of MV prolapse on 2D examination of this patient.

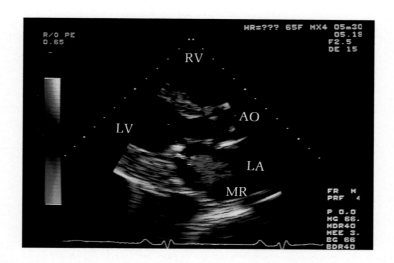

SECTION 3 MITRAL VALVE

Figure MV-43   Flail mitral valve. (A,B) Severe MR in a 77-year-old woman presents predominantly as red signals intermingled with mosaic-colored signals filling most of the LA in systole. The red signals represent antero-superior direction of the MR jet due to a flail posterior mitral leaflet. Because, in B, most of the LA is occupied by red signals and the mosaic-colored signals are confined to a small area under the mitral valve, MR severity would be grossly underestimated if the examiner mistook the red flow signals for prominent pulmonary venous flow. (C) Short axis view at the level of the high LVOT also shows a large area of red flow signals and a much smaller mosaic-colored area in the LA during systole. The small area of mosaic-colored signals in the RA represents associated mild TR. (D) Color M-mode study in the same patient shows mosaic-colored signals and more posteriorly located red signals in the LA throughout systole, indicating pansystolic MR.

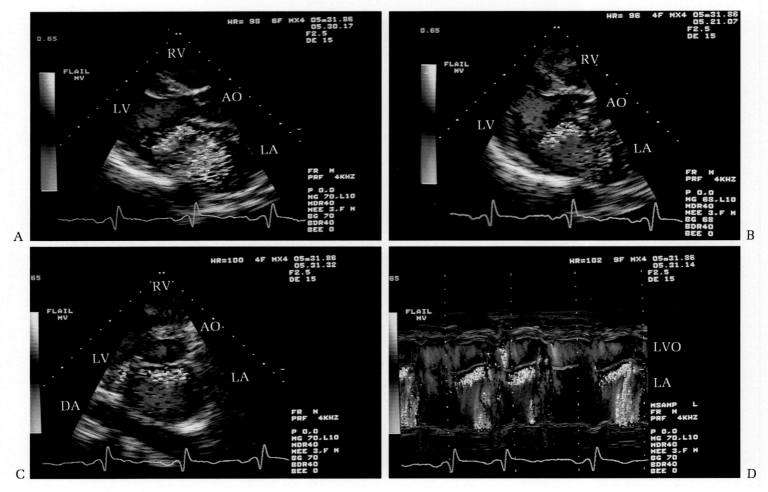

SECTION 3 MITRAL VALVE

Figure MV-44   **Flail mitral valve.** (A,B) Long axis and apical 4-chamber views in a 61-year-old man with mitral chordae rupture show prominent posterior leaflet prolapse (arrow) with clear-cut separation of the two leaflets in systole. PML=posterior mitral leaflet. (C,D) Color Doppler examination shows mosaic-colored signals moving through the area of leaflet separation and filling most of the LA, indicating severe MR. The aliased signals on the ventricular aspect of the MV represent flow acceleration (ACC). (E) Right parasternal examination in the same patient also shows mosaic-colored signals filling the whole LA. The continuous-wave Doppler cursor line was passed through these signals (right) and a high velocity of 4 m/sec was obtained (left). Because this imaging plane also represents one of the standard views in the evaluation of AS, great care has to be taken to delineate the true nature of the high-velocity signals obtained in this particular view in patients suspected to have both AS and MR. In this patient, the AV was structurally normal. F,G,H,I,J,K,L,M,N and O are color Doppler studies in a 74-year-old man with a flail MV and severe MR using two different color systems and various flow maps. The MR jet is directed anteriorly along the posterior wall of the aorta through the separation between the anterior and posterior leaflets. All are long axis views except H, which is an apical 4-chamber plane. The arrow shows the flail posterior mitral leaflet.

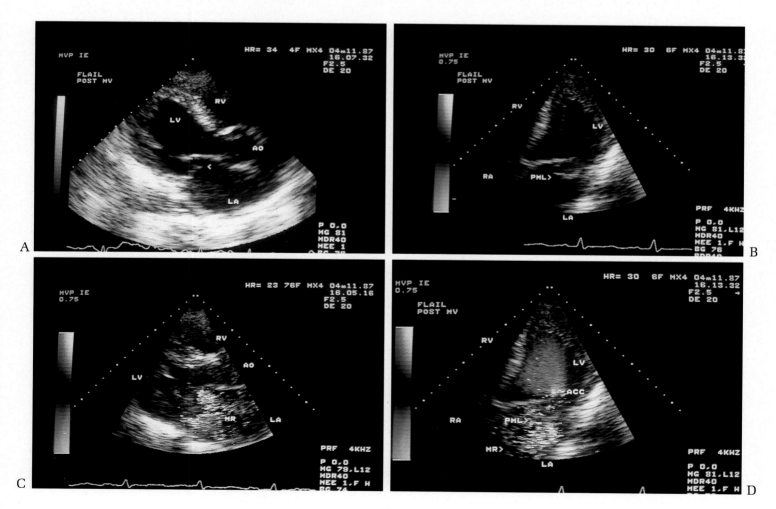

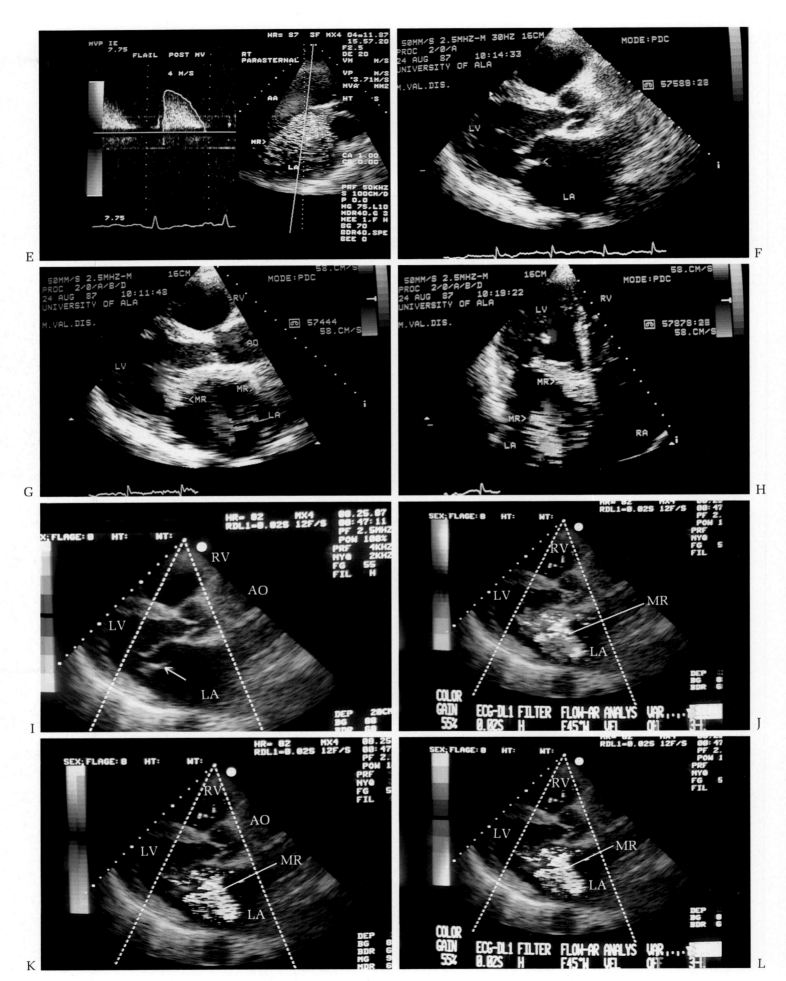

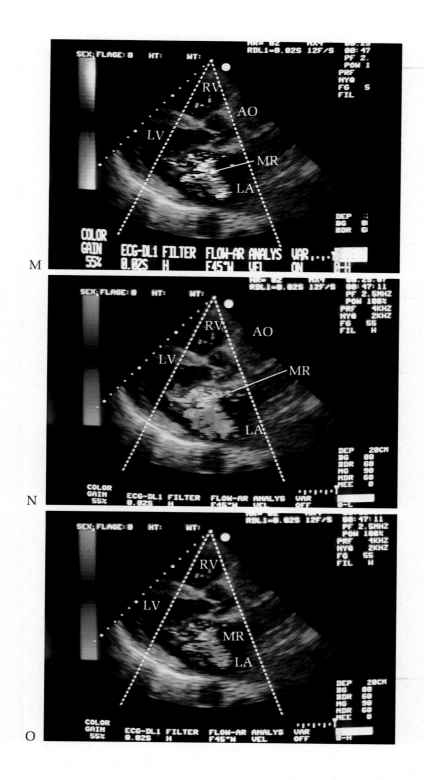

SECTION 3 MITRAL VALVE

Figure MV-45 **Mitral valve vegetations.** (A) Autopsy specimen shows a large vegetation (V) on the anterior mitral leaflet with chordae rupture (arrow), (B) Close-up of A. Multiple hemorrhagic mitral vegetations (V) and hemorrhagic vegetations (V) with MV perforation are shown in C and D.

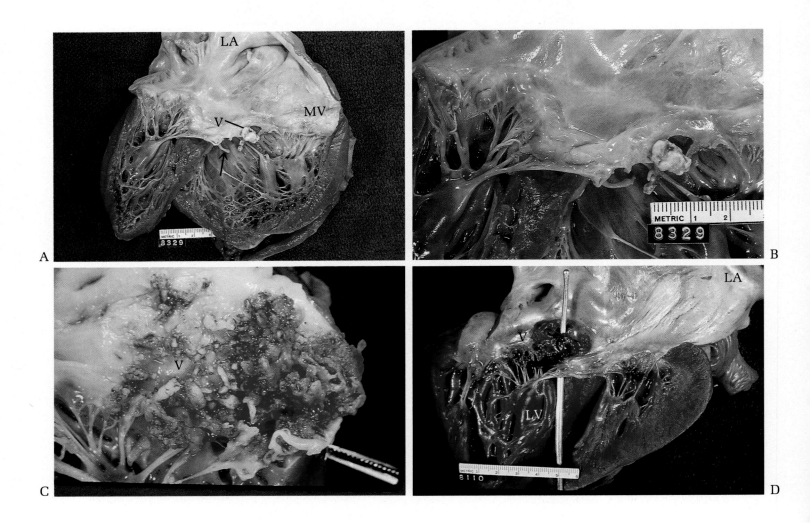

SECTION 3 MITRAL VALVE

Figure MV-46   Mitral valve vegetations. (A,B) Long axis views show mosaic-colored signals filling more than 40% of the LA during systole, indicating severe MR in a 46-year-old woman with bacterial endocarditis. The large vegetation (VEG) is clearly outlined. C is a schematic. D,E, and F are long axis and apical 4-chamber views in a 24-year-old woman with systemic lupus erythematosus, showing a huge vegetation on the MV prolapsing into the LA, indicating severe MR. The aliased red signals on the ventricular aspect of the MV represent flow acceleration. This patient died of intractable cardiac failure, and her autopsy specimen (G) shows a huge noninfective verrucous vegetation (Libman-Sacks endocarditis) and marked destruction of the MV. (H–K) Long axis views in a 29-year-old man with enterococcus bacterial endocarditis who presented with a left hemispheric cerebrovascular accident, chills and fever, angina, shortness of breath, and cardiac murmurs show mosaic-colored signals clearly moving during systole, from the LV into the LA through a 5 mm area of discontinuity (H, hole) seen in the proximal anterior mitral leaflet. Mosaic-colored signals of MR are also observed entering the LA from the coaptation area (tip) of the mitral leaflets during systole (K). J1 and J2 represent the two MR jets. The para-apical view (L) also shows the presence of severe MR. Diastolic long axis views (M,N) in the same patient show a linear vegetation (VEG) protruding into the LVO from the AV and mosaic-colored signals filling the entire extent of the LVO, indicating severe AR. Color M-mode examinations (O–R) show MR and AR as well as the fluttering vegetation (V). At surgery, a 7 mm perforation in the anterior mitral leaflet was closed and a Carpentier-Edwards annular ring inserted. The patient also underwent homograft AV replacement. S is a postoperative para-apical view showing very mild residual MR. There was no evidence of AR. The Rs represent parts of the Carpentier-Edwards ring.

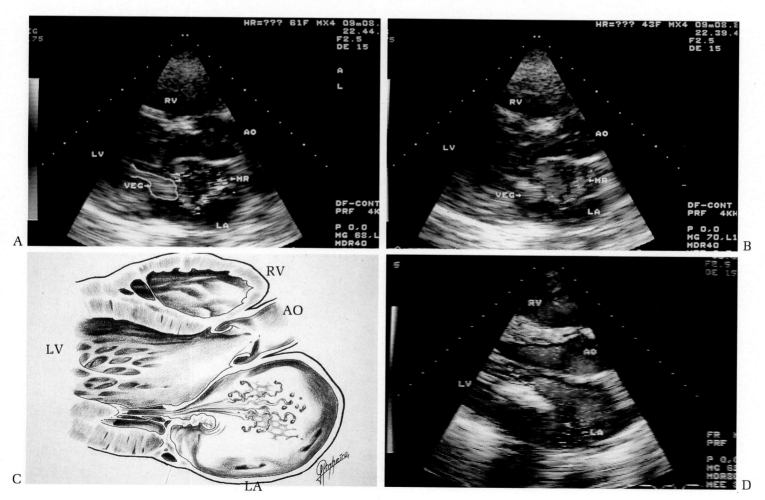

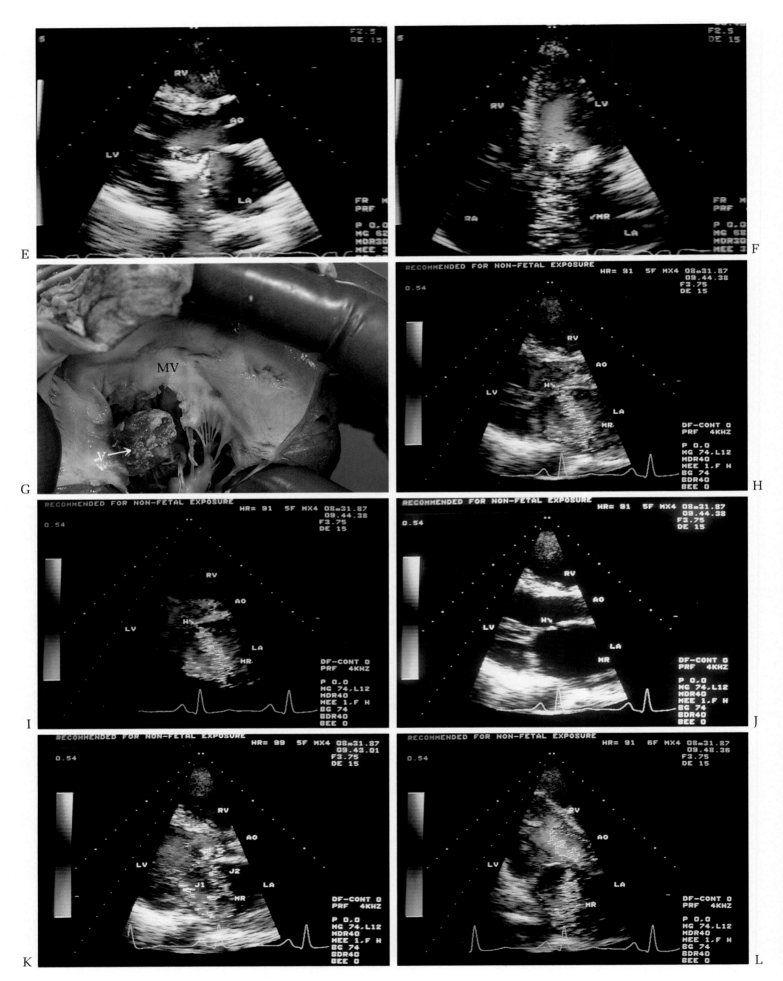

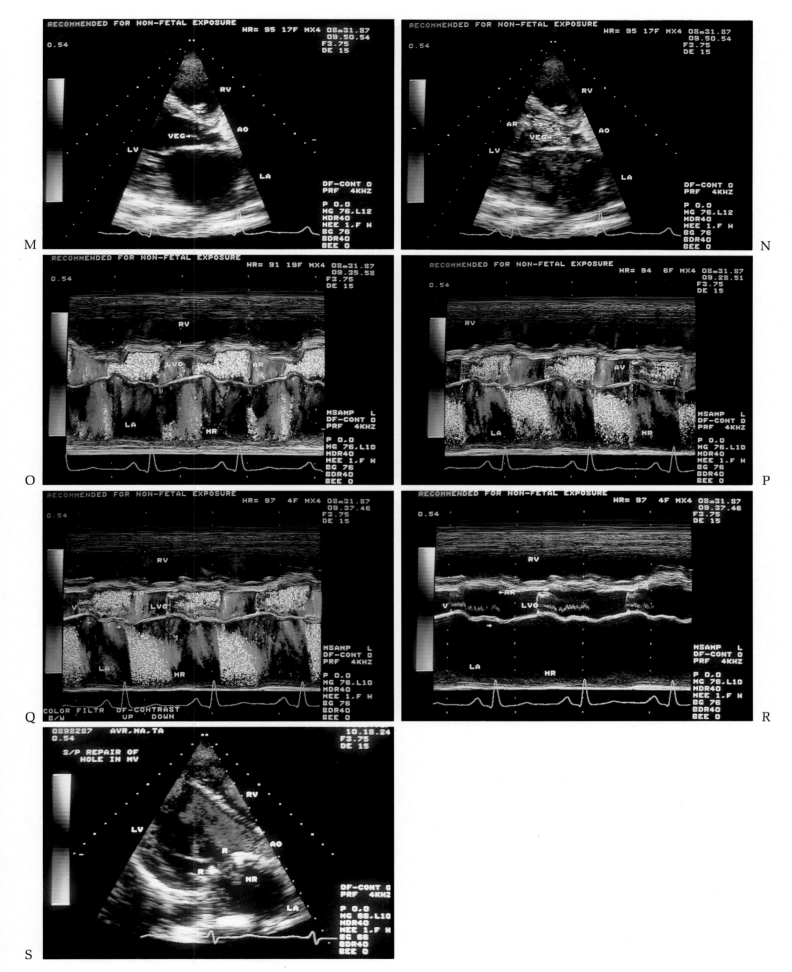

Figure MV-47   **Mitral regurgitation in acute rheumatic fever.** Aortic short axis view in a 15-year-old boy with acute rheumatic fever shows blue-colored signals in the LA in systole due to MR. This patient also has TR.

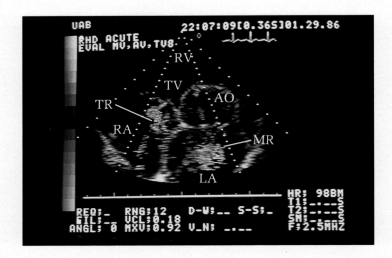

SECTION 3   MITRAL VALVE

Figure MV-48   **Mitral regurgitation due to papillary muscle dysfunction.** Apical 4-chamber view in a 68-year-old man with congestive cardiomyopathy shows inferior displacement of the mitral coaptation point and bluish-green flow signals in the LA originating from the MV, indicative of MR.

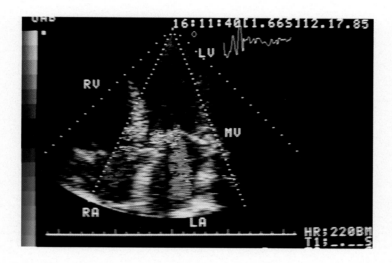

SECTION 3 MITRAL VALVE

Figure MV-49 **Mitral regurgitation due to acute rejection following cardiac transplantation.**
Apical view shows a narrow irregular band of blue signals in the LA during systole originating
from the MV consistent with mild MR. This patient did not have MR before the development of
acute rejection, and MR disappeared following resolution of rejection with immunosuppressive
therapy (biopsy proof). Development of MR after cardiac transplantation, in our experience, is a
good indicator of acute rejection.

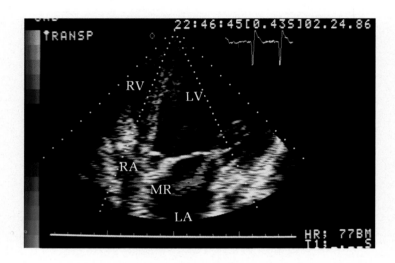

SECTION 3   MITRAL VALVE

Figure MV-50   **Mitral regurgitation induced by catheter.** (A,B,C) Apical 4-chamber views in a 69-year-old woman who underwent CA bypass surgery 3 years ago show bright linear echoes (C) in the LA and mitral orifice from a pressure monitoring line which apparently broke and could not be pulled out in the postoperative period. Color Doppler examination (D) demonstrates mild MR. The 2D directed M-mode (C) shows the catheter moving like the MV in diastole.

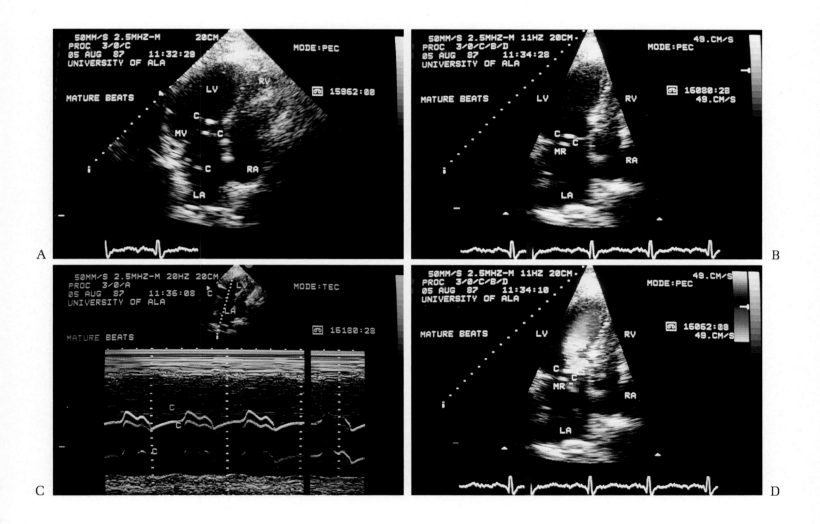

SECTION 3 MITRAL VALVE

Figure MV-51 Diastolic mitral regurgitation associated with severe AR. (A) Schematic shows diastolic MR (DMR) through a partially closed MV in a patient with significant AR and high left ventricular end diastolic pressure. (B) Color Doppler examination in a 33-year-old man with AV replacement shows a small area of mosaic-colored signals in the LA due to MR occurring in late diastole. The mosaic-colored signals filling up the entire LVOT in diastole represent severe AR in this patient. (C) Schematic shows DMR associated with severe AR. (D) Apical 4-chamber view (right) from the same patient shows diastolic mosaic-colored flow signals in the LA originating from the MV consistent with DMR. Color M-mode recording (left) confirms the occurrence of this regurgitation in late diastole.

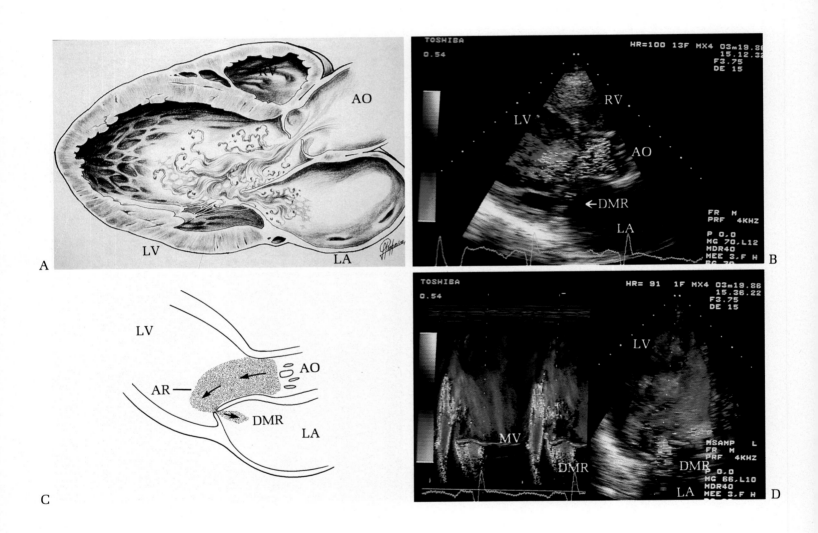

SECTION 3 MITRAL VALVE

Figure MV-52   **Diastolic mitral regurgitation associated with severe aortic regurgitation.** (A) The apical 4-chamber view in a 28-year-old male with severe AR shows flow signals moving through a partially closed MV into the LA following atrial systole. DMR is only mild in severity. The mosaic-colored signals in LV along the MV leaflet represent AR. (B) Color M-mode recording also shows the presence of late diastolic mitral regurgitation (DMR) in this patient. The mosaic-colored signals in front of the MV in diastole represent AR.

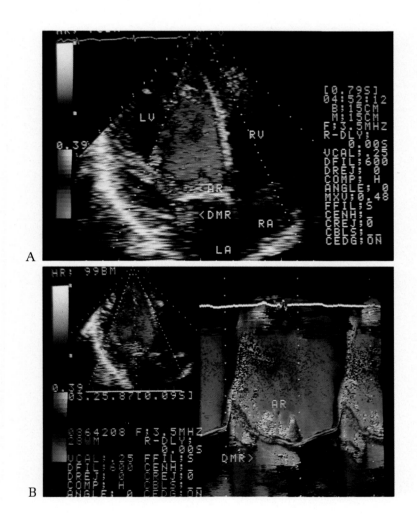

Figure MV-53 **Mitral regurgitation associated with tricuspid regurgitation.** (A) The apical 4-chamber view shows a small jet of MR and a larger and more extensive jet of TR. The mosaic-colored signals result from turbulence produced by the high-velocity regurgitant jets. B shows mild MR associated with mild TR in a 59-year-old man with multivalvular disease.

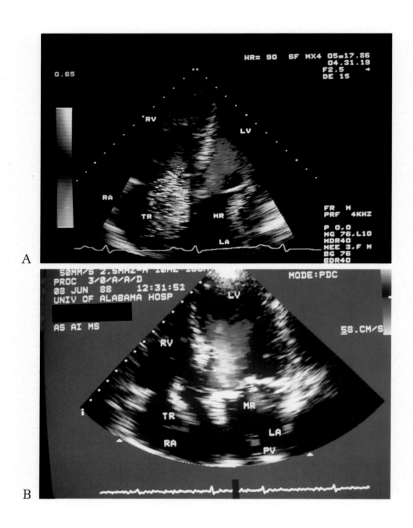

Section 4

AORTIC VALVE

AORTIC VALVE STENOSIS

Color Doppler supplements 2D echocardiography and conventional Doppler in the noninvasive assessment of aortic valve (AV) stenosis. 2D imaging identifies an abnormal AV by showing valve thickening and calcification and restriction of leaflet motion, but these findings do not always indicate the presence of significant stenosis. Continuous wave Doppler, which has been a major advance in the assessment of AV stenosis, allows the measurement of transaortic velocities. From these velocities, the peak and mean pressure gradients across the AV can be calculated using the Bernoulli equation. Recently, the continuity equation has been used to calculate the AV area. This equation is based on the premise that the volumetric flow across the LVOT (area by 2D echo times the velocity time integral) equals the volumetric flow moving through the AV (AV area times velocity time integral). Because the velocity across the AV and in the LVOT, as well as LVOT area, can be measured by CW Doppler, pulse Doppler, and 2D echocardiography, respectively, the AV area can be calculated noninvasively.

This technique is not without limitations, however. To obtain reliable measurements of velocity across the AV, it is necessary for the CW Doppler cursor to be parallel to the aortic stenotic jet; otherwise, significant underestimation of the velocity will occur. Because the flow is not visualized using either imaging or nonimaging CW Doppler, it is not possible to be certain that the cursor is aligned parallel to the aortic stenotic flow jet, which may be eccentrically directed. In practice, the examiner moves and angles the transducer so that the ultrasonic beam cuts the region of the AV in various planes. When a peak velocity is obtained, the examiner assumes that the Doppler cursor is parallel to the jet and uses that velocity for calculating a peak pressure gradient. This can lead to underestimation of peak flow velocity and the severity of AV stenosis because there is no way to confirm whether the cursor was indeed parallel to the flow direction or the jet was so eccentric that it was impossible to properly align the cursor originating from the apex of the wedge-shaped 2D sector image.

Color Doppler avoids this problem of determining the alignment of the Doppler cursor with the flow jet. With this technique, the aortic stenotic flow jet is readily visualized using the apical, suprasternal, or right parasternal view. In some cases, the aortic stenotic jet may be directed toward the posterior or anterior wall of the aorta, making it necessary to use the long axis view for optimal positioning of the Doppler cursor.

This visualization of the aortic stenotic flow jet provides a reference for the placement of the cursor parallel to the flow direction of the jet, and thus increases the confidence level of the examiner in assessing the severity of AV stenosis because the position of the Doppler cursor in relation to the aortic stenotic jet can be visualized and adjusted. It is important to emphasize that the aortic stenotic jet has three dimensions and therefore, even though the Doppler cursor may appear to be parallel to the stenotic jet in a given 2D echo plane, minor adjustments need to be made in its position to pass it through the central "core" of the jet to obtain the maximum velocity. (Fig. 4-1). In some patients, the aortic stenotic jet is so eccentric that the examiner is unable to properly align the Doppler cursor. Although the Doppler fails to measure peak velocities in such cases, the examiner is alerted to underestimation of the severity of AV stenosis. Studies in our laboratory have shown that color-guided CW Doppler measurements have higher correlation with AV area and mean transaortic pressure gradients obtained by cardiac catheterization than non-color-guided CW Doppler examination.

Color Doppler also provides an additional parameter for the estimation of aortic stenosis severity. We have found that the width of the stenotic jet at its origin is a

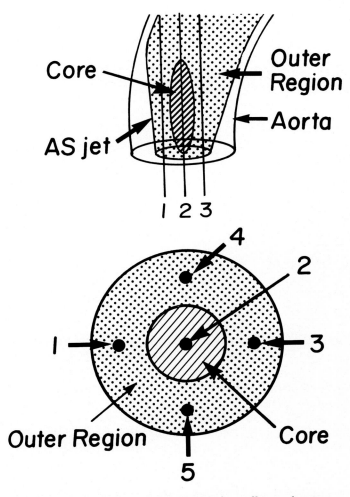

Figure 4-1 Because a stenotic jet consists of a small central region or "core" of high velocity and a larger outer region of lower velocity, the continuous wave Doppler cursor must be positioned in the jet "core" in addition to being aligned parallel to the jet direction to measure the maximum jet velocity. The three-dimensional structure of the jet may cause the continuous wave cursor to appear to be correctly positioned in the jet while, in reality, the cursor may not be properly placed in the jet "core." Therefore, after the initial alignment of the continuous wave cursor in the visualized jet, minimal transducer angulations are still required to interrogate the jet "core," which may be in the azimuthal plane. Failure to interrogate the "core" results in an underestimation of the peak transvalvar velocity and thus the severity of the stenotic lesion. In this illustration, the aortic stenosis (AS) jet is shown to consist of a central "core," which has the highest velocity, and this central "core" is surrounded by an outer region of lower velocity flows. The highest velocity is thus obtained if the continuous wave Doppler cursor is aligned parallel to the "core" of the jet (cursor 2), while lower velocities are recorded if the cursor is positioned outside the "core" (cursors 1, 3, 4, 5).

reliable indicator of the severity of AV stenosis. A narrow jet width indicates the presence of severe stenosis, and a wide jet indicates the absence of significant stenosis. In general, a jet width of 0.8 cm or less indicates critical aortic stenosis with an AV area of less than 0.75 cm² at cardiac catheterization. The jet width must be measured at the AV level because the jet widens considerably downstream due to the high driving pressure across the AV. In our laboratory, we have found that initially we were able to record the jet width in only 60% of patients with AV stenosis. We can now measure

the jet width in approximately 80% of the patients because of our increased experience in color flow mapping.

The aortic stenosis jet is optimally visualized most often in the right parasternal or suprasternal view, but in some cases it is viewed best in the apical or standard parasternal long axis view. In some patients, the measured peak aortic velocities are unreliable because of inability to obtain adequate quality Doppler spectral waveforms. This can result from the patient having either a small acoustic window or a very eccentrically directed aortic stenotic jet. A confident diagnosis of severe AV stenosis in these patients can still be made because of the narrow proximal jet width.

Flow acceleration on the ventricular aspect of the aortic stenotic jet can be seen in some patients. The presence of this flow acceleration suggests the existence of stenosis, but the use of the width of these signals near the AV to categorize the severity of AV stenosis has not yet been studied.

In some patients, especially those with small acoustic windows, the high velocities obtained from associated MR may be diagnosed as aortic stenosis because of inadequately recorded spectral waveform. Color Doppler may help in these cases because the Doppler cursor can be positioned parallel to the aortic stenotic flow jet rather than to the mitral regurgitant jet in both apical and right parasternal/suprasternal views.

Color Doppler can be used to assess the effects of balloon valvuloplasty in patients with AV stenosis. Considerable widening of the proximal jet width indicates significant relief of stenosis, while no changes in the jet width suggest unsuccessful valvuloplasty. Color-guided CW Doppler also provides reliable measurements of reductions in the peak and mean velocities and the peak and mean pressure gradients following catheter therapy. Any changes in the AV area can be assessed using these color-guided CW Doppler velocities in the continuity equation.

AORTIC REGURGITATION

A pulsed Doppler examination helps detect the presence of AR by showing aliased signals in the LVOT during diastole. It has comparable sensitivity to a color Doppler examination in the detection of the presence of AR, but limited ability in assessing its severity. The severity of AR is estimated with pulsed Doppler by measuring the distance in the LV that turbulent flow signals are seen. If a small area of high-velocity aliased signals is localized near the AV, the AR is classified as mild, and if these signals extend to the level of the anterior mitral leaflet, it is classified as moderate. Turbulent signals extending beyond the MV to the level of the papillary muscles or toward the left ventricular apex indicate severe AR. In many patients with an eccentrically oriented regurgitant jet, the diastolic turbulent signals may, however, be directed toward the anterior mitral leaflet or toward the ventricular septum and may not extend beyond the anterior mitral leaflet to the level of the papillary muscles in even severe AR. The aortic regurgitant jet may also extend past the level of the anterior mitral leaflet in patients with mild regurgitation because of a high diastolic pressure gradient across the AV, such as occurs in patients with systemic hypertension.

A color Doppler examination overcomes these limitations of a pulsed Doppler examination, making it currently the technique of choice in the noninvasive assessment of the severity of AR. This lesion is detected by color Doppler when mosaic signals originating from the AV are located in the LVOT during diastole. The width or height of these signals at their origin from the AV is a good indicator of the severity of AR. When the proximal jet width (height) occupies less than 25% of the width of the LVOT at the same location, the regurgitation correlates with mild or Grade I regurgitation found by angiocardiography using Hunt's criteria. When the jet width (height) is between 25 and 46% or 47 and 64% of the width of the LVOT, the AR is classified as moderate or Grade II, or moderately severe or Grade III regurgitation, respectively, by angiocardiography. A regurgitant jet width (height) greater than 64% of the width of the LVOT indicates severe or Grade IV and V AR by angiocardiography. These criteria for estimating the severity of AR are based on the rationale that the width (height) of the aortic regurgitant jet signals moving through the AV is related to the size of the defect in the aortic valve. For example, if the defect is very small, the width (height) of the regurgitant signals moving into the LV at its origin from the AV is small; if the defect is large and occupies a significant proportion of the AV, the flow signals moving through that defect also have a larger width (height).

It is important to remember that the aortic regurgitant jet produces turbulence and "entrainment" in the blood already present in the LVOT, and therefore the width of the turbulence is usually greater than the width of the defect in the AV. This has been documented by our in vitro studies with a flow model reproducing AR. Also, the aortic regurgitant jet has three dimensions, and therefore measuring only two dimensions of the jet as in the long axis imaging plane may not be adequate to determine its size. To eliminate this problem, the aortic regurgitant jet must also be examined in the short axis imaging plane taken at the high LVOT just proximal to the level of the AV. This view gives the exact shape of the jet as it originates from the AV, allowing for its area and the amount of the LVOT it occupies to be accurately measured or the severity of the AR present to be estimated. In this short axis view at the level of the high LVOT, the severity expressed as a ratio of the areas of the regurgitant signals to the LVOT ranges from 0 to 3%, 4 to 24%, 25 to 59%, and 60 to 100% to correspond to angiographic gradings of Grades, I, II, III, IV, and IV–V, respectively, using Hunt's criteria. These ratios correlate better with the angiographic grading than the long axis measurements because in the short axis view, an

estimate of the jet area at its origin from the AV can be obtained in all three dimensions. This is technically more difficult to perform, however, because the 2D echo "slice" at the level of the LVOT has to be perpendicular to the jet or an overestimation of the severity of AR may occur. Also, to obtain this view in many patients is very difficult, and if the view is obtained below the level of the high LVOT, the jet appears to be much larger because the aortic regurgitant jet frequently widens immediately after its origin from the AV due to the driving pressure across the AV during diastole. Therefore, when assessing the severity of AR in short axis view, only high LVOT planes, preferably those in which the AV elements are also imaged, must be used. This guarantees an accurate measurement of the regurgitant jet area at its origin from the AV. Although the aortic regurgitant jet appears circular in the short axis view, in most patients with AR, especially mild, it can appear elliptical or irregular in other patients. The width of the aortic regurgitant jet may also be measured in the apical long axis view, and the severity of this regurgitation expressed as a percent ratio of the widths of the regurgitant jet to LVOT width can be estimated using this view.

In our experience, expressing the width of the jet at the level of the high LVOT in the long axis view as a ratio to the width of the LVOT is an adequate method for estimating the severity of AR in most patients. The severity of AR can be reliably estimated using our criteria even when there is coexisting mitral stenosis because, at its origin from the AV, the jet is clearly distinguishable from the mitral stenotic jet. The two jets, however, may merge farther downstream, making it difficult to distinguish between them and to measure the maximum area of AR in the LV in many cases. We have found this to be true even in patients who do not have mitral stenosis because the prominent normal mitral inflow signals mix with the lower-velocity AR signals farther downstream in the LV, making the exact aortic regurgitant area difficult to delineate. The area, unlike the proximal width of the aortic regurgitant jet, also depends on the diastolic pressure gradient across the AV. For example, when the size of the anatomical defect in the AV remains constant, the aortic regurgitant area is much larger in a patient with systemic hypertension than in one with normal blood pressure (Fig. 4-2).

The measured width of aortic regurgitant signals in a patient may vary when the patient is examined on different color Doppler systems because of the different instrument settings available on each system. These differences are generally not significant enough to alter the grading of the AR in the most patients. In assessing the presence and severity of AR, however, it is recommended to use a set of standard optimal instrument settings and to move and angle the transducer in small increments and multiple directions to obtain the maximum proximal width of the aortic regurgitant jet.

Occasionally, a localized area of flow acceleration is seen on the aortic side of the AV, directly opposite the origin of the aortic regurgitant jet during diastole. This

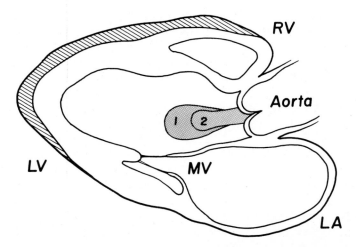

Figure 4-2 Effect of systemic hypertension on aortic regurgitation. The area and not the proximal width of the aortic regurgitant jet depends on the diastolic pressure gradient across the AV. For example, the aortic regurgitant area is much larger in the parasternal long axis view of a patient with systemic hypertension (1) than in one with normal blood pressure (2), even though approximately the same size defect is present. The depth that the regurgitant jet extends into the LV also depends on the diastolic pressure gradient across the AV. In general, the observed depth is larger in a patient with systemic hypertension.

flow acceleration often indicates the site of the defect in the AV and may provide an estimate of the size of the defect because this flow acceleration tends to take the shape of the defect in the valve.

We have encountered difficulties in assessing the severity of AR in some specific clinical situations. For example, we have found that, if the aortic root is aneurysmally enlarged, the jet width in the long axis underestimates the severity of AR. This is probably because the wide LVOT and aortic root tend to cause a small width ratio despite even a large jet width. In patients with AV vegetations also, we have sometimes underestimated the severity of aortic regurgitation. This may have occurred because the vegetation causes dispersion of the aortic regurgitant jet and resultant difficulty in measuring its width at the level of the AV.

In patients with moderate or severe AR, color Doppler examination of the aorta frequently shows prominent retrograde flow in both the ascending and descending aortas during diastole. In our experience, these prominent retrograde flow signals in the descending aorta during diastole indicate the presence of severe AR. It is, however, important to emphasize that the presence of a few retrograde flow signals in the ascending aorta in diastole does not necessarily imply the presence of AR.

Color Doppler has also been found useful in diagnosing the presence of diastolic MR. This regurgitation may be associated with severe AR when the high left ventricular end diastolic pressure exceeds the left atrial pressure during late diastole. Usually this diastolic regurgitation is mild in severity, but whenever it is detected, it signifies the presence of severe AR. This is true only in

the absence of first-degree or complete atrioventricular block, because if the P wave occurs much earlier during diastole. mitral diastolic regurgitation may occur even in the absence of AR.

The aortic regurgitant jet signals may be directed centrally into the LV, posteriorly along the anterior mitral leaflet, or anteriorly toward the ventricular septum (VS). In some patients, we have observed this jet to move posteriorly, striking the anterior mitral leaflet and then being deflected by the leaflet anteriorly toward the VS. We have also seen this regurgitant jet directed anteriorly toward the VS until it is deflected posteriorly toward the MV. This appears as a characteristic inverted "U" shape. The jet, which strikes the MV and then is deflected anteriorly toward the septum, produces a characteristic "J" shape or "hockey stick" appearance. An occasional aortic regurgitant jet may first be directed centrally into the LV until it suddenly changes its direction anteriorly toward the septum or posteriorly toward the anterior mitral leaflet. In some instances, especially with bicuspid AVs, the jet may originate anteriorly or posteriorly near the junction of the aortic wall with the VS. The AR jet has also been noted to bifurcate, with one portion moving posteriorly toward the left ventricular wall and the other moving anteriorly toward the VS. Two distinct jets of AR may also sometimes be seen directed toward the VS and toward the anterior mitral leaflet. In our experience, most patients have an aortic regurgitant jet originating centrally from the coaptation point of the aortic leaflet. Occasionally, in the parasternal long axis view, an apparently wide jet originating from the anterior aspect of the aortic valve may be observed to be directed posteriorly along the AV, leading to the conclusion of the presence of severe AR, but if the origin of the regurgitant jet is examined, it may be discovered that an erroneous diagnosis of severe AR has been made. In other words, even when the AR is mild, the jet may originate eccentrically near the junction of the anterior aortic wall with the VS causing it to move posteriorly along the AV, and this posterior direction of the jet may be misinterpreted as a wide aortic regurgitant jet filling the entire width of the LVOT. To avoid this misinterpretation, the examiner must pay careful attention to delineating the width of the aortic regurgitant jet at its origin from the AV. In numerous patients with mild AR, the width of the aortic regurgitant jet at its origin from the AV does not seem to change significantly as the jet moves downstream into the LV. In other patients, the jet appears to widen considerably downstream in the LVOT. The aortic regurgitant jet often loses its mosaic color pattern deep into the LV because its velocity decreases to below the Nyquist limit for that particular examination.

Color Doppler studies in patients with AR also facilitate the parallel placement of the continuous wave Doppler cursor to the direction of the aortic regurgitant jet so that reliable diastolic spectral velocity waveforms may be obtained. Inspection of deceleration of the peak velocity in patients with AR has been found useful in providing some information regarding the left ventricular end diastolic pressure and in estimating the severity of AR using the pressure half-time method. If the velocity deceleration during diastole is fast, it suggests the presence of an increased left ventricular diastolic pressure, and if it is slow, a normal left ventricular diastolic pressure exists.

Careful attention should be paid to the timing in the cardiac cycle when assessing patients for AR. For example, anteriorly directed signals appearing to originate from the AV may sometimes be seen near the VS during systole. These signals can be easily mistaken for AR if careful attention is not paid to the timing of the cardiac cycle. Because these signals are present during systole and consistently absent during diastole, they possibly result from a ghosting artifact from the motion of the VS.

For timing the onset and duration of AR, color M-mode is more accurate than 2D color Doppler because of its increased frame rate. The slower frame rate of the 2D color Doppler may cause errors in timing because it may cause overlapping of flow information from two adjacent areas. Using color M-mode, we have found that even with mild AR, the regurgitant jet is pandiastolic, although clinically the murmur is audible by auscultation only during early diastole.

In patients with AR and a "bowing" or "bent knee" deformity of the anterior mitral leaflet, color Doppler examination generally shows moderate to severe AR with the aortic regurgitant jet impinging on the anterior mitral leaflet at the site of the deformity. In our experience, this deformity is not seen in patients in whom the aortic regurgitant jet is not directed toward the anterior mitral leaflet. This deformity is thus shown by color Doppler to probably result from the high-velocity aortic regurgitant jet impinging on the anterior mitral leaflet.

AORTIC ANEURYSMS AND DISSECTION

In patients with ascending aortic aneurysms, color Doppler examination frequently shows swirling of blood flow in the aneurysmal ascending aorta with antegrade or forward flow during early to middle systole and retrograde or backflow during late systole and diastole. Color Doppler examination of aneurysms in the descending thoracic aorta also shows swirling of the blood flow with antegrade flow during systole and retrograde flow during late systole and diastole.

Color Doppler is useful in detecting the presence of associated AR and assessing its severity. It shows the width of the aortic regurgitant signals at their origin from the AV and allows this width to be compared to the width of the LVOT. In our experience, color Doppler evaluation of the severity of associated AR generally correlates well with angiocardiography. In some patients with ascending aortic aneurysms and angiographically documented severe AR, however, the width of the aortic regurgitant signals in the high LVOT may be small in relation to the size of the enlarged LVOT. This finding is misleading because it suggests that the AR is not severe. In such cases, examination of the descending aorta for prominent retrograde flow during diastole can be used to obtain a correct assessment of severity. Significant AR is also indicated by the presence of prominent diastolic retrograde or backflow in the nonaneurysmal portion of the aorta, such as occurs in the ascending aorta in a patient with aneurysmal descending aorta and in the descending aorta in a patient with an ascending aortic aneurysm, or in peripheral vessels such as brachiocephalic branches and femoral arteries. The presence of a clot can also be well delineated by color Doppler because the flow signals are prominently displayed in the nonclotted lumen but not in the area of the clot.

Color Doppler supplements 2D echocardiography and pulsed Doppler in the assessment of an aortic dissection. A simultaneous recording of oppositely directed flows as shown by red and blue signals separated by a linear echo indicates a dissection. This flow pattern allows a confident diagnosis of the presence of a dissection to be made, especially in patients in whom the intimal dissection flap is not mobile and when it is unclear whether the linear echo is caused by an artifact or a dissection. If the dissection flap is highly mobile, a confident diagnosis of aortic dissection can be made on the basis of a 2D examination alone.

In the proximal ascending aorta, the lumen which is in direct communication with the AV is the true lumen, but identification of the true lumen in the aortic arch and in the descending thoracic aorta is difficult. Also, in some patients, the false lumen may be the perfusing conduit and the true lumen may be clotted. The site of the origin of the dissection and its extent determine the classification of the dissection. When the dissection originates from the ascending aorta and extends by varying degrees in the descending thoracic and abdominal aorta or is restricted to the ascending aorta and aortic arch, it is classified as DeBakey I and II, respectively. A DeBakey III dissection indicates that the dissection is confined to the descending thoracic and abdominal aorta. In our experience, most patients have DeBakey I. Some patients with DeBakey III, have been observed, but so far only one patient with DeBakey II has been observed.

A color Doppler examination also shows the site of communication or a gap between the two lumina by clearly displaying flow signals moving from one lumen into the other through an area of discontinuity in the dissection flap in the ascending aorta, aortic arch, descending thoracic aorta, or abdominal aorta. A back-and-forth movement of the flow during the cardiac cycle may be seen at the site of communication between the two lumina. Flow signals are observed moving from the true lumen into the false lumen during one portion of the cardiac cycle, usually systole. During diastole, flow signals are seen moving back into the true lumen from the false lumen. In some patients, however, the site of communication between the two lumina may not be visualized by color Doppler directly, but can still be indirectly deduced. For example, in one patient we have observed flow signals moving toward the transducer in only one of the two lumina in the ascending aorta during early systole. During late systole, we observed flow signals still present in the first lumen and additional oppositely directed flow signals in the second lumen. These flow patterns indicated that the site of communication between two lumina was in the aortic arch, and this was later confirmed at surgery. Simultaneous opacification of the two lumina in the proximal ascending aorta with flow signals moving in the same direction suggests that the communication is located in the proximal ascending aorta, although it may not be clearly outlined using 2D imaging, and color Doppler may not display the flow moving from one lumen into the other. The presence of flow in one lumen and its absence in the other lumen may alert the examiner to the presence of a clot in the nonopacified lumen.

Color Doppler identifies the site of communication between the two lumina with accuracy comparative to that of angiocardiography, although both techniques complement each other because, in some patients, the site of communication is detected by color Doppler and missed by angiocardiography and vice versa. One of the aims of the surgeon operating on a patient with aortic dissection is to close the site of communication between the two lumina. This causes one lumen to become clotted and to serve as a buttress to the other lumen, thus reducing the possibility of extending the dissection and rupturing the dissected aorta.

Color Doppler is also very useful in assessing the presence and severity of associated AR by noting the width of the aortic regurgitant signals at their origin from the AV and comparing it to the LVOT width measured at the same location. In our experience, color Doppler evaluation of the severity of regurgitation in the presence of dissection is as accurate as angiocardiography.

In patients with aortic dissection and dilatation of the descending aorta or aneurysms of the descending aorta, the lung is often displaced so that posterior intercostal spaces can be used for acoustic access to the descending thoracic aorta. This can best be accomplished by placing the patient in the lateral decubitus position, applying the transducer in the posterior intercostal spaces, and angling it to view the descending thoracic aorta in the long and short axis planes.

In patients with a surgically closed communication between the two lumina of an aortic dissection, color Doppler is useful in showing the absence of flow in one of the lumina. A successful closure of the communication between the true and the false lumen is indicated by color Doppler showing flow signals in one lumen and none in the other. Color Doppler is also useful in examining patients in whom an intraluminal tube graft and AV prosthesis have been surgically placed because it displays the presence of any leak through the intraluminal tube graft into the native aneurysm and facilitates the parallel positioning of the continuous wave Doppler cursor to the flow through the aortic prosthesis to accurately obtain pressure gradients across it. For example, we found in one patient that color Doppler accurately showed a leakage into the native aneurysm, its location in the posterior aspect, and a large hematoma. This patient underwent surgery to repair the site of the leak, and a repeat study in the postoperative period showed absence of communication between the intraluminal tube graft and the native aortic dissecting aneurysm. The intraluminal tube graft may be easily identified, using 2D echocardiography, by the presence of rugae or corrugations in its walls, which are made of Teflon. The leak between the intraluminal tube graft and the native aneurysm usually occurs at the suture line, which may need to be repaired surgically. Color Doppler is also useful in assessing the presence and severity of aortic prosthetic regurgitation.

REFERENCES

Aortic Valve Stenosis

1. Hatle, L., Angelsen, B.A., and Tromsdal, A.: Noninvasive assessment of aortic stenosis by Doppler ultrasound. Br. Heart J. 43:284, 1980.
2. Currie, P.J., Seward, J.B., Reeder, C.S., Viletstra, R.E., Bresnahan, D.R., Bresnahan, J.F., Smith, H.C., Hagler, D.J., and Tajik, A.J.: Continuous wave Doppler echocardiographic assessment of severity of calcitic aortic stenosis: A simultaneous Doppler catheter correlative study in 100 adult patients. Circulation 71:1162, 1985.
3. Switzer, D.F., and Nanda, N.C.: Limitations of pulsed and continuous-wave Doppler echocardiography (Editorial). Echocardiography: A Review of Cardiovascular Ultrasound 2:207, 1985.
4. Zoghbi, W.A., Farmen, K.L., Soto, J.G., Nelson, J.G., and Quinones, M.A.: Accurate noninvasive quantification of stenotic aortic valve area by Doppler echocardiography. Circulation 73:452, 1986.
5. Panidis, I.P., Mintz, G.S., and Ross, J.: Value and limitations of Doppler ultrasound in evaluation of aortic stenosis: A statistical analysis of 70 consecutive patients. Am. Heart J. 12:150, 1986.
6. Hsiung, M.C., Moos, S., Woo, R., Yoganathan, A.P., and Nanda, N.C.: Correlation of color Doppler guided continuous wave Doppler velocities with catheterization pressures and laser Doppler velocities in an in vitro aortic stenosis model (Abstract). Clin. Res. 34:308A, 1986.
7. Come, P.C., Riby, M.F., McKay, R.C., and Satian, R.: Echocardiographic assessment of aortic valve area in elderly patients with aortic stenosis and of changes in valve area after percutaneous balloon valvuloplasty. J. Am. Coll. Cardiol. 10:115, 1987.
8. Fan, P.H., Kan, M.N., Helmcke, F., Cooper, J.W., and Nanda, N.C.: Color Doppler assessment of aortic valve stenosis (Abstract). J. Am. Coll. Cardiol. 9:65A, 1987.
9. Villa Costa, I., Aggarwal, K.K., Bulle, T., Dean, L., Baxley, W., and Nanda, N.C.: Color Doppler flow imaging in balloon valvotomy. (Abstract). Circulation 72 (Suppl IV): IV-1987.

Aortic Regurgitation

1. Bommer, W.J., Mapes, B.S., Miller, L., Mason, D.T., and DeMaria, A.N.: Quantitation of aortic regurgitation with two-dimensional Doppler echocardiography. Am. J. Cardiol. 47:412, 1981.
2. Esper, R.J.: Detection of mild aortic regurgitation by range gated pulsed Doppler echocardiography. Am. J. Cardiol. 50:1037, 1982.
3. Omoto, R., Yokote, Y., Takamoto, S., Kyo, S., Ueda, K., Asano, H., Namekawa, K., Kasai, C., Kondo, Y., and Koyano, A.: The development of real-time two-dimensional Doppler echocardiography and its clinical significance in acquired valvular disease: With specific reference to the evaluation of valvular regurgitation. Japan. Heart J. 25:325, 1984.
4. Touche, T., Prasquier, R., Nitenberg, A., DeZuterre, D., and Gourgon, R.: Assessment and follow-up of patients with aortic regurgitation by an updated Doppler echocardiographic measurement of the regurgitant fraction in the aortic arch. Circulation 72:819, 1985.
5. Kitabatake, A., Ito, H., Inove, M., Tanouchi, J., Ishihara, K., Morita, T., Fujii, K., Yoshida, Y., Masuyama, T., Yoshima, H., Hori, M., and Kamada T.: A new approach to noninvasive evaluation of aortic regurgitant fraction by two-dimensional Doppler echocardiography. Circulation 72:523, 1985.
6. Byard, C.E., Perry, G.J., Roitman, D.I., and Nanda, N.C.: Quantitative assessment of aortic regurgitation by color Doppler (Abstract). Circulation 72 (Suppl. III): III, 146, 1985.
7. Rokey, R., Sterlin, L.L., Zoghbi, W.A., Sartori, M.P., Limacher, M.C., Kuo, L.C., and Quinones, M.A.: Determination of regurgitant fraction in isolated mitral or aortic regurgitation by pulsed Doppler two-dimensional echocardiography. J. Am. Coll. Cardiol. 7:1273, 1986.
8. Masuyama, T., Kodama, K., Kitabatake, A., Nanto, S., Sato, H., Clematsu, M., Inoue, M., and Kamada, T.: Noninvasive evaluation of aortic regurgitation by continuous-wave Doppler echocardiography. Circulation 73:460, 1986.
9. Perry, G.J., and Nanda, N.C.: Diagnosis and quantitation of valvular regurgitation by color Doppler flow mapping. Echocardiography: A Review of Cardiovascular Imaging 3:493, 1986.
10. Switzer, D.F., Yoganathan, A., Nanda, N.C., Woo, Y.R., and Ridgway, A.J.: Calibration of color Doppler flow mapping during extreme hemodynamic conditions in vitro: A foundation for a reliable quantitative grading system for aortic incompetence. Circulation 75:837, 1987.
11. Beyer, R.W., Ramirez, M., Josephsan, M.A., and Shah, P.M.: Correlation of continuous-wave Doppler assessment of chronic aortic regurgitation with hemodynamic and angiography. Am. J. Cardiol. 60:852, 1987.
12. Perry, G.J., Helmcke, F., Nanda, N.C., Byard, C., and Soto, B.: Evaluation of aortic insufficiency by Doppler color flow mapping. J. Am. Coll. Cardiol. 9:952, 1987.
13. Perry, G.J., and Nanda, N.C.: Color Doppler evaluation of left-sided valvular regurgitation. Dynam. Cardiovasc. Imag. 1:28, 1987.
14. Perry G.J., and Nanda, N.C.: Recent advances in color Doppler evaluation of valvular regurgitation. Echocardiography: A Review of Cardiovascular Imaging 4:503, 1987.
15. Wong, M., Matsumura, M., Suzuki, K., and Omoto, R.: Technical and biologic sources of variability in the mapping of aortic, mitral and tricuspid color flow jets. Am. J. Cardiol. 60:847, 1987.
16. Becher, H., Grube, E., and Luderitz, B.: Evaluation of aortic valve insufficiency using color Doppler echocardiography. Z. Kardiol 76:8, 1987.
17. Perry, G.J., Helmcke, F., Kan, M.N., Tracy, W., Kirklin, J.K., Moos, S., and Nanda, N.C.: Determination of regurgitant volume by combined color and continuous wave Doppler in a dog model of aortic insufficiency (Abstract). Circulation 72 (Suppl. IV), 1987.
18. Goyal, R.G., Hsiung, M.C., Perry, G.J., Helmcke, F., Nanda, N.C., and Kan, M.N.: Extended experience in color Doppler evaluation of aortic regurgitation (Abstract). Clin. Res. 35:282A, 1987.

Aortic Aneurysms and Dissection

1. De Maria, A., Bommer, W., Neumann, A., Weinert, L., Borgen, H., and Mason, D.T.: Identification of aneurysm of ascending aorta by cross-sectional echocardiography. Circulation 59:755, 1979.
2. Victor, M.F., Mintz, G.S., Kotler, M.N., Wilson, A.R., and Segal, B.L.: Two-dimensional echocardiographic diagnosis of aortic dissection. Am. J. Cardiol. 48:1155, 1981.
3. Iliceto, S., Antonelli, G., Biasco, G., and Rizzon, P.: Two-dimensional echocardiographic evaluation of aneurysms of the descending thoracic aorta. Circulation 66:1045, 1982.
4. Iliceto, S., Ettorre, G., Francioso, G., Antonelli, G., Biasco, G., and Rizzon, P.: Diagnosis of aneurysm of the thoracic aorta: Comparison between two non-invasive techniques: two-dimensional echocardiography and computed tomography. Eur. Heart J. 5:545, 1984.
5. Miller, J.L., Nanda, N.C., Singh, R.P., Mathew, T., Iliceto, S., and Rizzon, P.: Echocardiography diagnosis of aortic aneurysms and dissection. Echocardiography: A review of cardiovascular ultrasound 1:507, 1984.
6. Mathew, T., and Nanda, N.C.: Two-dimensional and Doppler echocardiographic evaluation of aortic aneurysm and dissection. Am. J. Cardiol. 54:379, 1984.
7. Omoto, R., Yokote, Y., and Takamoto, S.: Diagnostic significance of real-time two-dimensional Doppler echocardiography (2-D Doppler) in congenital heart diseases, acquired valvular diseases, and dissecting aortic aneurysms. J. Cardiogr. 14:103, 1984.
8. Granato, J.E., Dee, P., Gibson, R.S.: Utility of two-dimensional echocardiography in suspected ascending aortic dissection. Am. J. Cardiol. 56:123, 1985.
9. Dagli, S.V., Nanda, N.C., Roitman, D., Moos, S., Hsiung, M.C., Nath, P.H., and Soto, B.: Evaluation of aortic dissection by Doppler color flow mapping. Am. J. Cardiol. 56:497, 1985.
10. Mohr-Kahaly, S., Erbel, R., Borner, N., Drexler, M., Wittlich, N., Iversen, S., Oelert, H., and Meyer, J.: Combination of Color Doppler and transesophogeal echocardiography in emergency diagnosis of type I aortic dissections. Z. Kardiol. 75:616, 1986.
11. Iliceto, S., Nanda, N.C., Rizzon, P., Hsuing, M.C., Goyal, R.C., Amico, A., and Sorino, M.: Color Doppler evaluation of aortic dissection. Circulation 75:748, 1987.

SECTION 4   AORTIC VALVE

The usefulness of color Doppler flow imaging in the assessment of AV stenosis, AV regurgitation, aortic aneurysm, and aortic dissection is demonstrated in this section.

Figure AV-1   **Rheumatic aortic valve stenosis.** Autopsy specimen shows a narrowed aortic orifice and thickened leaflets.

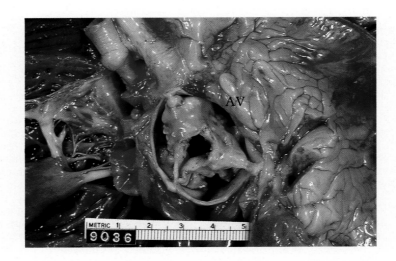

SECTION 4   AORTIC VALVE

Figure AV-2   **Degenerative aortic valve stenosis.** (A) In this autopsy specimen, the AV is viewed from the aortic side and shows a markedly narrow orifice with fibrocalcific deposits in the leaflets. The AV is tricuspid in nature, but one of the commissures is indistinct because of fusion of the two adjacent leaflets. (B) Another autopsy specimen from an elderly patient shows severe bicuspid AV stenosis with a slit-like orifice and heavy calcification.

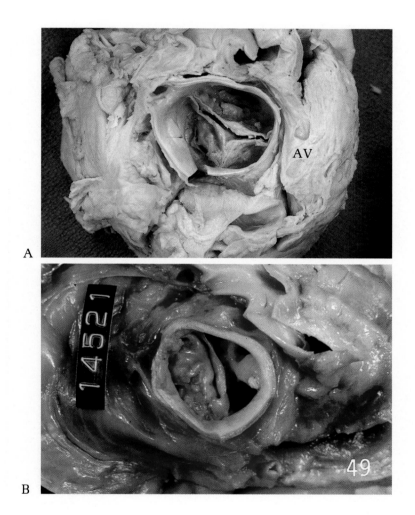

SECTION 4   AORTIC VALVE

Figure AV-3   **Aortic valve stenosis.** (A) Schematic illustrates thickening of the aortic leaflets and a stenotic aortic orifice (arrow). This view corresponds to the 2D echocardiographic examination of the AV from the suprasternal or right parasternal approach. (B) Second schematic shows that the thickened and stenotic AV shown on the left produces a narrow jet, while a wide jet originates through the normal valve, as shown on the right. (C) Third schematic illustrates turbulent flow across a stenotic aortic orifice during systole. The flow acceleration (FA) on the ventricular side of the aortic leaflets is clearly represented (arrow).

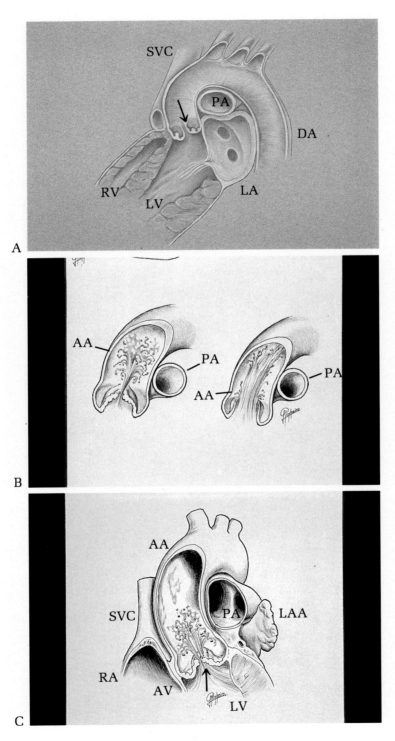

SECTION 4   AORTIC VALVE

Figure AV-4   **Aortic valve stenosis: Calculation of aortic valve area.** (A) The right parasternal view in a 60-year-old man shows a narrow jet of mosaic signals at the AV. These turbulent signals spread out immediately and extend to the entire width of the AA, which is also shown schematically in B. The width of these signals at the AV indicates the severity of AS. For example, with increasing stenosis, the width of the jet decreases. A larger jet width will be obtained if the jet is measured above the AV, and thus the severity of AS will be underestimated. A continuous wave Doppler cursor (C) aligned parallel to the aortic stenotic jet records a peak velocity of 4.28 m/sec, which translates into a peak pressure gradient of 73 mm Hg using the Bernoulli equation. This is schematically illustrated in D. The pulse Doppler sample volume (E) placed in the blue signals in the LVOT just proximal to the AV records a peak velocity of 0.75 m/sec. Schematic (F) demonstrates this technique. The long axis view (G) shows the LVOT. Its inside diameter is measured at almost the same location where the peak velocity is measured by pulse Doppler, and in this patient, the diameter is equal to 22 mm. Schematic (H) illustrates this position. With use of the continuity equation, the AV area in this patient has been calculated as 0.66 cm².

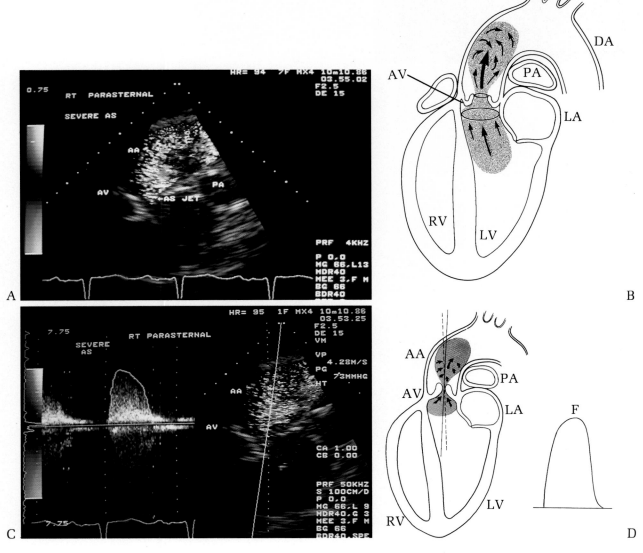

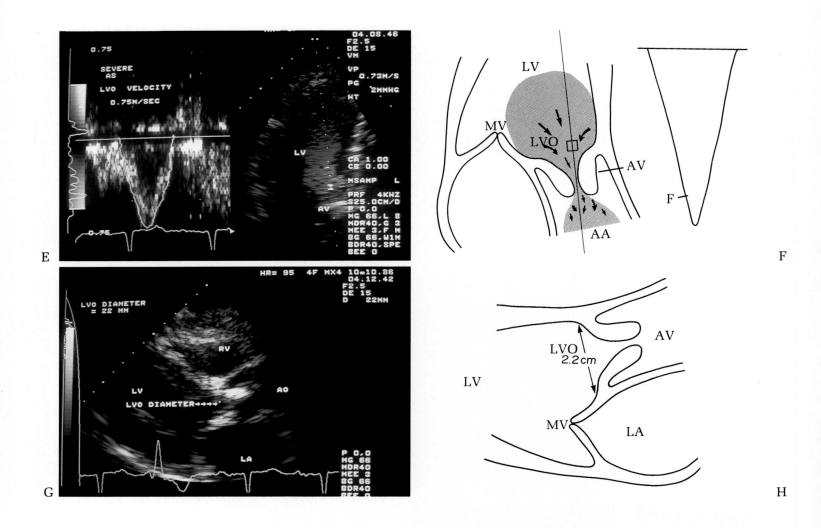

E

F

G

H

SECTION 4 AORTIC VALVE

Figure AV-5 **Aortic valve stenosis.** (A) The right parasternal view in a 67-year-old woman with clinical evidence of AS shows two narrow jets of mosaic signals at the origin of the AV. These signals of AS merge further upstream in the proximal AA. The entire AA and a part of the aortic arch are filled with mosaic turbulent signals. The continuous wave cursor (B) placed parallel to the flow signals in the proximal AA records a peak velocity of 3.96 m/sec, which translates into a peak instantaneous pressure gradient of 63 mm Hg. Visualization of the AS flow signals facilitates optimal alignment of the continuous wave cursor with the actual direction of the AS flow, and thus increases the confidence with which reliable peak velocities and pressure gradients can be estimated. Without color flow signals, the continuous wave cursor is placed arbitrarily in the center of the aorta and parallel to its wall. The transducer is then angulated in various directions until maximum velocity and the best spectral waveform are achieved.

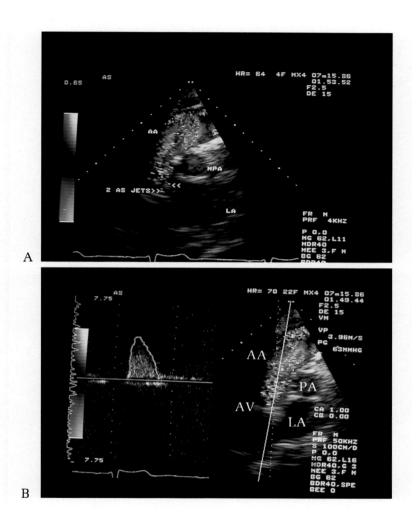

SECTION 4 AORTIC VALVE

Figure AV-6 **Aortic valve stenosis.** Right parasternal views (A and B), using different color Doppler machines, show narrow mosaic jets of AS originating from the AV and spreading out in the proximal AA. C and D represent parasternal long axis views using two different flow maps in a 77-year-old man showing a narrow (5 mm) flow jet moving through the heavily calcified and immobile AV during systole. In this patient, continuous wave Doppler examination was unsuccessful in obtaining adequate velocity waveforms from the apex and the right parasternal/suprasternal transducer approaches, and the diagnosis of critical AS (AV area less than 0.75 cm) was made on the basis of the narrow proximal AS jet seen best in the long axis view. Subsequent cardiac catheterization demonstrated an AV area of 0.6 cm². Balloon valvotomy was attempted in this patient, but no significant increase in the proximal jet width or AV area was achieved.

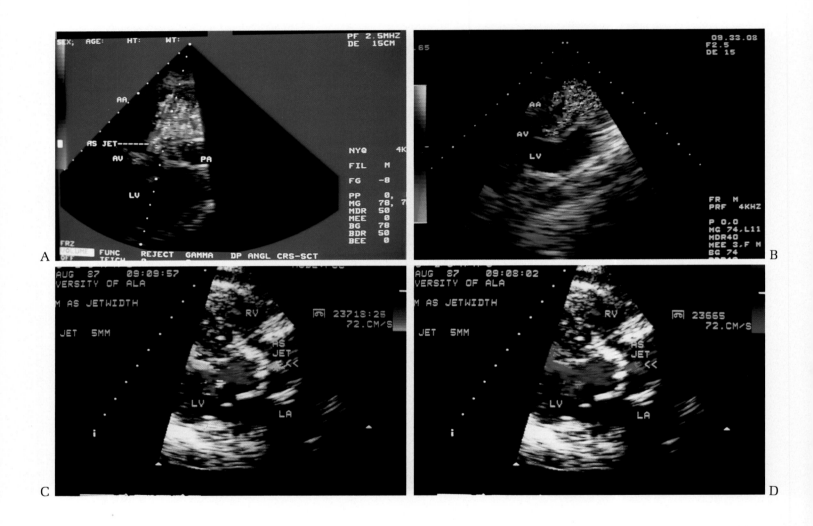

SECTION 4 AORTIC VALVE

Figure AV-7 **Aortic valve stenosis and regurgitation.** (A) Suprasternal view in a 54-year-old woman who has predominant AR and mild AS reveals mosaic turbulent signals during systole in the AA and the aortic arch. These signals are wide at the origin, indicating mild AS. The continuous Doppler cursor (B) is placed parallel to the flow jet and records a peak pressure gradient of only 23 mm Hg. This low gradient can result from AR and thus does not imply significant AS. C and D also demonstrate wide mosaic-colored signals at the AV level in a 59-year-old man with mild AS (AV area 1.4 cm²). This study was performed from the right parasternal approach.

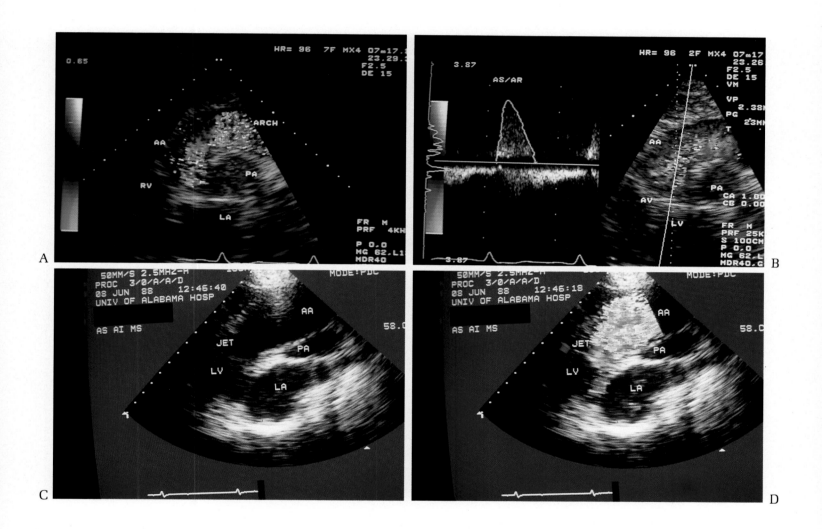

SECTION 4   AORTIC VALVE

Figure AV-8   **Aortic valve stenosis.** Right parasternal view in a 72-year-old woman shows an apparently wide jet of mosaic signals in the proximal AA. When the transducer is angled appropriately, however, the narrow jet of significant AS at the AV can be easily obtained. The continuous wave cursor placed in the mosaic signals records a peak pressure gradient of 56 mm Hg, implying moderately severe AS.

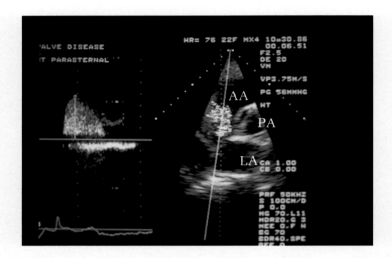

SECTION 4   AORTIC VALVE

Figure AV-9   **Aortic valve stenosis: Eccentric jet.** The continuous wave cursor is not placed parallel to the flow jet in the right parasternal view in a 56-year-old woman with critical AS and, in fact, appears to be perpendicular to the jet direction. In this type of case, the peak velocities obtained and the severity of AS are significantly underestimated. A color Doppler examination provides a reference to determine if the continuous wave cursor is placed parallel to the flow, while a conventional Doppler examination provides no reference to indicate that reliable velocities are being recorded and the actual severity of AS is being determined.

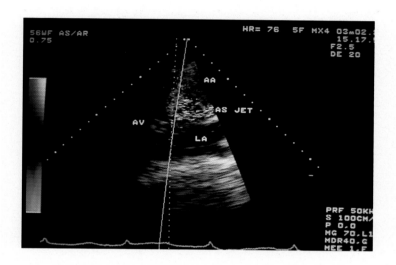

SECTION 4 AORTIC VALVE

Figure AV-10   **Eccentric aortic stenotic flow jet.** (A and B) Schematics illustrate the eccentric direction of the AS mosaic jet. In A, this jet moves toward the medial wall of the aorta, while in B, it moves toward the lateral wall. Because of the eccentric direction of the jet, the continuous wave cursor is not aligned parallel to it. An angle correction in the Doppler equation may be used to correct for this nonparallel orientation. In our experience, however, the angle correction tends to overestimate the severity of AS, and thus we angle the transducer in various directions in an attempt to achieve parallel orientation.

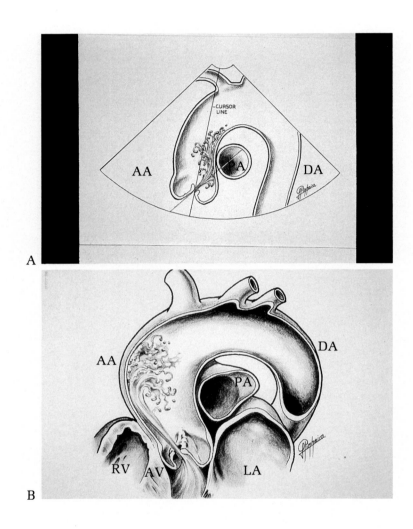

SECTION 4 AORTIC VALVE

Figure AV-11 **Aortic valve stenosis: Long axis plane.** (A) Schematic illustrates a thickened AV with a narrow aortic orifice (arrow), a hypertrophied LV, and the AA in the long axis view. The long axis view (B) in an adult patient with AS and AR shows mosaic turbulent signals in the AA, originating from the thickened AV. The schematic (C) illustrates the AS flow jet moving posteriorly through the AV and striking the posterior wall of the AA. Reliable estimation of the peak pressure gradient across the AV may be obtained by placing the continuous wave Doppler cursor as parallel as possible to the posteriorly directed AS flow signals (D). E and F represent parasternal long axis views in a 26-year-old man with congenital AS and post-aortic coarctation repair in childhood showing the AS flow signals directed eccentrically toward the anterior aortic wall. This facilitates placement of the continuous wave Doppler cursor line parallel to the AS jet in the long axis plane to obtain a peak pressure gradient of 46 mm Hg. Other views such as apical, right parasternal, and suprasternal recorded considerably smaller pressure gradients. Note that the width of the stenotic jet at its origin from the domed AV is also narrow (9 mm), indicating the presence of significant AV stenosis in this patient.

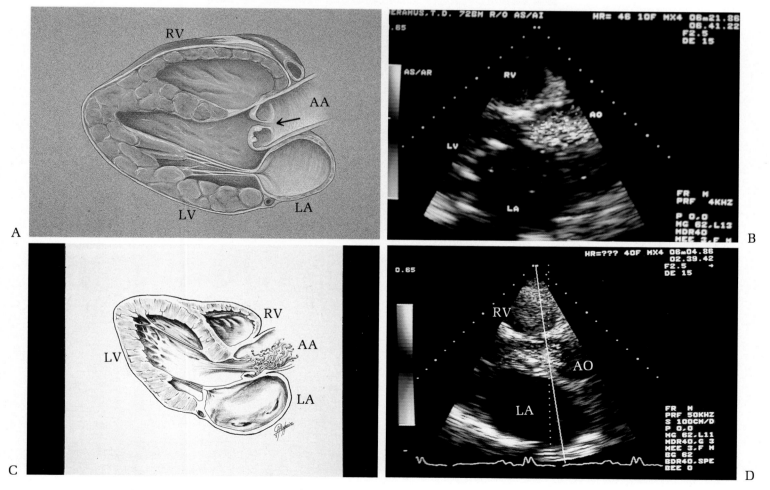

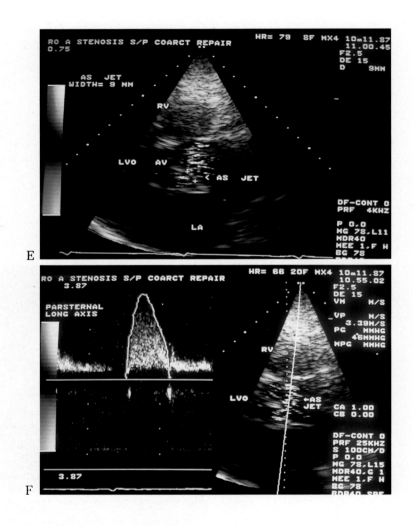

SECTION 4   AORTIC VALVE

Figure AV-12 **Aortic valve stenosis: Long axis plane.** (A) Parasternal long axis view shows a narrow jet of mosaic signals originating from a thickened and calcified AV. This narrow jet implies the presence of significant AS. The width of the stenotic jet should be evaluated in the view in which the jet is best visualized. For example, in B, the jet width is only 8 mm. In our experience, jet widths of 8 mm or less correspond to critical AS (AV area of 0.75 cm² or less by cardiac catheterization), and jet widths of more than 10 mm correspond to less severe AS. The bluish-green signals on the ventricular aspect of the AV in B represent FA. C demonstrates a very narrow jet width at the AV level, also viewed in long axis plane, in a 56-year-old man with critical AS. Note marked calcification of the AV leaflets.

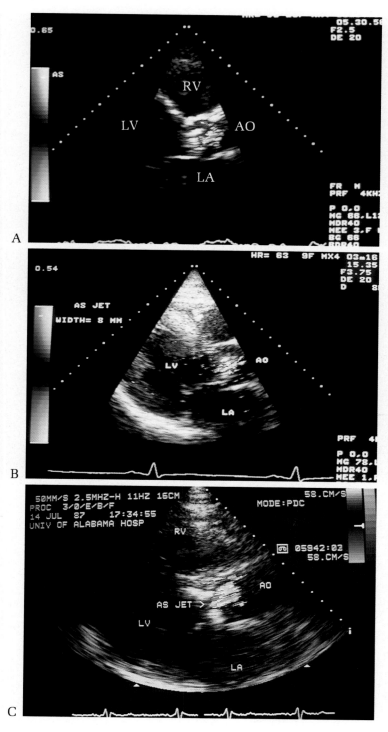

SECTION 4   AORTIC VALVE

Figure AV-13   **Aortic valve stenosis.** Right parasternal views (A–D) in a 33-year-old man show mosaic signals originating from the AV and occupying the entire width of the AA. The red signals on the ventricular aspect of the AV represent flow acceleration (FA). Slight angulations of the transducer (B–D) cause some of the flow signals to disappear at the origin of the AV, causing a smaller jet width at the AV than in A. Therefore, the AS in B, C, and D appears to be more severe than in A. This patient, however, does not have severe AS; thus the jet width depends strongly on the angulation of the transducer. Many views with different transducer angulations must be examined and the maximum width of the jet at the AV in these views used to evaluate AS severity.

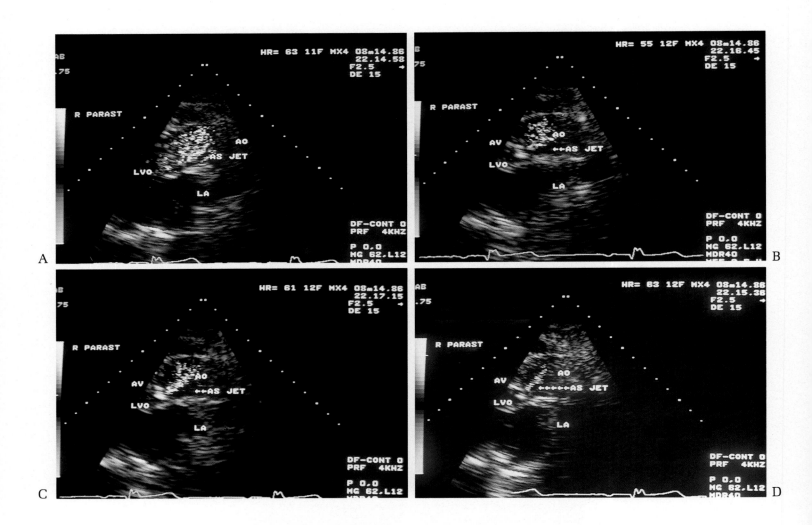

SECTION 4   AORTIC VALVE

Figure AV-14   **Aortic valve stenosis.** (A) Schematic of the apical long axis view illustrates a thickened AV with a restricted opening and left ventricular hypertrophy. The color Doppler examination from the apical view (B) shows mosaic signals due to turbulence in the dilated AA, originating from the AV. The blue signals in the LVOT represent FA (arrow). A continuous wave cursor (C) passed across a calcified AV through the flow signals in the AO from the apical view in another adult patient records a peak velocity of 2.1 m/sec, which translates into a peak pressure gradient of 19 mm Hg, implying only mild AS.

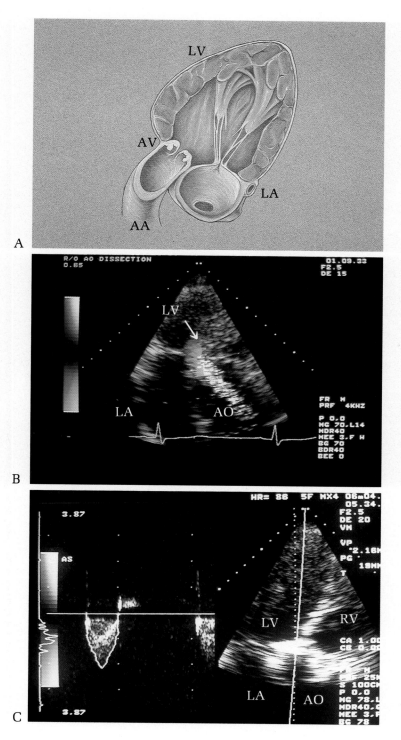

SECTION 4   AORTIC VALVE

Figure AV-15   **Aortic valve stenosis associated with mitral regurgitation.** (A) Apical 4-chamber view in a 72-year-old man shows mosaic signals of MR during systole. A continuous wave cursor (A) passed through the AV records a peak pressure gradient of 28 mm Hg, and the continuous wave cursor (B) passed through the mitral regurgitant jet records a peak pressure of 130 mm Hg. While both the spectral waveforms in A and B are systolic and below the baseline, the mitral regurgitant waveform in B has an earlier onset, a longer duration, and a more rounded peak than the aortic stenotic waveform obtained in A. This differentiation may not be possible when the spectral waveforms are not sharply outlined or when they are superimposed because of the continuous wave cursor passing through portions of both the AS and MR flow jets. Therefore, in the presence of MR, a misdiagnosis of severe AS can result from the apical view. The problems in differentiating AS and MR spectral waveforms are also demonstrated in another patient (C and D).

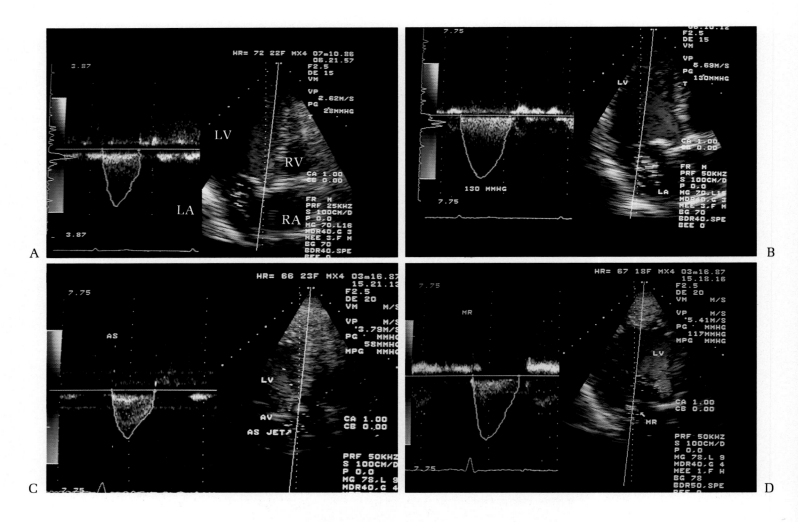

SECTION 4 AORTIC VALVE

Figure AV-16 **Aortic regurgitation.** (A) Diastolic frame of the long axis view in a 39-year-old man shows a wide jet of mosaic signals in the LVOT, originating from the AV and directed toward the LV posterior wall. The width of regurgitant jet at its origin from the AV is a good indicator of the severity of AR. When the jet width (height) occupies less than 25%, 25 to 46%, 47 to 64%, and 65% or more of the width of the LVOT, the AR is mild (grade 1), moderate (grade 2), moderately severe (grade 3), and severe (grade 4 & 5, Hunt's angiographic criteria), respectively. In this patient, the mosaic signals at the origin completely fill the LVOT, and thus the AR is severe. The short axis view at the level of the high LVOT (Reproduced with permission from Nanda, N.C., Color Doppler Echocardiography, International Journal of Cardiac Imaging, in press, 1988) (B) shows mosaic signals in a crescent shape occupying a large area of the LVOT, also implying severe AR.

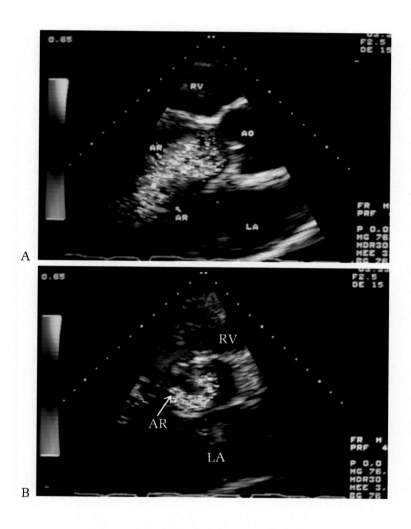

Figure AV-17   **Severe aortic regurgitation.** (A) Long axis view shows diastolic mosaic signals originating from the AV and completely filling the LVOT, implying severe AR. The blue signals seen in the LA indicate the presence of mild diastolic MR. This regurgitation is occasionally observed in patients with severe AR. Color M-mode examination (B and C) using different color Doppler machines shows diastolic fluttering of the anterior MV leaflet and mosaic signals in front of this leaflet throughout diastole.

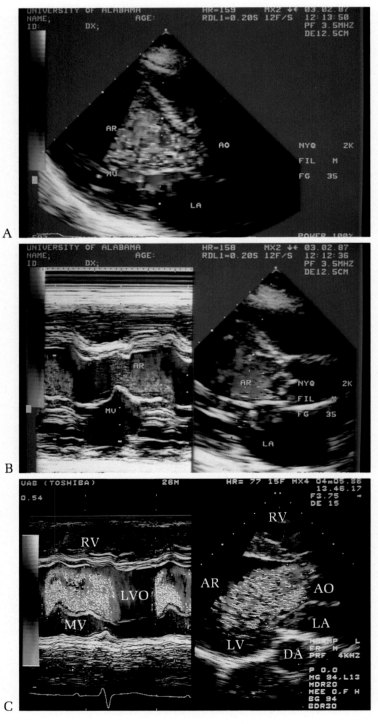

SECTION 4 AORTIC VALVE

Figure AV-18 **Severe aortic regurgitation.** (A–C) Long axis views in a 32-year-old woman from three different color Doppler machines show diastolic mosaic signals originating from the AV and completely filling the LVOT, indicating severe AR. The patterns of color differ on these three machines because of their different Nyquist limits for the same PRF and depth. These varying patterns are also seen in the short axis views of the high LVOT (D–F) in this patient and using the same three machines. Despite the varying color patterns, the area occupied by the turbulent signals in both the long and short axis views is almost the same on all three machines.

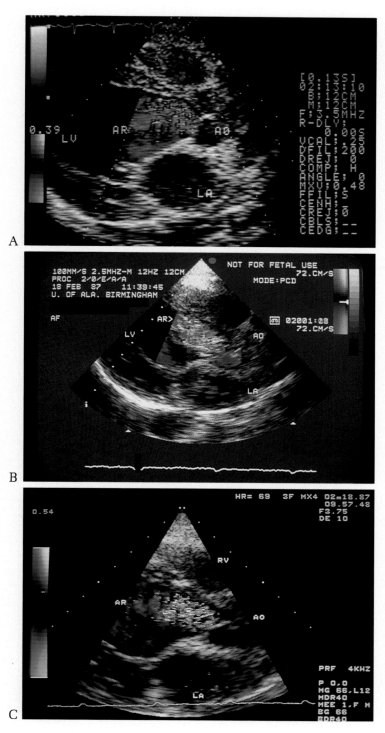

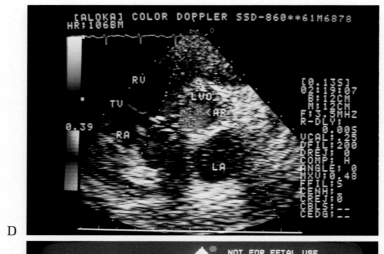

D

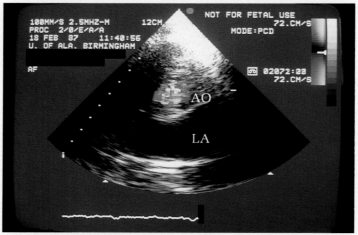

E

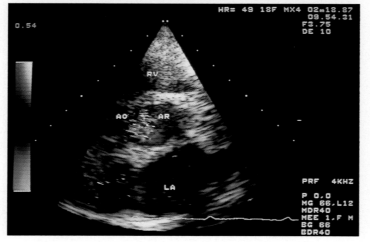

F

SECTION 4 AORTIC VALVE

Figure AV-19   **Severe aortic regurgitation.** Parasternal long axis view (A) and apical view (B) in a 43-year-old woman show mosaic signals of severe AR which completely fill the entire LVOT in diastole. The tiny area of yellow signals on the aortic side of the AV in B represents flow acceleration, and the red signals in the left ventricular cavity originating from the MV, also in B, result from mitral inflow.

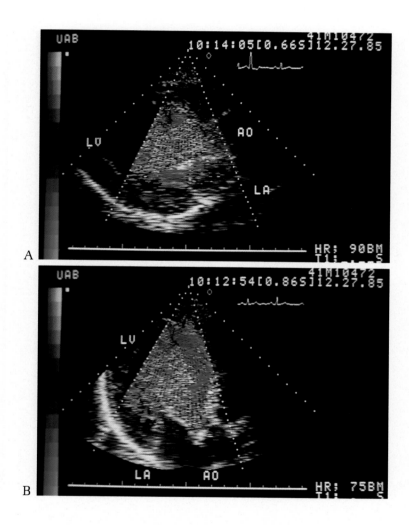

SECTION 4   AORTIC VALVE

Figure AV-20   **Severe aortic regurgitation.** (A) Parasternal long axis view in a 39-year-old man shows mosaic signals of severe AR completely filling the LVOT. The blue signals in the LA in this late diastolic frame represent mild diastolic regurgitation, which implies an elevated LV end-diastolic pressure with severe AR. The short axis view at the level of the MV (B) also shows mosaic signals in front of the anterior MV leaflet during diastole. The relationship between the AV and the MV in the short axis view during diastole is schematically illustrated in C.

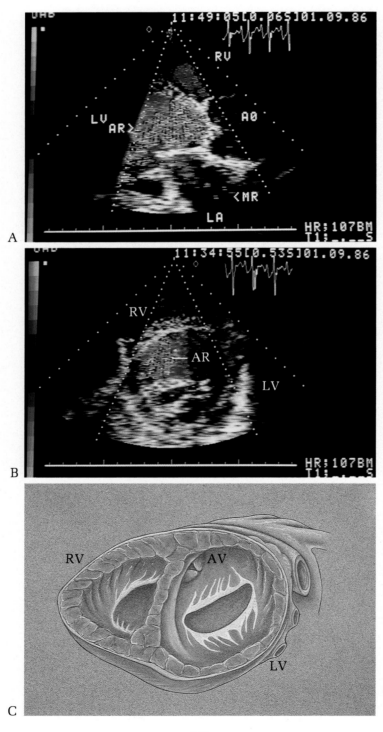

SECTION 4 AORTIC VALVE

Figure AV-21 **Severe aortic regurgitation.** (A) Parasternal long axis view in a 33-year-old man shows mosaic signals of severe AR occupying the entire LVOT. The continuous wave cursor (B) placed parallel to the mosaic AR signals in the apical view records a peak velocity of 5.49 m/sec, which translates into a peak pressure gradient of 121 mm Hg. The sharp deceleration of the peak velocity in the spectral waveform is related to increased LV diastolic pressure.

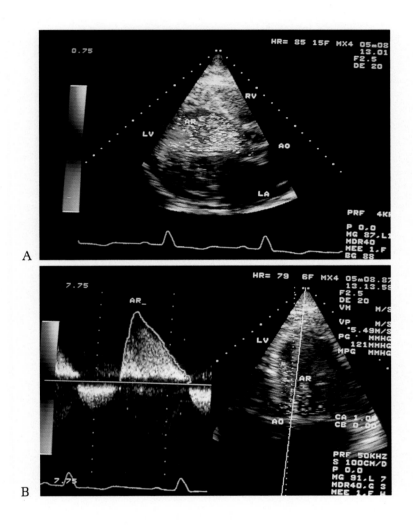

SECTION 4 AORTIC VALVE

Figure AV-22 **Aortic regurgitation.** Parasternal long axis view in an 18-year-old man with AS shows a jet of mosaic signals originating from the thickened AV and directed toward the anterior MV leaflet. The small width of the jet at the origin suggests mild AR. The blue signals on the aortic side of the AV represent flow acceleration (ACC).

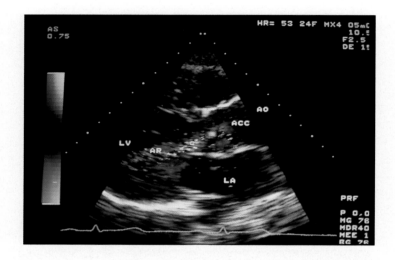

SECTION 4   AORTIC VALVE

Figure AV-23   **Mild aortic regurgitation.** (A) Parasternal long axis view in a 21-year-old man shows a narrow mosaic jet of mild AR originating from the AV and directed toward the anterior MV leaflet. The jet widens considerably downstream in the LV. The short axis view (B) also shows the presence of very mild AR. The apical long axis view (C) shows a narrow mosaic jet of AR, which also broadens farther in the LVOT. These mosaic signals farther downstream turn red in color because the velocity of the jet decreases.

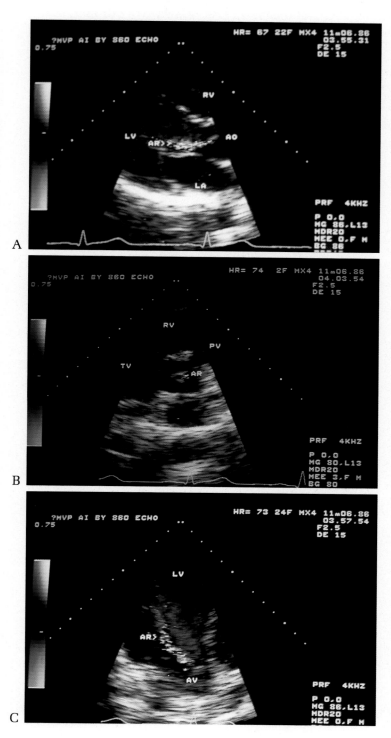

SECTION 4 AORTIC VALVE

Figure AV-24 **Aortic regurgitation: Estimation of severity.** (A) Schematic illustrates the technique for estimating the severity of AR. The width of the aortic regurgitant jet is taken proximally at its origin and expressed as a percentage of the LVOT width taken at the same location. The percentage ranges of 1 to 24%, 25 to 46%, 47 to 64%, and 65 to 100% represent grades 1, 2, 3, and 4/5 AR, respectively, when compared with Hunt's criteria on angiography. (Reproduced with permission from Perry et al., J. Am. Coll. Cardiol. 9:952, 1987.) The parasternal long axis views (B and C) demonstrate, in a 77-year-old man with congestive heart failure, the measurement of the jet and LVOT widths, respectively. The jet width is 5 mm and the LVOT width is 17 mm. The percentage of the jet width to the LVOT width equals 29.4%, indicating moderate or grade 2 AR. The aortic regurgitant jet is viewed in the short axis at the high LVOT (D and E). The jet area measured is 0.62 cm², and the LVOT area is 5.2 cm². The ratio of the two areas is 12%. In the short axis view, the ranges of the area ratios of 0–3%, 4–24%, 25–59%, and 60–100% correspond to angiographic gradings of grades 1, 2, 3, and 4 AR respectively using Hunt's criteria. Thus, this patient has moderate (Grade 2) AR shown by both methods. (In A, LVOH=LVO height, JH=jet height or width.)

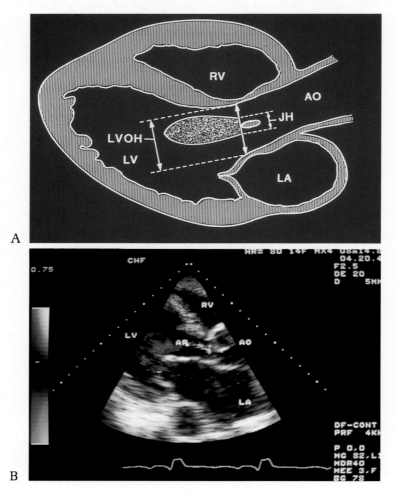

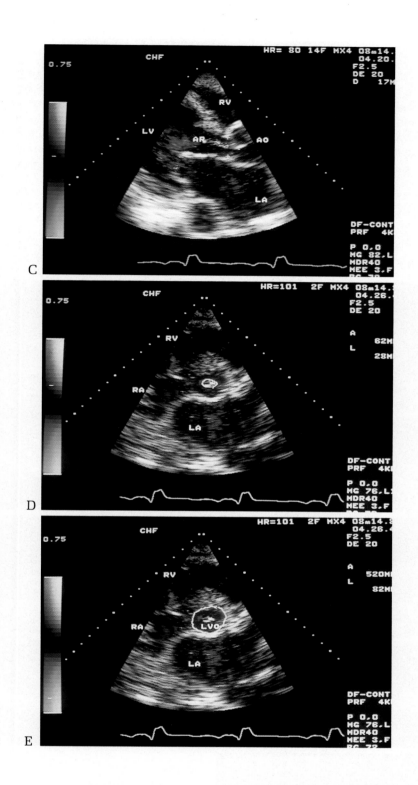

SECTION 4 AORTIC VALVE

Figure AV-25 **Aortic regurgitation: Estimation of severity.** (A) Long axis view in a 43-year-old woman with cardiomyopathy shows a relatively narrow mosaic jet of AR originating from the AV and widening downstream in the LVOT. The short axis views of the AR jet at the LVOT level (B–D) demonstrate a ratio of 11.7% when the jet area and the LVOT area are planimeterized and compared, indicating the presence of grade 2 AR. The short axis view (E) taken at the level of MV shows a relatively large area of mosaic signals in front of the anterior MV leaflet. This area cannot be used to estimate severity because the jet signals have broadened at the level of the MV.

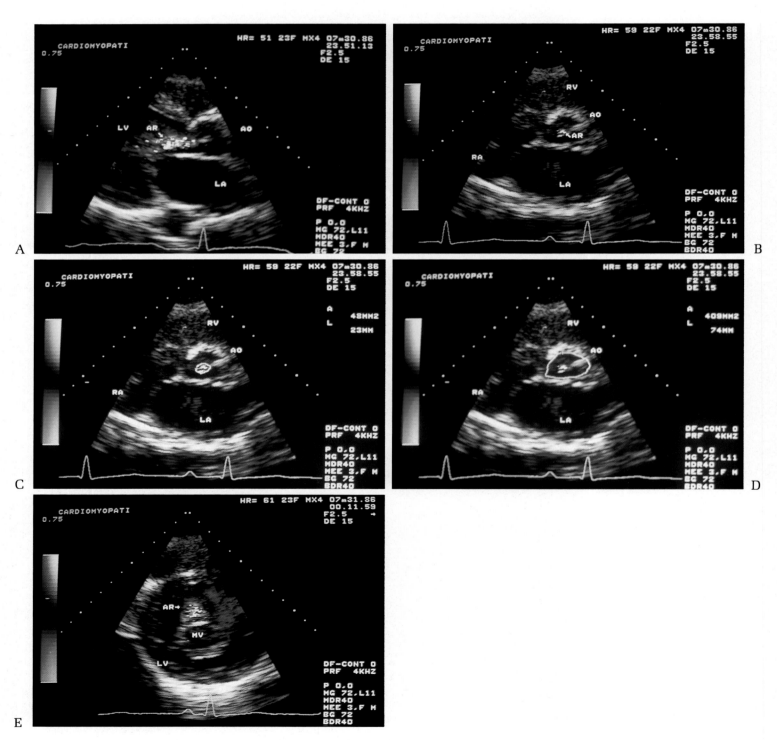

Figure AV-26 **Aortic regurgitation.** The short axis views (A–C) at the level of the LVOT in three different patients show mosaic signals of mild to moderate AR in the LVOT, using different color Doppler systems. The mosaic signals are crescent-shaped and larger in C.

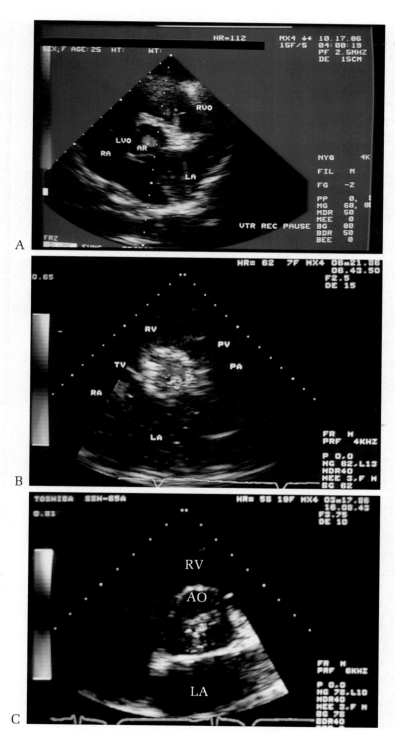

SECTION 4   AORTIC VALVE

Figure AV-27   Aortic regurgitation. Short axis view (A) at the level of the AV in an 83-year-old man shows a small mosaic jet of AR, while view B, taken at a slightly lower level in the LVOT, shows an eccentrically located and larger jet of AR. In assessing the severity of AR from short axis views, it is important to consider only high LVOT planes, preferably those in which the AV elements are also imaged. This ensures accurate measurement of the AR jet area at its origin from the AV. C shows a small area of mosaic-colored AR signals at the level of the high LVOT, viewed in short axis in a 53-year-old man with hypertensive heart disease. The long axis plane (D) also shows a narrow AR jet at its origin from the AV. These findings suggest the presence of only mild AR in this patient. E is a short axis view at the level of the high LVOT, showing a circular AR jet in another adult patient.

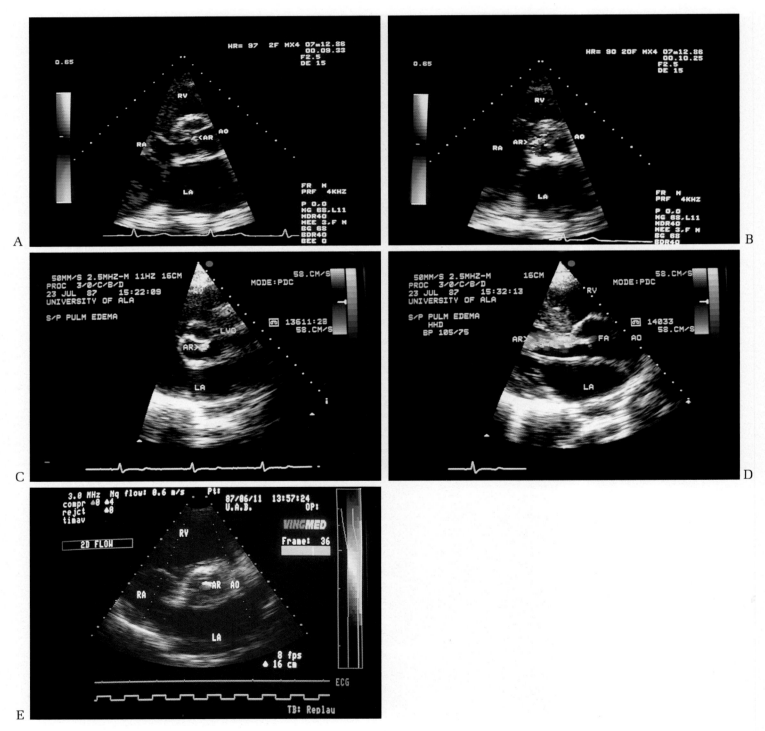

SECTION 4   AORTIC VALVE

Figure AV-28 **Aortic regurgitation.** (A) Apical long axis view shows a relatively narrow jet of AR originating from the AV. The color of the jet is reddish-yellow at the origin, indicating high velocity, but further in the LV, it turns deep red, indicating a decrease in the velocity of the jet. B shows two discrete jets of AR (J_1 and J_2) in the apical plane in a 31-year-old man with AV, MV, and TV prolapse. MF=mitral inflow.

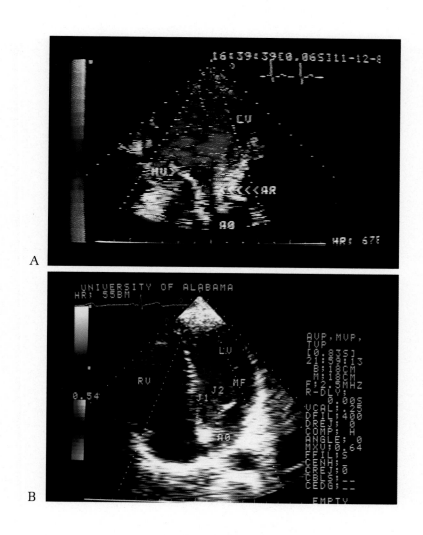

SECTION 4 AORTIC VALVE

Figure AV-29 **Aortic regurgitation.** (A) Early diastolic frame of low parasternal long axis view shows a narrow red jet (J) of mild AR originating at the AV and broadening downstream in the LV. The distinct red signals of mitral inflow (DI) are easily distinguishable from the red signals of AR. Later in diastole, however, the two jets merge, making delineation of the aortic regurgitant area difficult.

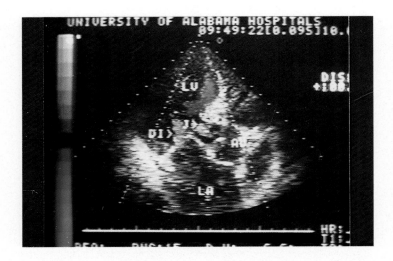

SECTION 4   AORTIC VALVE

Figure AV-30   Aortic regurgitation. Apical long axis views (A–C) in a patient with systemic hypertension show a relatively narrow mosaic jet of AR. A jet of red signals representing the mitral inflow (MF) is seen moving from the LA to the LV. Further in the LV, these jets merge, making the delineation of the aortic regurgitant area difficult. The width of the AR jet at its origin is well defined, however, and thus the AR jet width rather than the jet area is used to semi-quantify the severity of AR. A continuous wave cursor (D) passed through the AV appears to be nonparallel to the AR jet. Angling the transducer, however, places the continuous wave cursor (E) parallel to the AR signals, and a high velocity of 5.13 m/sec is recorded. The spectral waveform obtained shows a slow deceleration during diastole, implying mild AR and a normal left ventricular end-diastolic pressure.

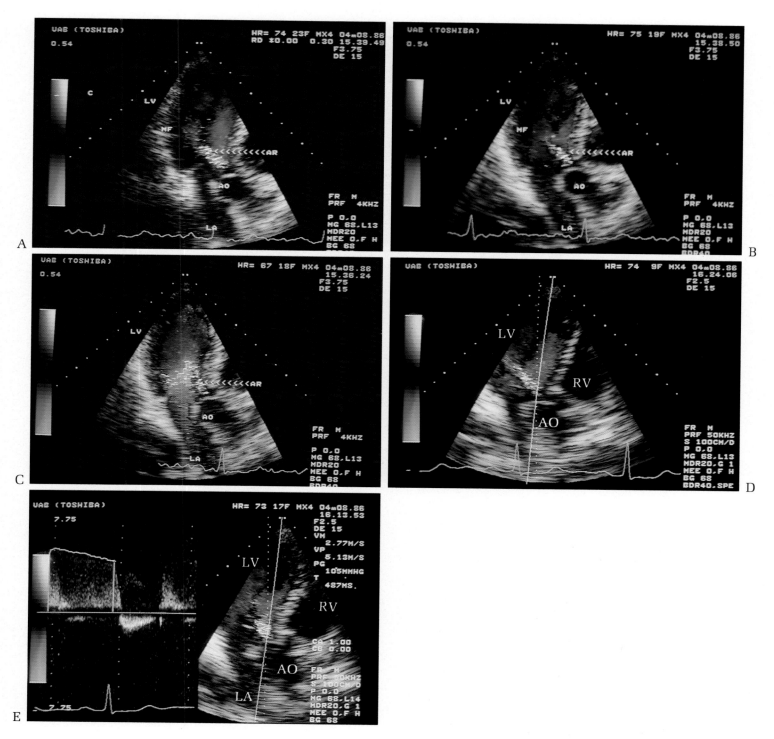

SECTION 4   AORTIC VALVE

Figure AV-31   **Erroneous aortic regurgitation.** The systolic frame of an apical long axis view shows red signals along the VS which appear to originate from the AV. These signals may be mistaken for aortic regurgitant signals if careful attention is not paid to their timing in the cardiac cycle. They may possibly be caused by a ghosting artifact (ART) from the motion of the VS or by aliasing of the LVO signals due to a low Nyquist limit. Mosaic signals of MR are seen in the LA.

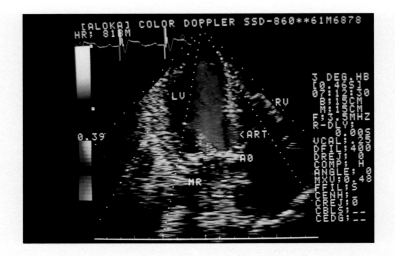

SECTION 4   AORTIC VALVE

Figure AV-32   **Aortic regurgitation associated with mitral stenosis.** The diastolic frames of apical views (A and B) in two different patients show mosaic signals of AR and MS. These signals can be easily differentiated near their respective valves. Further downstream, however, these signals merge, making it difficult to distinguish between them. The red signals of FA on the atrial aspect of the mitral leaflet (B) help to separate the proximal portions of the AR and MS signals.

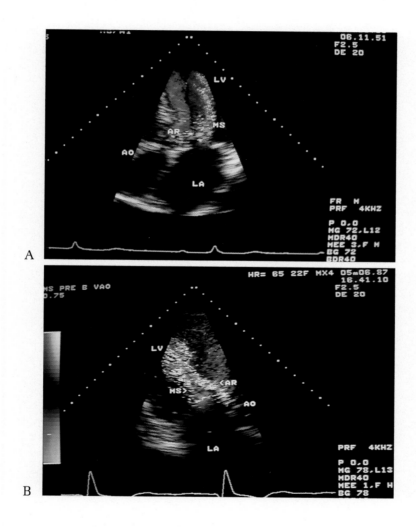

SECTION 4   AORTIC VALVE

Figure AV-33   **Two jets of aortic regurgitation.** (A) Long axis view in a 55-year-old woman shows two distinct red jets of AR. One of the jets is located along the VS (1) and the other along the anterior mitral leaflet (2). (B) Long axis view in another patient (26-year-old woman) shows development of two small jets (arrowheads) of AR, one anteriorly along the VS and the other posteriorly along the anterior mitral leaflet following aortic valvotomy. AI=Aortic regurgitation.

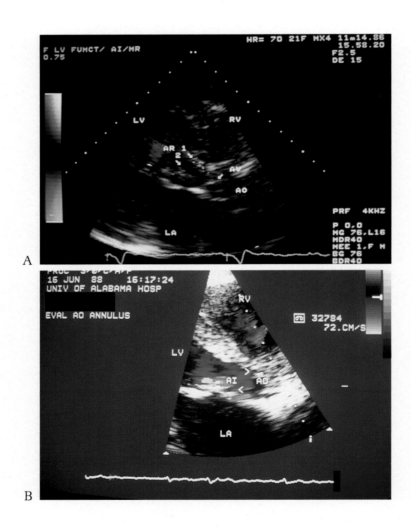

SECTION 4   AORTIC VALVE

Figure AV-34   **Varying shapes of the aortic regurgitant jet.** (A–K) Long axis views illustrate variations in the shape of the AR jet. In A, a relatively narrow red jet of AR is seen directed toward the LV apex (arrow), while in B, a central red jet (arrow) originating from the valve turns blue in color as it moves toward the LV posterior wall. Another central jet originating from the valve in C bifurcates (arrow) and turns blue as it moves toward the LV wall, then turns red as it moves toward the VS. In D, E, and F, the mosaic AR jet is directed toward the VS, but in E and F, after striking the septum, the jet swirls and turns blue as it moves posteriorly toward the anterior AV leaflet. A schematic (G) illustrates this type of AR jet. The long axis view (H) shows the AR jet moving from the AV posteriorly along the posterior cusp as blue signals. When it reaches the base of the anterior MV leaflet, it turns red as it swirls anteriorly toward the VS, thus giving a "J" shape as illustrated in I. The jet width can be overestimated in this case because the blue signals appear to occupy 50% of the LVOT. The jet, however, is very narrow at the origin. The long axis view (J) shows a relatively large mosaic jet of AR originating from the noncoronary cusp and directed along the anterior MV leaflet as also shown on the color M-mode (K). The schematic (L) illustrates the AR jet directed toward the anterior MV leaflet (top) and the VS (bottom).

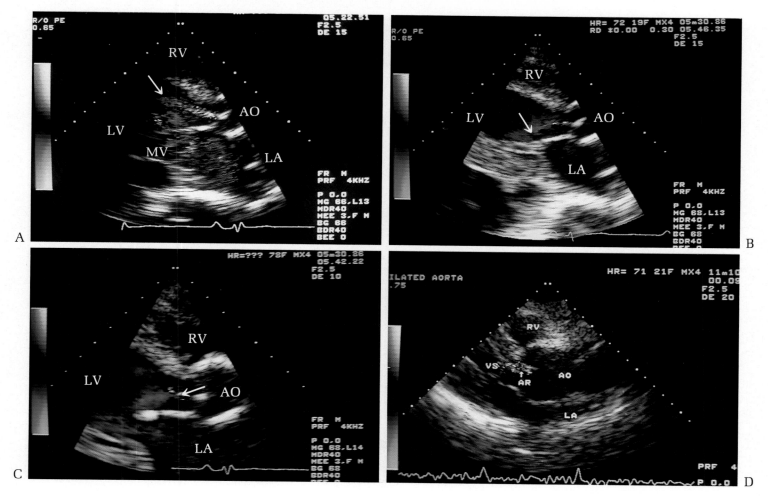

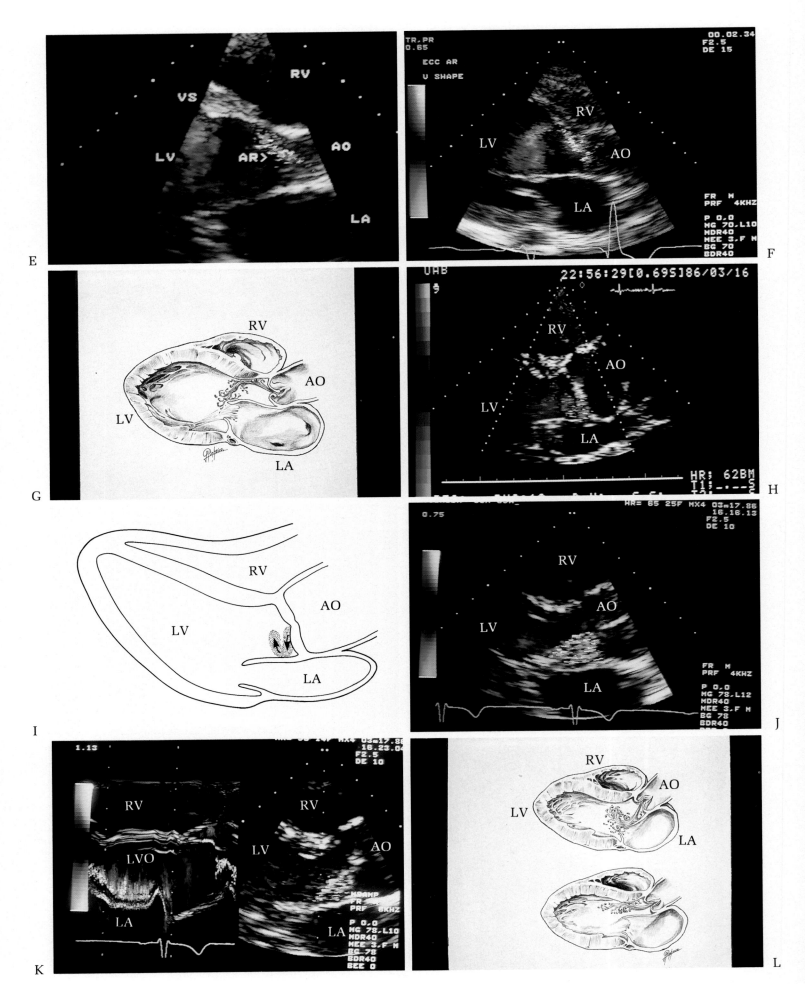

SECTION 4 AORTIC VALVE

Figure AV-35 **Aortic valve prolapse and aortic regurgitation.** (A) Long axis view shows marked prolapse of the aortic leaflet (arrow). M-mode recording (left) shows an eccentric diastolic closure and diastolic fluttering due to a flail AV. Color Doppler examination (B,C) shows mosaic-colored signals filling a large area of the LVOT during diastole, indicating severe AR.

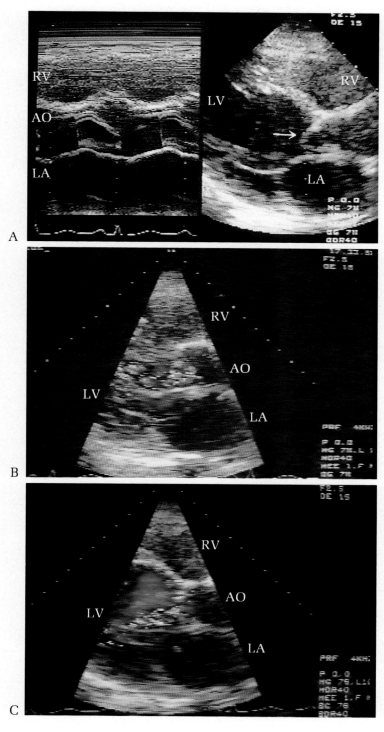

SECTION 4   AORTIC VALVE

Figure AV-36   **Mitral valve deformity produced by aortic regurgitation.** Long axis (A) and short axis (B) views in a 28-year-old man show a reverse doming (D) of the anterior MV leaflet. This deformity (D), as shown by color Doppler examination (C–F) could result from the mosaic AR jet impinging on the anterior leaflet. In our experience, this deformity is seen only in patients with this type of AR jet, and more often in patients with moderate to severe AR. The continuous wave cursor (G) placed parallel to the AR signals records a high velocity with a slow deceleration slope, implying AR with relatively normal LV end-diastolic pressure. Color M-mode examination (H) reveals pandiastolic AR. Blue signals on the aortic aspect of the AV represent flow acceleration (ACC). I and J demonstrate similar findings seen in long axis view in another patient (31-year-old man) with AR. K is a schematic showing diastolic deformity of the anterior mitral leaflet produced by AR. An autopsy specimen (L) in another patient shows thickening and fibrosis of the anterior MV leaflet (arrow) because of AR.

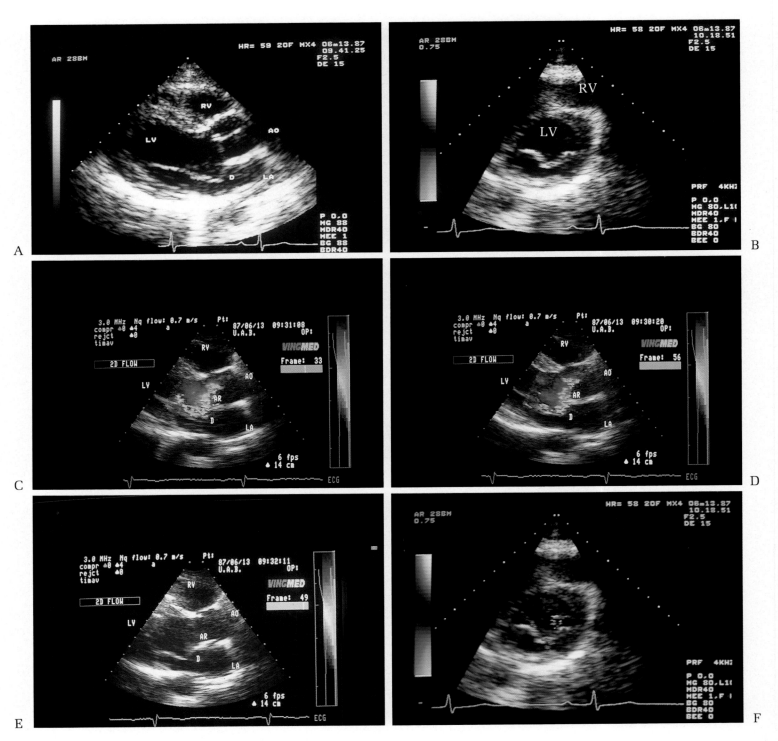

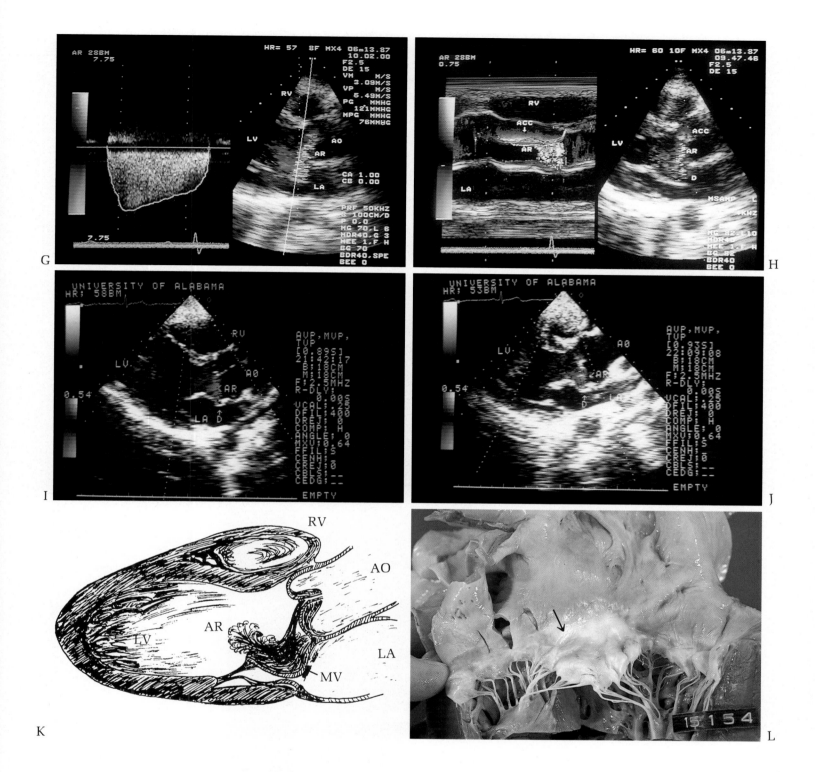

SECTION 4 AORTIC VALVE

Figure AV-37   **Aortic valve vegetation.** (A and B) Autopsy specimens show large vegetations (arrows) on the AV which extend down to destroy a portion of MV leaflet. Another autopsy specimen (C) shows a large vegetation on the aortic leaflets and two small vegetations (arrows) near the tip of the anterior MV leaflet.

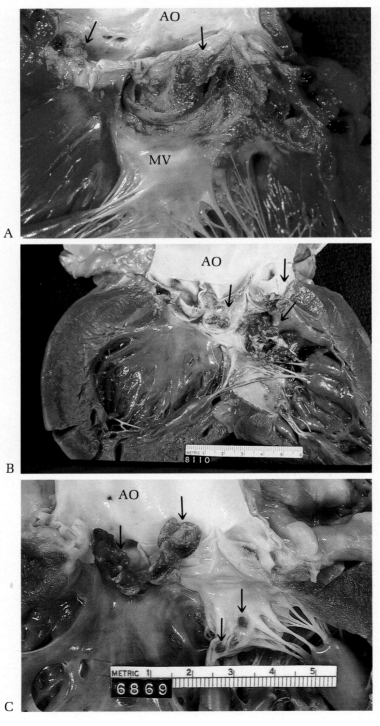

SECTION 4   AORTIC VALVE

Figure AV-38   **Aortic valve vegetation.** (A) Long axis view in a 28-year-old man shows a large vegetation on the AV. Color Doppler examination (B) shows mosaic signals of severe AR filling the entire LVOT. Mild diastolic MR is also seen.

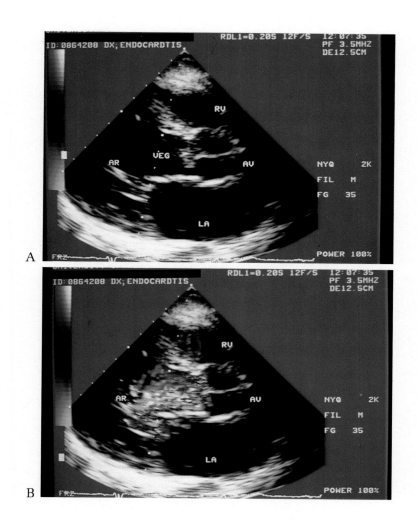

SECTION 4   AORTIC VALVE

Figure AV-39   **Aortic valve vegetation.** (A) Long axis view in a patient with bacterial endocarditis shows severe AR. The aortic root is not enlarged. (B) Short axis view also shows mosaic signals of severe AR in the LVOT.

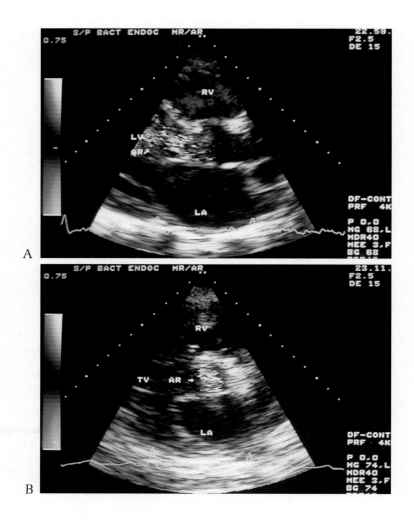

SECTION 4   AORTIC VALVE

Figure AV-40   **Aortic valve vegetation.** (A) M-mode recording of the AV in a 9-year-old child with bacterial endocarditis shows diastolic fluttering (arrows) typical of flail AV. (B) Color M-mode recording, besides showing the diastolic fluttering, also shows mosaic signals of AR during diastole. In addition, color M-mode recording (C) of the MV shows high-frequency diastolic fluttering of the anterior MV leaflet and mosaic signals of AR in front of this leaflet.

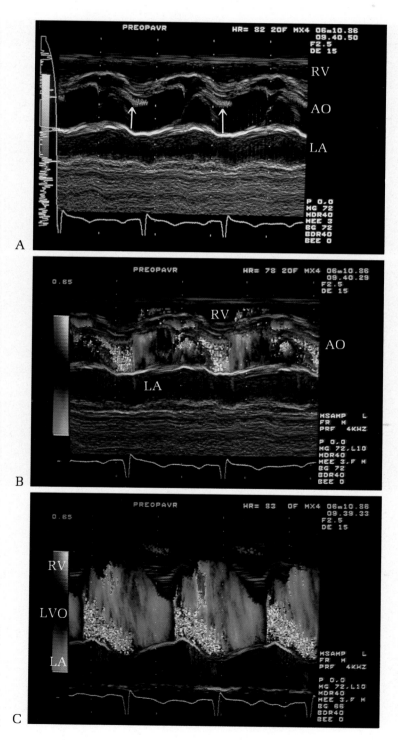

SECTION 4   AORTIC VALVE

Figure AV-41   **Aortic regurgitation.** Color M-mode recordings (A,B) of the MV in 2 different patients show AR signals in front of the anterior MV leaflet and a diastolic fluttering (F) of this leaflet. C is a color M-mode recording of the AV in a 74-year-old woman, showing pandiastolic AR even though mild in severity. D shows pandiastolic AR in the LVOT in a 43-year-old woman with congestive cardiomyopathy. Associated MR is also seen in A and D.

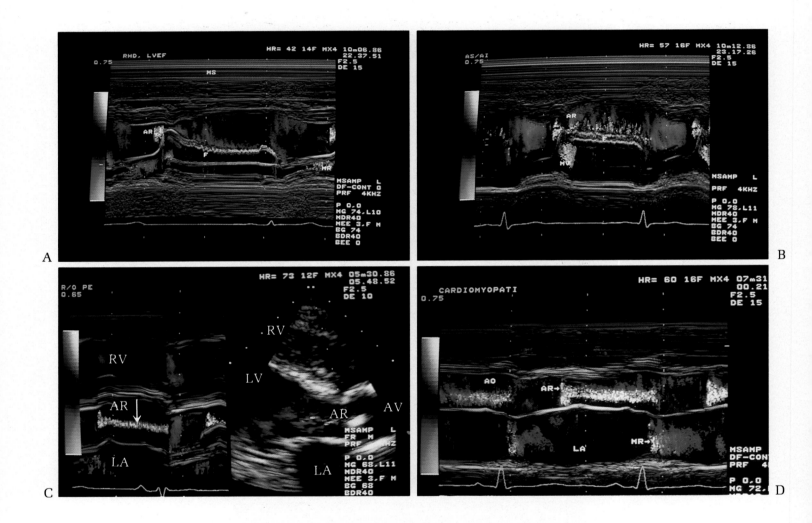

SECTION 4   AORTIC VALVE

Figure AV-42   **Diastolic mitral regurgitation associated with aortic regurgitation.** (A) Late diastolic frame of the long axis view in a 47-year-old man with severe AR shows mosaic signals of AR in the LVOT and blue signals of diastolic (D) MR in the LA. (B) Color M-mode examination shows mosaic signals of AR in front of blue signals of late DMR present behind the MV.

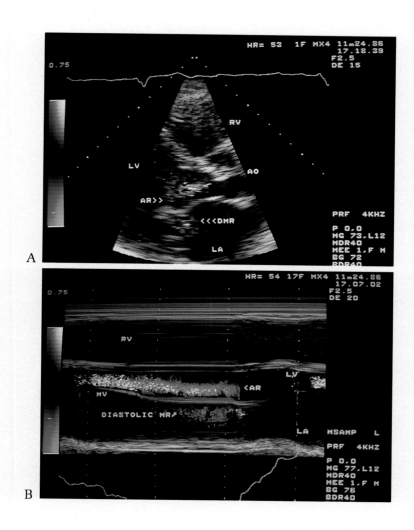

SECTION 4   AORTIC VALVE

Figure AV-43   Aortic regurgitation. A perforation of one of the cusps of an AV is shown (arrows) in an autopsy specimen (A) taken from an elderly patient with degenerative atherosclerosis and illustrated in the schematic (B). This is one of the causes of AR in the elderly. Right parasternal examination (C) in a 55-year-old man shows mild thickening of the AV and mosaic signals of significant AR moving through an apparent defect in the AV and along the anterior mitral leaflet. The red signals on the aortic aspect of the AV represent flow acceleration (ACC). The continuous wave cursor (D) placed parallel to the mosaic signals records a high velocity of 4.2 m/sec. (MF, MIF=mitral inflow).

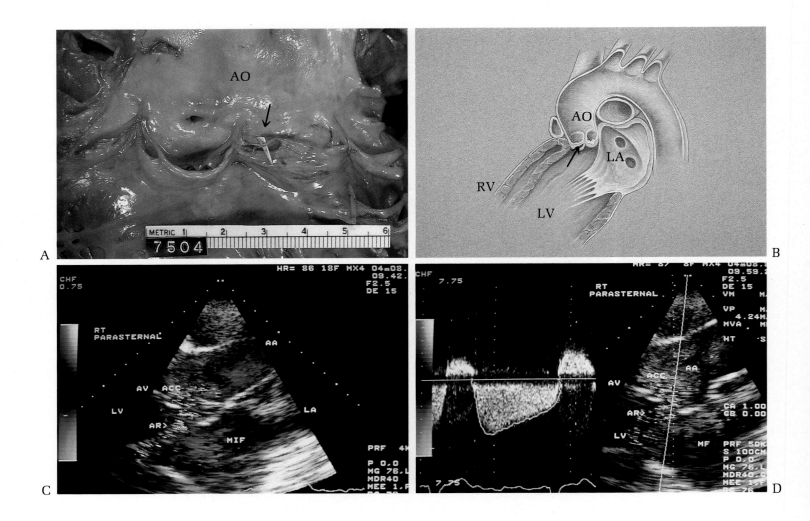

SECTION 4   AORTIC VALVE

Figure AV-44   Aortic backflow in aortic regurgitation. Color M-mode examinations (A and B) from the right parasternal approach in 2 different patients with AR show backflow or retrograde flow in the AA during diastole, implying significant AR. The mosaic signals in A and the red signals in B during systole represent normal or antegrade flow. The diastolic frame in C (same patient as in B) shows blue signals in the AA which are seen during diastole on the color M-mode shown on the left. Examination of the DA in 3 other patients (D,E,F) demonstrates retrograde flow during diastole in this vessel as red signals. The systolic blue signals in E and F represent antegrade flow in the DA, while the red color within them represents aliasing. Demonstration of prominent retrograde flow in the DA during diastole is a good indicator of severe AR. BF=backflow.

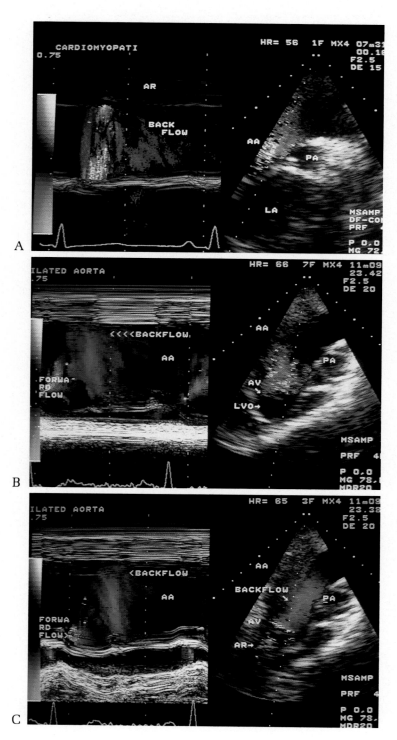

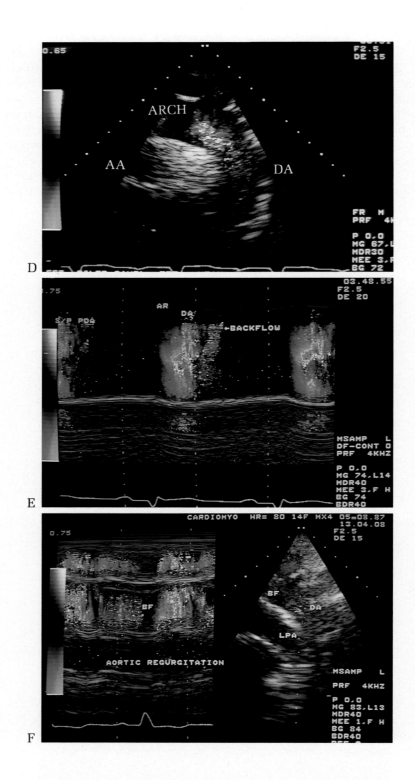

SECTION 4   AORTIC VALVE

Figure AV-45   **Ascending aortic aneurysm.** (A) Color Doppler examination from the right parasternal view shows swirling and backflow in the aneurysmal AA in an adult patient. The red signals represent antegrade or normal flow into the AA, while the blue signals represent retrograde or backward flow. These flow patterns are also illustrated in the schematic (B).

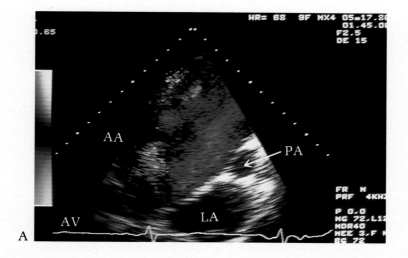

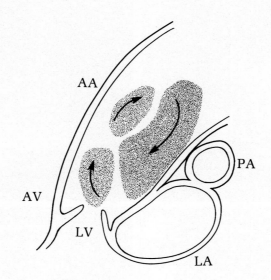

SECTION 4   AORTIC VALVE

Figure AV-46   **Ascending aortic aneurysm.** 2D echo and color Doppler examination (A,B) from the right parasternal approach in a 25-year-old man shows swirling and backflow in the aneurysmal AA. The red signals represent antegrade flow into the AA, while the blue signals represent retrograde flow. Suprasternal examination (C–F) during systole shows antegrade flow in the AA, arch (red with some blue and greenish-yellow within it due to aliasing and turbulence) and DA (predominantly blue signals). During diastole (G,H,I), prominent retrograde or backward flow (BF) is noted in the DA (yellowish-red with some blue due to aliasing) and AA (blue), indicating the presence of severe AR. Parasternal long axis (J,K,L) and short axis (M,N,O) views show mosaic-colored signals due to AR in the LV body and LVOT. Note that, despite the presence of angiographically documented torrential AR, the width of the AR signals at their origin from the AV (M,N,O) is small in relation to the LVO size. This misleading finding, which would suggest that AR is not severe, is probably related to the aneurysmal dilatation of the aorta. In such cases, pulsed Doppler examination of the AA and DA for the presence of prominent diastolic backward flow (AR) is useful in correctly assessing the severity of AR (P,Q). FF=forward flow. Prominent backward flow (AR) is also observed in a cephalic branch, CB(R). The abdominal aorta (AB AO) and the femoral artery (FA) in this patient are only mildly dilated, but show prominent diastolic backflow (AR,BF) when interrogated by pulse Doppler (S,T,U). FF=forward flow; L=liver. These findings also indicate the presence of severe AR. (Frames K and O are similar to J and N, respectively, except for the use of a different color flow map.) Repeat examination (V,W) after surgical repair of the aneurysm shows closely spaced linear echoes representing the rugae of the teflon aortic graft (G). Autopsy specimen (X) from another patient shows an ascending aortic aneurysm.

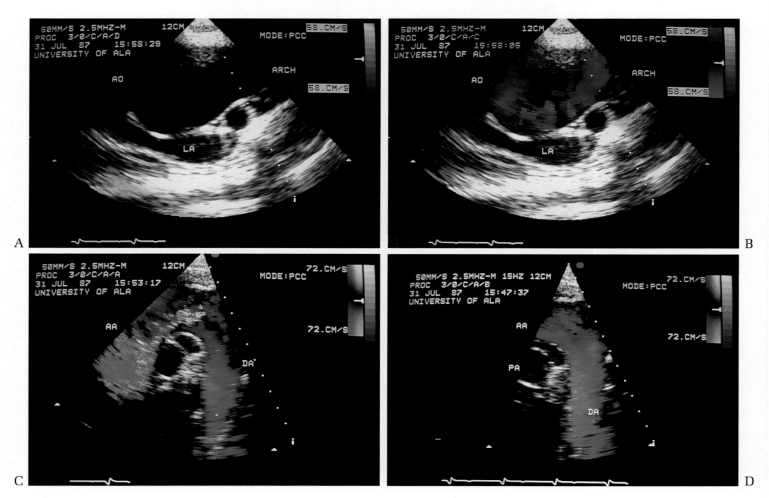

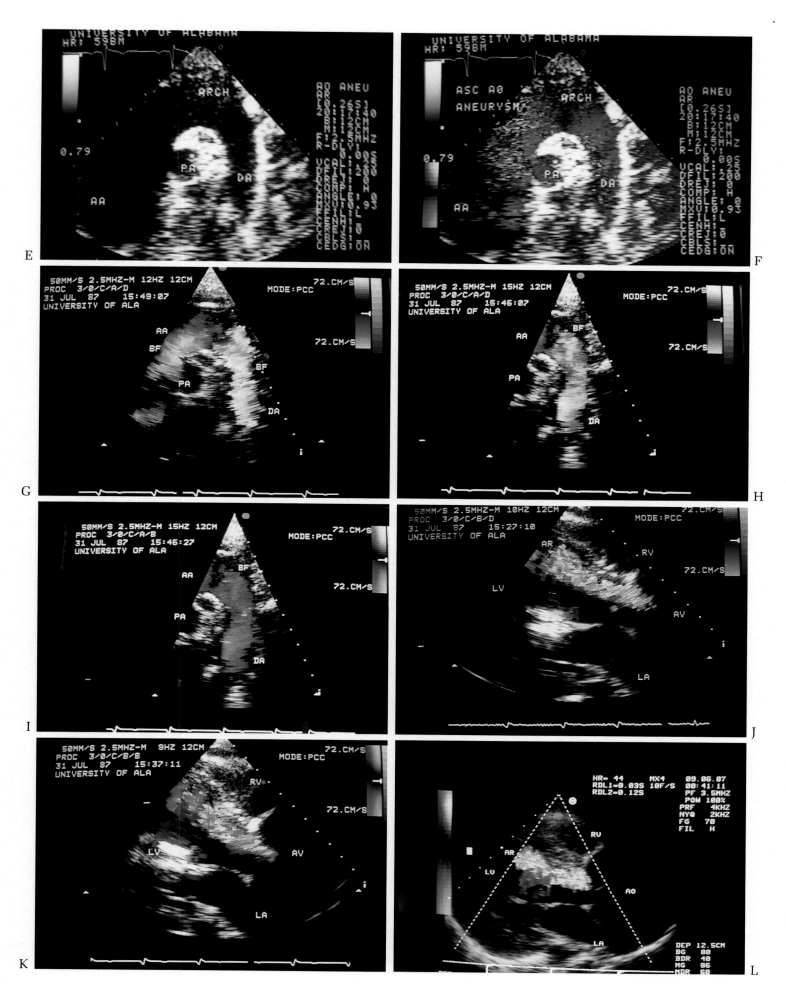

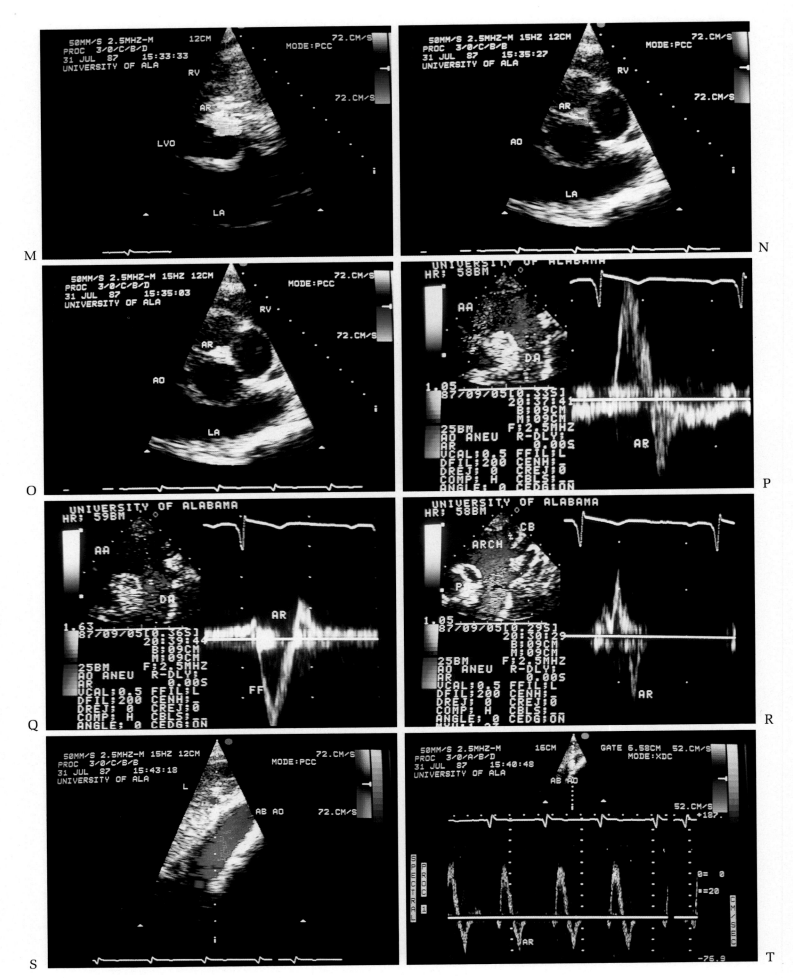

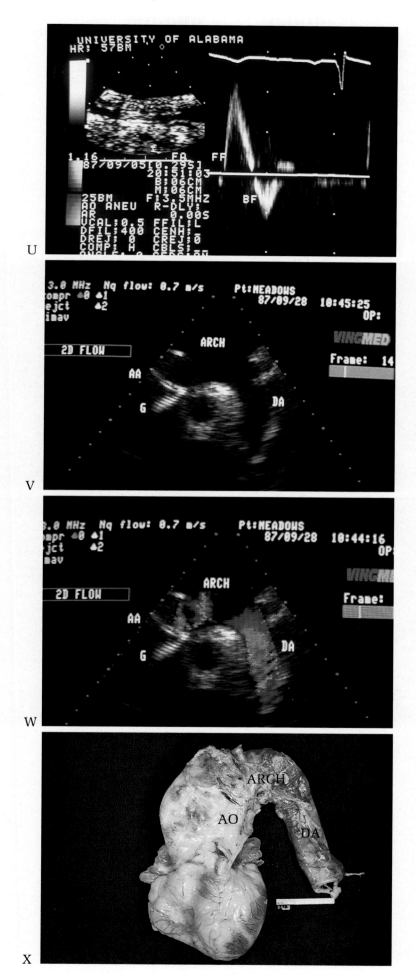

U

V

W

X

173

SECTION 4 AORTIC VALVE

Figure AV-47 **Descending aortic aneurysm.** Suprasternal examination of (A–D) in a 79-year-old woman shows aneurysmal dilatation of the DA with a large clot lining its lateral wall. Antegrade systolic flow (B, blue) and swirling in diastole (C, red and blue signals) are noted. Similar findings are also demonstrated on the color M-mode study (D).

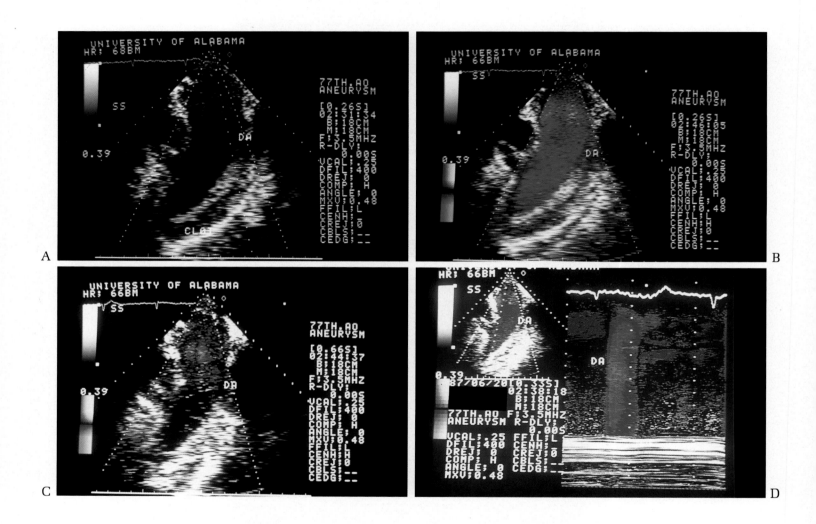

Figure AV-48 **Traumatic descending aortic aneurysm.** Suprasternal examination in a 24-year-old man with a post-traumatic aortic aneurysm shows a dilated proximal descending aorta (DESC). The blue signals represent antegrade flow in the DA, and the red signals within them are due to aliasing.

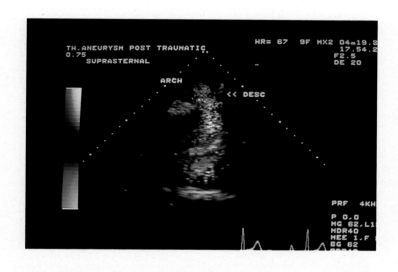

Figure AV-49 **Abdominal aortic aneurysm.** (A,B) Abdominal examination demonstrates an aneurysmally dilated proximal abdominal aorta (AA) in both long axis (A) and short axis (B) views in an 80-year-old man. A large clot lining the wall of the aneurysm is also shown (B). L=liver

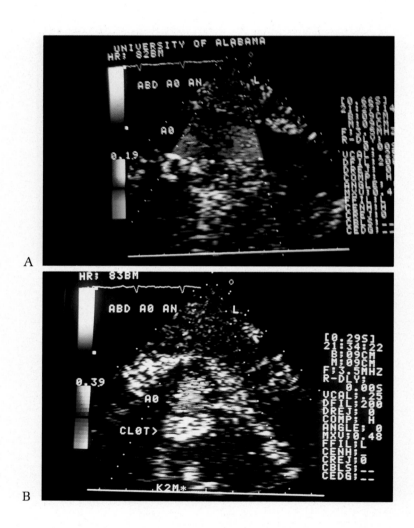

SECTION 4   AORTIC VALVE

Figure AV-50   **Aortic Dissection.** (A) Autopsy specimen shows an extensive dissection (arrows) of the aortic root which extends to the descending thoracic and abdominal aortas. (B) Autopsy specimen shows a dissecting hematoma (arrow) in the DA. This specimen has been cut open to show the false lumen (arrow) more clearly (C). The short axis view in the schematic (D) shows noncoaptation (N) of the AV produced by the dissecting hematoma (DH) compressing the aortic root. The resulting AR is shown in the long axis view on the right. The long axis view on the left shows a rupture of the dissecting hematoma into the LVOT, causing regurgitation (REG) into the LV. This regurgitation simulates AV regurgitation.

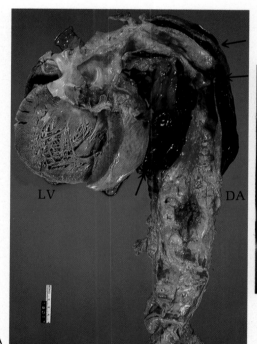

A

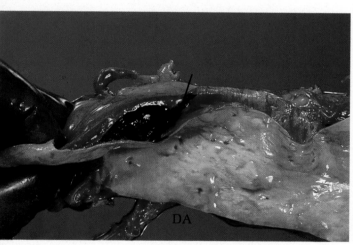

B

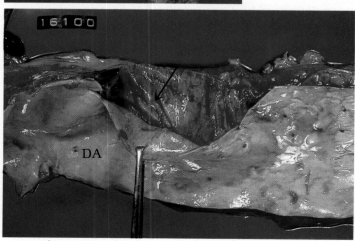

C

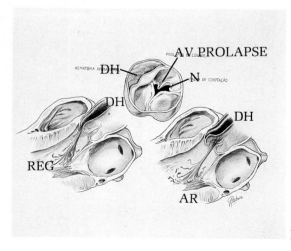

D

SECTION 4 AORTIC VALVE

Figure AV-51 **Aortic dissection.** The figures in this schematic illustrate a dissection flap in the AA and an opening between the true and false lumens near the aortic cusps (top) and in the aortic arch (bottom). AR is also shown in the bottom figure.

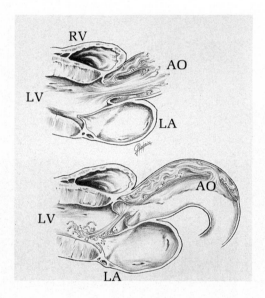

Figure AV-52 **Aortic dissection: Site of communication in the proximal ascending aorta.** (A) Parasternal long axis view in a 47-year-old man with DeBakey Type I dissection shows part of the aortic flow (vertical arrow) channelling into the false lumen (horizontal arrow) through the dissection flap. The long axis view (B) shows simultaneously the oppositely directed flows in the true and false lumens as red and blue signals (arrows) respectively, and the diastolic frame of the long axis view (C) shows blue signals of moderately severe AR in the LVOT. The schematic (D) illustrates flow in the true lumen entering the false lumen through an opening in the dissection flap. The color Doppler examination from the suprasternal view (E) shows simultaneous occurrence of oppositely directed flows in the two lumens of the distal AA and proximal arch (bidirectional flow). The red signals represent antegrade or forward flow in the true lumen, while the blue signals represent retrograde flow or backflow in the false lumen. F=dissection flap. (Reproduced with permission from Iliceto, S., Nanda, N.C., Rizzon, P., et al: Circulation 75:748–755, 1987.)

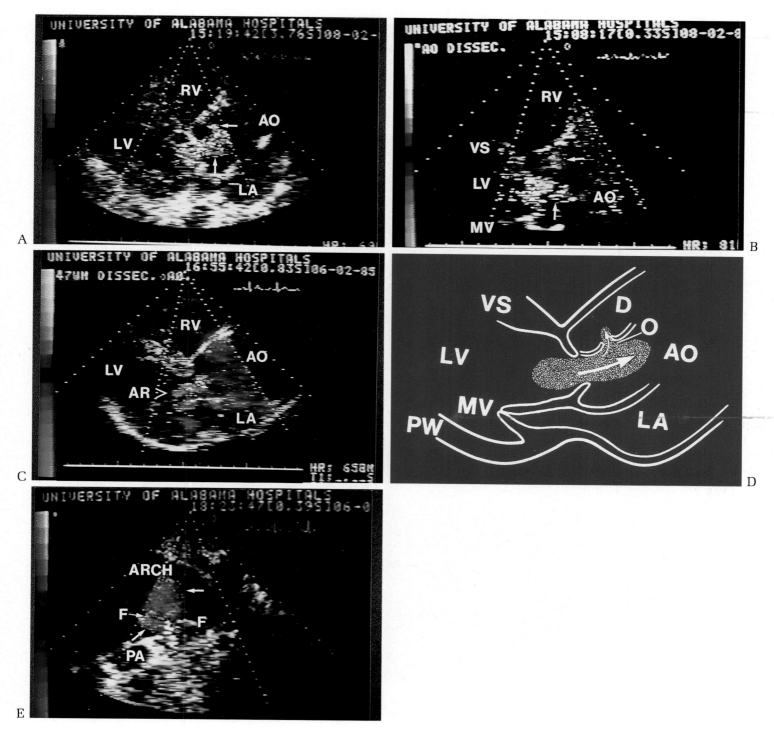

Figure AV-53   **Aortic dissection: Site of communication in the proximal ascending aorta.** (A) Suprasternal view of the AA in a patient with a DeBakey Type I dissection shows a dissection flap with an opening between two lumens in the AA. Red signals are seen during early systole in one of the lumens (L1), while flow signals in the other lumen (L2) are not visualized. This is shown schematically in B. In the late systolic frame (C), red signals are seen moving toward the dissection flap and entering into the other lumen. The schematic (D) illustrates this flow pattern. (Reproduced with permission from Iliceto, S., Nanda, N.C., Rizzon, P., et al: Circulation 75:748–755, 1987.) E,F,G and H represent right parasternal views in a 64-year-old man with DeBakey Type I dissection showing mosaic-colored turbulent flow signals moving through a large (2.5 cm) communication (C) into the false lumen during systole (E,F,G). During diastole (H), the flow signals (blue) move back into the true lumen, which is identified by its continuity with the AV. The color Doppler study also showed the presence of severe AR. This patient has had no evidence of chest pain or other clinical evidence of dissection, and was referred to us for evaluation of AR, which he was known to have for several years. All 2D and color Doppler echocardiographic findings were subsequently confirmed by angiography and surgery, during which the AV was replaced and an intraluminal tube graft inserted.

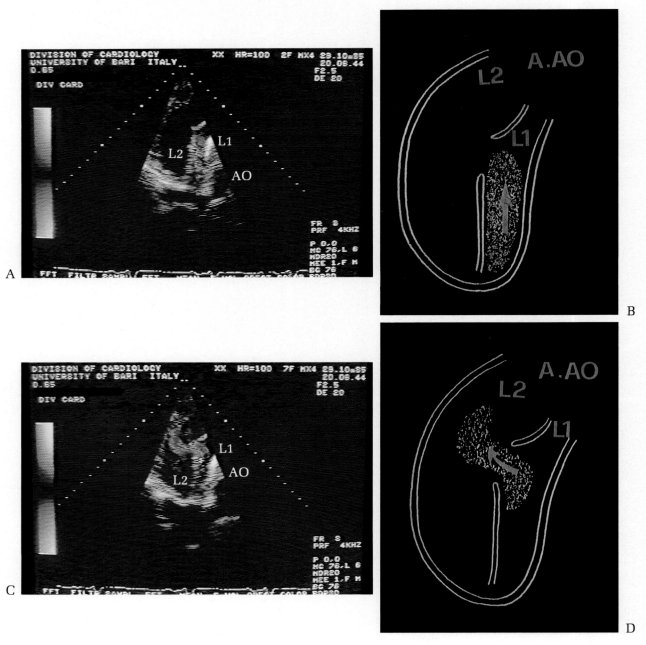

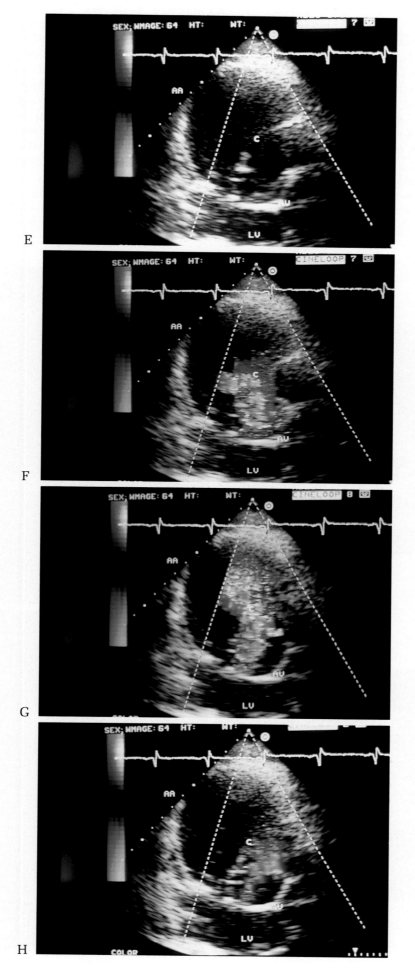

Figure AV-54   Aortic dissection. DeBakey Type I dissection with site of communication between the two lumina in the aortic arch. (A) Suprasternal long axis view of the ascending aorta (AA,A.AO). In early systole, flow is noted in one of the two lumina (L1) and is directed toward the transducer (predominantly red with some backward flow due to swirling shown in blue). The other lumen (L2) remains unopacified. (B) Schematic. (C) In late systole, flow signals in the first lumen (L1) are still present and predominantly directed toward the transducer, while flow signals appear in the second lumen (L2) and are directed in the opposite direction (downward and away from the transducer, blue). These findings indicate that the site of communication between the two lumens is in the aortic arch. (D) Schematic (Reproduced with permission from Iliceto, S., Nanda, N.C., Rizzon, P., et al: Circulation 75:748–755, 1987.)

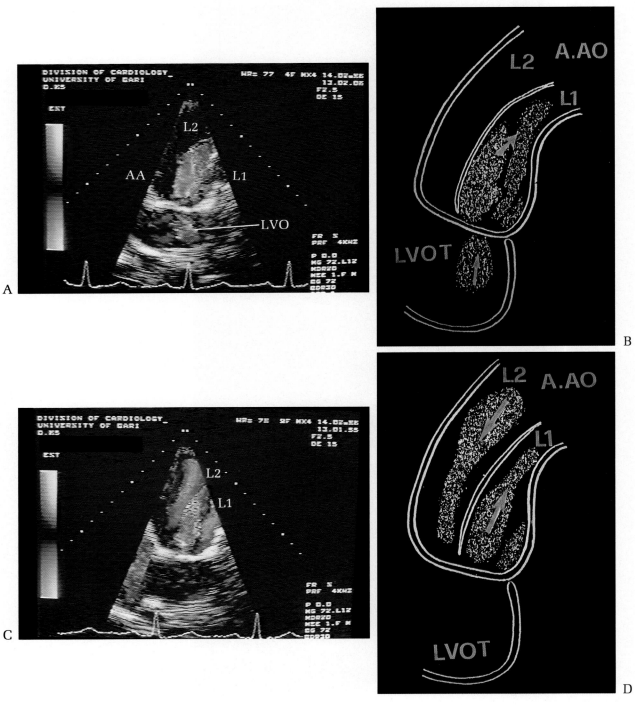

SECTION 4   AORTIC VALVE

Figure AV-55   **Aortic dissection: Site of communication in the descending thoracic aorta.** (A) On the left, the systolic frame of a suprasternal view in a patient with DeBakey Type III aortic dissection shows blue signals in the inner lumen representing antegrade flow in the DA. The red signals marked with an arrow represent flow from the inner lumen to the outer lumen through an opening in the dissection flap. In the diastolic frame shown on the right, red signals in the outer lumen imply upward flow in the DA. The blue signals marked with an arrow indicate flow from the outer lumen to the inner lumen through the dissection flap. These flow patterns are schematically illustrated in B and C respectively. (DTA=descending thoracic aorta; IL=inner lumen; OL=outer lumen.) (Reproduced with permission from Iliceto, S., Nanda, N.C., Rizzon, P., et al: Circulation 75:748–755, 1987.) Right parasternal examination (D,E,F) of the AA in a 79-year-old man with chronic DeBakey Type II aortic dissection shows prominent flow signals (red) moving from the true lumen into the false lumen through a large communication during systole (D,E). Backward flow (blue) into the true lumen is seen during diastole (F). The dissection flap is located 5 to 6 cm above the AV level. There was no evidence of dissection in the aortic arch or DA.

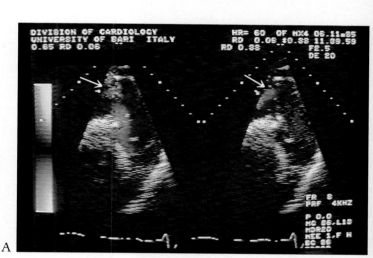

A

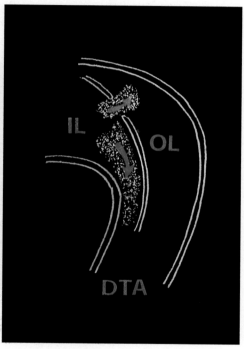

B

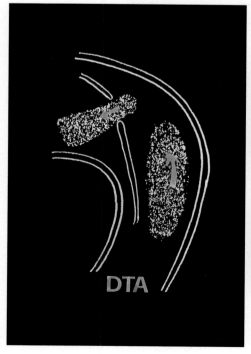

C

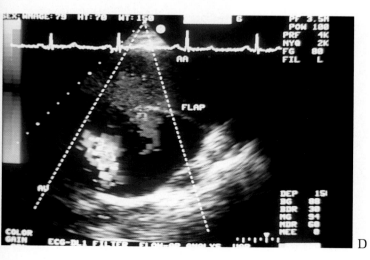

D

183

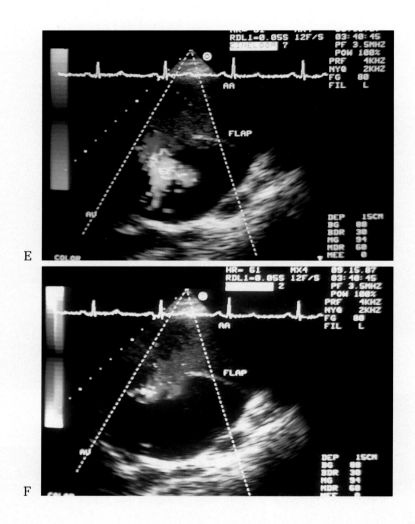

E

F

SECTION 4   AORTIC VALVE

Figure AV-56 **Aortic dissection.** A 38-year-old man with Marfan's syndrome had a composite intraluminal tube graft for a dissecting aneurysm of the aorta. The modified left supraclavicular view (A) in this patient shows blue signals moving from the false lumen (L2) to the true lumen (L1) during diastole through an opening or communication (C) in the dissection flap. During systole (B and C), the mosaic signals move from the true to the false lumen. L1 is well delineated by the presence of aliased flow signals. The site of the communication, however, is not clear on 2D examination (D). Color M-mode examinations (E and F) show flow signals moving from L1 to L2 during systole and in the reverse direction during diastole. The short axis views (G and H) of the DA from a posterior intercostal space show a dissection flap and flow signals in both lumens. The color M-mode recording (I) shows flow in the true lumen (L1) during systole and very faint flow signals in the false lumen (L2) during diastole. Moving the transducer to a lower posterior intercostal space (J) shows flow in the narrowed true lumen (L1) and a clotted false lumen (L2). TH=thrombus. Rotating the transducer to visualize the DA in the long axis (K and L) shows prominent flow signals in true lumen (L1) with only faint signals in the clotted false lumen (L2).

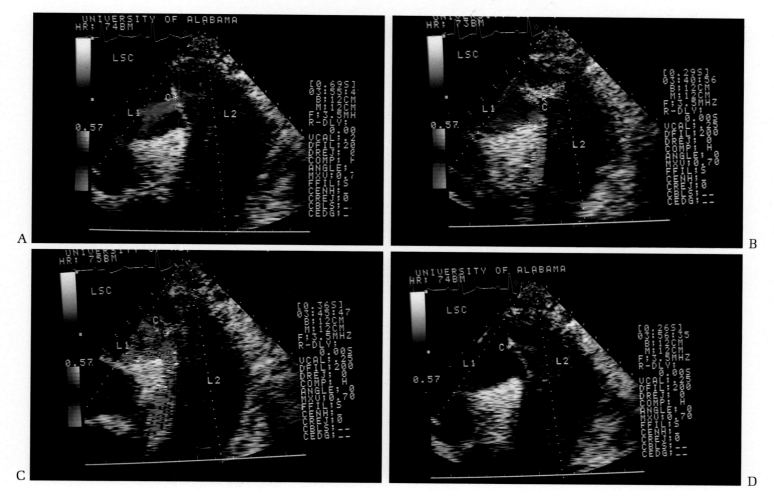

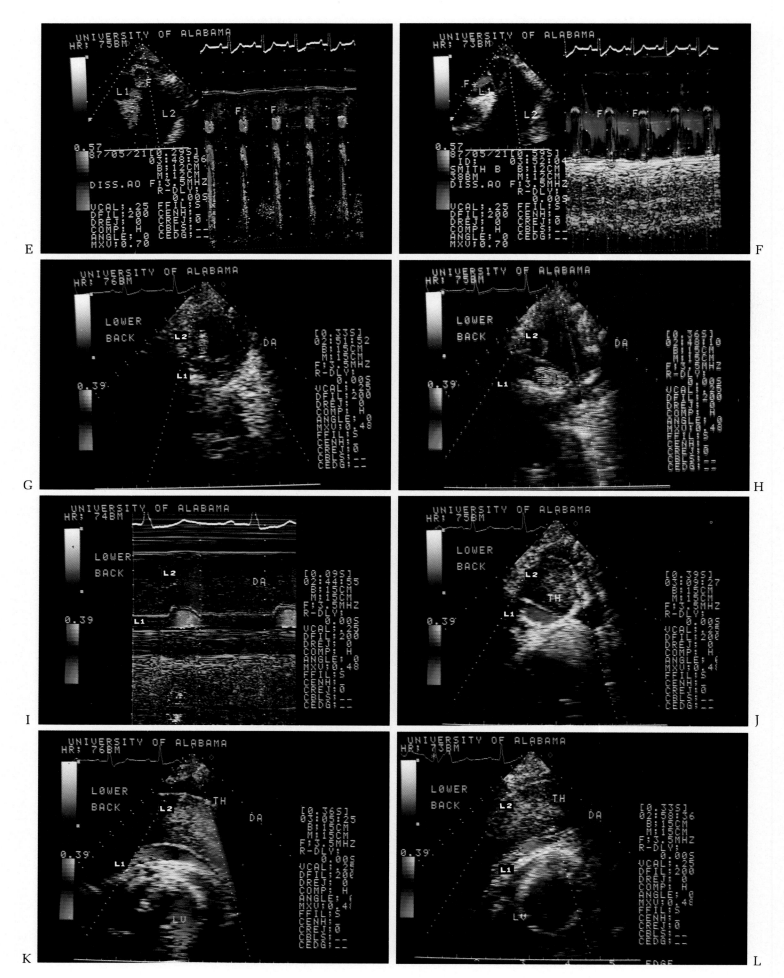

SECTION 4 AORTIC VALVE

Figure AV-57 **Repair of aortic dissection.** (A) 2D examination performed from the right parasternal approach in the 38-year-old man examined in Figure AV-56 clearly shows in the AO the intraluminal tube graft (TG), identified by the presence of rugae or corrugations in its walls (arrows). Color Doppler study (B) shows mosaic signals in the tube graft (TG), as well as the St. Jude's aortic prosthesis (AP). The blue signals below the graft represent a leak through the graft into the native aortic aneurysm (AN). Color Doppler examination (C) performed after the leak was repaired shows mosaic signals in the graft but no flow signals at the site of the previous leak.

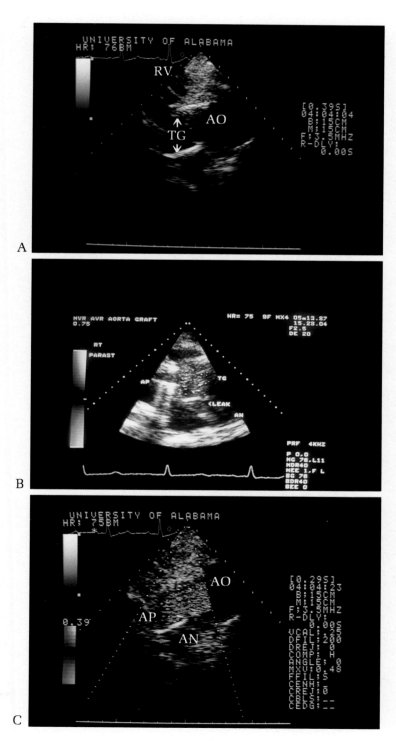

Figure AV-58　**Repair of aortic dissection.** (A and B) Autopsy specimens show a synthetic intraluminal TG in the AA with preservation of the native AV. The dissection channel (D) is also seen. (C) Autopsy specimen shows a resection of the proximal aorta and its replacement with a tube graft. The dissection channel distal to the graft is clearly delineated.

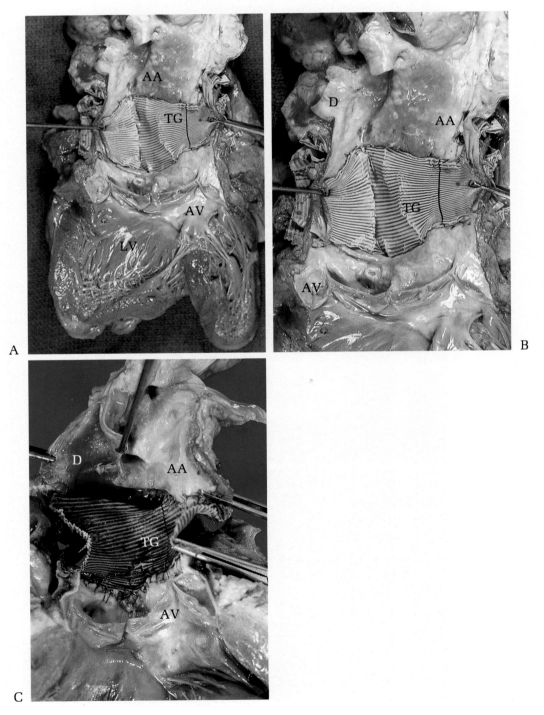

SECTION 4 AORTIC VALVE

Figure AV-59 **Repair of aortic dissection.** A 27-year-old man had an intraluminal tube graft (ILTG) for repair of a dissecting ascending aortic aneurysm. The modified parasternal long axis view in this patient shows a narrow band of mosaic signals originating from the anterior part of the tube graft and moving through the aneurysm (AN) into the RVOT. This represents a small leak, which was subsequently repaired surgically.

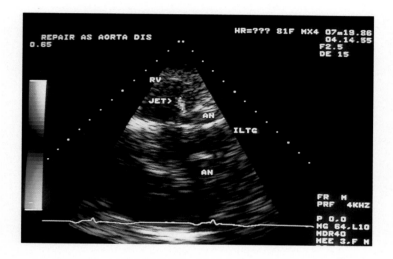

SECTION 4 AORTIC VALVE

Figure AV-60 **Repair of aortic dissection.** Right parasternal view in a 43-year-old man who had a repair of a dissection shows mosaic signals in the outer or true lumen (OL) and no flow signals in the inner or false lumen (IL). This implies a successful closure of the opening between the true and the false lumens. In repairing a dissection, one of the aims is to stop flow into the false lumen, causing it to clot to provide additional support and prevent further extension of the dissection. F=Dissection flap.

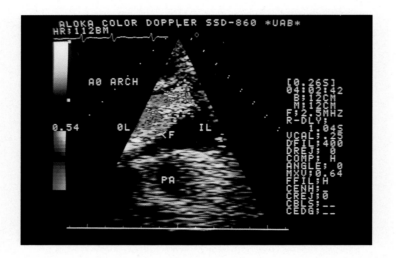

Section 5

TRICUSPID VALVE

TRICUSPID REGURGITATION

Color Doppler echocardiography provides a better evaluation of tricuspid regurgitation (TR) than pulsed Doppler echocardiography because this type of regurgitation can be viewed in multiple imaging planes in a much shorter period of time with color Doppler than with pulsed Doppler.

A color Doppler examination of TR using either the aortic short axis, right ventricular inflow, or apical 4-chamber view shows mosaic signals originating from the tricuspid valve (TV) and extending into the RA during systole. In some patients, however, TR is best visualized using the right parasternal imaging plane combined with suitable transducer angulations because it produces a larger view of the right atrial cavity. TR may also be seen using the apical right ventricular 2-chamber view or, in younger patients, subcostal views such as 4-chamber views.

The tricuspid regurgitant jet in the RA is initially mosaic in color because of turbulence and aliasing. It may, however, become laminar farther in the RA as its velocity decreases below the Nyquist limit, causing it to be shown as either red or blue depending on the direction of the flow in relation to the transducer. Diastolic frames may show prominent inflow signals moving into the RV from the RA, representing increased flow across the TV during diastole. This increased flow occurs because the tricuspid regurgitant flow combines with right atrial inflow. In some patients, the tricuspid regurgitant jet may not show any aliasing or obvious turbulence because of a nonparallel orientation of the Doppler beam to the tricuspid regurgitant flow or, in some cases, because of a small difference between the right ventricular and right atrial systolic pressures.

The tricuspid regurgitant signals in some imaging planes may not appear to originate from the TV, but careful manipulation of the transducer clearly defines the TV as the origin of these flow signals. The TR jet must also be distinguished from a thin linear vertical band of high-frequency signals which may be seen at the closure point of the TV during color M-mode examination. The tricuspid regurgitant signals are broader than the ghosting artifact signals that result from rapid closing movement of the TV.

Tricuspid regurgitant signals may be oriented laterally, centrally, or medially toward the atrial septum (AS). In the latter case, the jet may be located very close to the AS and, when pulsed Doppler is used, may be mistaken for a mitral regurgitant jet because of its proximity to the AS. Color Doppler, however, clearly displays no signals in the left atrial cavity and shows the tricuspid regurgitant jet limited by the AS and originating from the TV. In patients with right ventricular pacemakers, the tricuspid regurgitant jet may have a markedly eccentric direction because of the presence of a pacemaker lead in the TV orifice. In patients with moderate or severe TR and a nondilated right atrial cavity, the TR flow may swirl back toward the TV after impacting the back wall of the RA. When it hits the back wall and swirls back toward the TV, the regurgitant jet loses kinetic energy; that is, its velocity decreases, causing it to be displayed by mainly laminar flow signals. These laminar signals occur during systole and can be distinguished as a part of the tricuspid regurgitant flow by their continuity with the mosaic-colored tricuspid regurgitant jet. In the presence of a dilated right atrial cavity, we have noticed this phenomenon of swirling only in patients with severe TR.

Two distinct mosaic jets of TR may be seen in some patients originating from the same leaflet or from two different leaflets. These two jets may not merge with each other or may merge downstream in the RA. We have sometimes seen one jet of TR that bifurcates farther upstream in the right atrial cavity.

The exact site of the defect in the TV may sometimes

be pinpointed by noting the location of the flow acceleration on the ventricular aspect of the TV. Flow acceleration is shown as an increase in the color brightness of the retrograde flow signals or as aliasing. It may also take on a shape that can reflect the size of the defect in the TV. Occasionally, multiple sites of flow acceleration or regurgitation are observed in the TV because of the presence of multiple anatomic defects.

No real "gold standard" for estimating the severity of TR exists. Cardiac catheterization cannot be used to evaluate this lesion because the catheter passing through the TV for right ventricular injection interferes with the closure of the TV leaflets, causing artifical TR. In our experience, the severity of TR is best estimated with use of color Doppler by planimeterizing the maximum tricuspid regurgitant jet obtained, using the available multiple imaging planes and transducer angulations. This jet area is expressed as a percentage of the area of the right atrial cavity, obtained by using the frame in which the maximum tricuspid regurgitant jet was noted. A ratio of 20% or less indicates the presence of mild TR and a ratio between 20 and 34% indicates the presence of moderate TR. Severe TR is indicated by a ratio greater than or equal to 35%. These color Doppler criteria have been indirectly validated. We recently assessed the presence and severity of TR by color Doppler in patients who were scheduled to undergo MV or AV replacement and correlated our results with intraoperative assessment of TR. In approximately 90% of patients judged by the surgeon to have TR severe enough to require TV annuloplasty, the maximum tricuspid regurgitant jet area by color Doppler occupied 35% or more of the right atrial area. On the other hand, the maximum tricuspid regurgitant jet area by color Doppler occupied less than 35% of the right atrial area in about 90% of patients judged by the surgeon not to have severe TR and therefore not candidates for TV repair or replacement. Therefore, color Doppler can be used to identify patients with severe TR who would require TV repair in conjunction with AV or MV replacement. It is important to realize that intraoperative assessment of TR is not absolutely reliable, and the surgeon often uses both intraoperative and the clinical findings to make a judgment on whether or not to replace the TV. Color Doppler can also be used to estimate the severity of residual TR after TV annuloplasty repair.

When tricuspid regurgitant signals are observed moving into the IVC and hepatic veins during systole, the regurgitation is not classified as mild but as moderate to severe. This flow pattern can be best visualized by interrogating a vertical hepatic vein so that the Doppler beam is parallel to the flow patterns in this vein. Severe TR is indicated when systolic retrograde flow is observed moving into the SVC. Although this finding is specific for severe TR, it lacks sensitivity and is rarely observed. Tricuspid regurgitant signals may also be occasionally seen moving into the coronary sinus in patients with severe TR. This is best observed using the right parasternal imaging plane, but it may also be observed in the right ventricular inflow view.

After color Doppler identifies the presence of TR, the systolic pulmonary artery pressure can be estimated using the results obtained from color-guided continuous wave Doppler. The mosaic signals of TR displayed by color Doppler help to provide a reference for the positioning of the continuous wave Doppler cursor parallel to the regurgitant flow and to record reliable peak velocities during systole. The Bernoulli equation then can be used to calculate the pressure gradient across the TV using these velocities. Adding an assumed right atrial pressure of 10 mm Hg to this calculated pressure gradient, the pulmonary artery systolic pressure can be estimated. We have found this estimation technique extremely useful in assessing the severity of pulmonary hypertension in patients with both AV and MV disease and in patients being considered for cardiac transplantation.

Although color Doppler allows diagnosis of TR, its etiology is often determined by 2D echocardiography. For example, a mass on the TV in a patient with a febrile illness alerts the examiner to the presence of bacterial endocarditis. Patients with rheumatic involvement show TV thickening, and patients with papillary muscle dysfunction due to ischemic heart disease show an inferiorly displaced coaptation point of the TV below its annulus. The TV may appear to be flail in patients with chordae rupture due to endocarditis or trauma. In many other patients, however, the etiology of TR is not clear even though the dilatation of the RA, tricuspid annulus, and RV suggest the presence of "functional" TR, or regurgitation due to right heart enlargement. It should be emphasized also that minimal TR may occur in apparently normal healthy individuals and thus may not necessarily be pathologic.

TRICUSPID VALVE STENOSIS

TV stenosis, an uncommon lesion often associated with mitral stenosis, can be evaluated by color Doppler. The width of the signals observed at the level of the TV during diastole provides a reliable estimate of the severity of TV stenosis. A narrow width implies severe stenosis and a larger width mild stenosis. Prominent flow acceleration may also be seen on the atrial aspect of a stenotic TV. A continuous wave Doppler cursor placed parallel to diastolic TV inflow signals obtains an accurate estimate of the mean and peak pressure gradients across the TV in patients with tricuspid stenosis.

REFERENCES

TRICUSPID REGURGITATION

1. Waggoner, A.D., Quinones, M.A., Young, J.B., Brandon, T.A., Shah, A.A., Verani, M.S., and Miller, R.R.: Pulsed Doppler echocardiography detection of right sided valve regurgitation. Am. J. Cardiol. 47:279, 1981.

2. Hatle, L., Angelson, B.A.J., and Tromsdal, A.: Non-invasive estimation of pulmonary artery systolic pressure with Doppler ultrasound. Br. Heart J. 45:157, 1981.

3. Miyatake, K., Okamoto, M., Kinoshita, N., Ohta, M., Kozuka, T., Sakakibara, H., and Nimura, Y.: Evaluation of tricuspid regurgitation by pulsed Doppler and two-dimensional echocardiography. Circulation 66:4, 1982.

4. Yock, P.G., and Popp, R.L.: Non-invasive estimation of right ventricular systolic pressure by Doppler ultrasound in patients with tricuspid regurgitation. Circulation 70:657, 1984.

5. Suzuki, Y., Kambara, H., Kadoya, K., Tamaki, S., Yamazoto, A., Nohara, R., Osakada, G., Kawai, C., Kubo, S., and Karaguchi, T.,: Detection and evaluation of tricuspid regurgitation using a real-time, two-dimensional, color coded, Doppler flow imaging system: Comparison with contrast two dimensional echocardiography and right ventriculography. Am. J. Cardiol. 57:811, 1986.

6. Konstadt, S., Thys, D., Mindich, B., Kaplan, J., and Goldman, M.E.: Validation of quantitative intraoperative transesophageal echocardiography. Anesthesiology 65:418, 1986.

7. Goldman, M.E., Fuster, V., Guarino, T., and Mindich, B.P.: Intraoperative echocardiography for the evaluation of valvular regurgitation: Experience in 262 patients (Abstract). Circulation 74: (Supp. I) I:143, 1986.

8. Goyal, R.G., Kan, M.N., Helmcke, F., and Nanda, N.C.: Color Doppler/2-dimensional echo identification of severe tricuspid regurgitation requiring surgery (Abstract). Clin. Res. 35:282A, 1987.

TRICUSPID VALVE STENOSIS

1. Quinones, M.A., and Nelson, J.G.: Doppler evaluation of right sided lesions and pulmonary hypertension. In: Nanda, N.C. (Ed): Doppler Echocardiography, New York, Igaku-Shoin Medical Publishers, Inc., 1985.

SECTION 5   TRICUSPID VALVE

Many examples in this section clearly demonstrate the value of color Doppler in all types of pathologies affecting the TV.

Figure TV-1   **Tricuspid regurgitation.** (A) Schematic of the aortic short axis view illustrates incomplete coaptation of a thickened TV during systole. The aortic short axis view (B) shows mosaic signals originating from a slightly thickened TV and filling approximately 20% of the RA, implying mild TR. Color M-mode examination (C) shows mosaic signals in the RA throughout systole, indicating pansystolic regurgitation. During diastole, the red signals below the TV represent right atrial flow, while the blue signals in front of the TV represent pulmonic regurgitant flow moving toward the RV inflow in this patient.

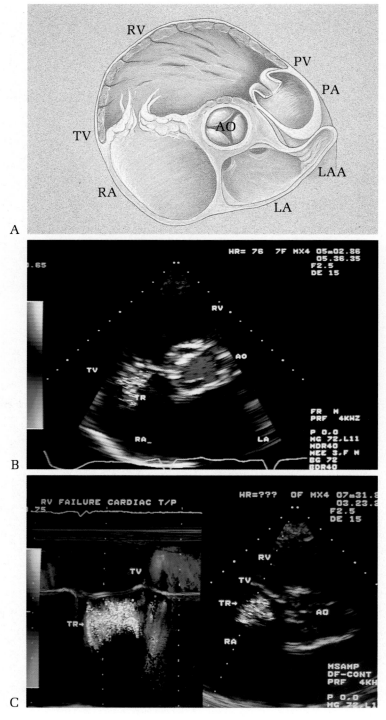

SECTION 5   TRICUSPID VALVE

Figure TV-2   **Mild tricuspid regurgitation.** (A and B) Aortic short axis views in 2 patients show small areas of mosaic and blue signals originating from the septal leaflet of the TV and occupying less than 20% of the RA. This indicates mild TR. The red signals seen in B represent the IVC flow moving into the RA.

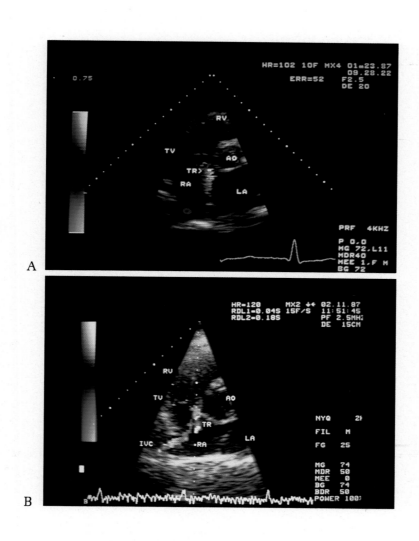

SECTION 5   TRICUSPID VALVE

Figure TV-3   **Tricuspid regurgitation.** (A and B) Short axis views at the level of the high LVOT in a 59-year-old woman show mosaic signals during systole occupying 25 to 30% of the RA, implying moderate TR. Further in the RA, these mosaic signals become blue because their velocity decreases below the Nyquist limit of 0.54 m/sec. Color M-mode examination (B) shows the mosaic and blue signals to be present below the TV throughout systole. The red signals in diastole represent tricuspid inflow, while the blue signals behind the TV result from the swirling of blood flow in the dilated RA.

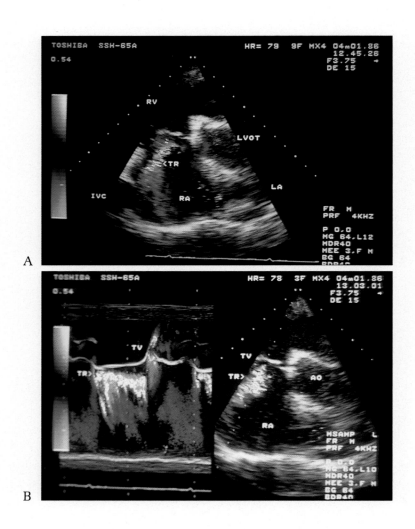

SECTION 5   TRICUSPID VALVE

Figure TV-4   **Tricuspid regurgitation.** (A) Systolic frame of the aortic short axis view in a 31-year-old woman shows mosaic signals of moderate TR in the RA. (B) Diastolic frame shows prominent red signals representing increased flow across the TV during diastole. This increased flow occurs because the tricuspid regurgitant flow combines with the right atrial inflow. The bluish-white color seen within these red signals represents aliasing.

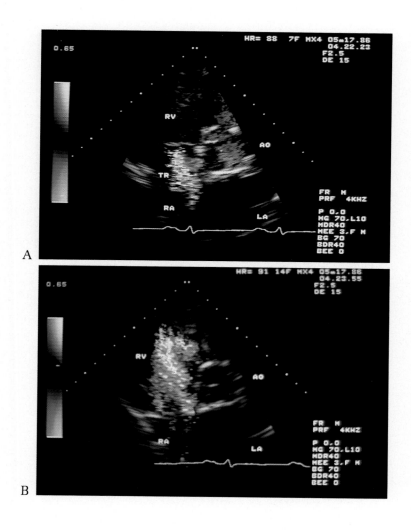

SECTION 5   TRICUSPID VALVE

Figure TV-5   **Tricuspid regurgitation.** Aortic short axis view as shown on the right shows mosaic and blue signals of moderate TR within the RA. Color M-mode as shown on the left shows pansystolic regurgitation and diastolic red signals moving across the TV. These red signals represent tricuspid inflow, and the blue color within them results from aliasing. The deep blue signals observed behind the TV during end diastole (arrow) may represent diastolic TR resulting from a prolonged PR interval.

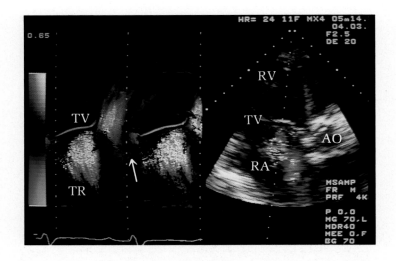

SECTION 5 TRICUSPID VALVE

Figure TV-6 **Tricuspid regurgitation** (A and B) Short axis views in 2 different patients show mosaic signals of TR which occupy 25 to 30% of the dilated right atrial cavity, implying moderate TR. Further in the RA in B, the mosaic signals turn blue because the velocity of the regurgitant jet decreases below the Nyquist limit of 0.75 m/sec. CRISTA = crista supraventricularis. C and D are autopsy specimens showing the relationship of the TV to RV muscle bands and papillary muscles. The trabeculo septo-marginalis (TSM) branches into a superior arm (SA, septal band) and a posterior arm (PA). The infundibular septum (IS), together with portions of superior and posterior arms and the ventricular infundibular fold (not shown), form the crista supraventricularis (CS, dotted line). The portion of the IS attached to RV free wall represents its parietal extension (also called the parietal band, PB). The TSM is connected to the anterior papillary muscle (APM) through the moderator band (MB) located near the RV apex. The small muscle arising from the PA is the medial papillary muscle or the muscle of Lancisi (ML).

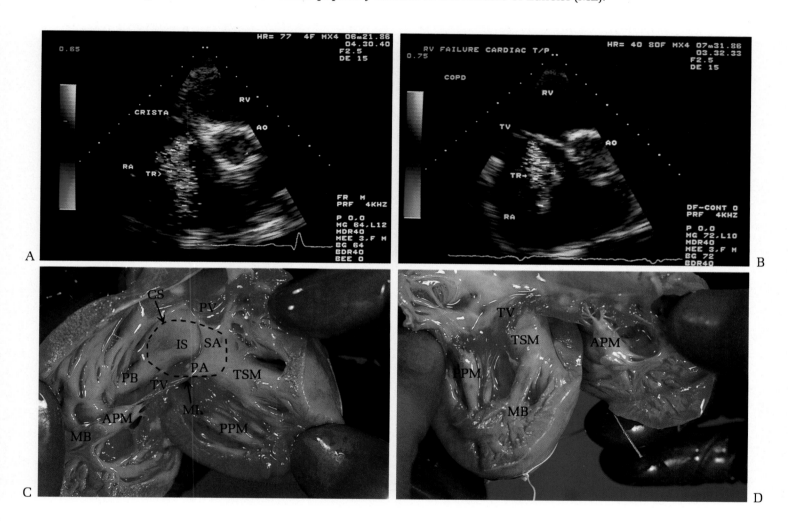

SECTION 5 TRICUSPID VALVE

Figure TV-7 **Tricuspid regurgitation.** (A and B) Apical views show significant right ventricular and atrial dilatation and prominent mosaic and blue signals of TR which completely fill the RA, indicative of severe TR. Schematic C shows a thickened TV in the apical 4-chamber view, while schematic D illustrates noncoaptation of the tricuspid leaflets, significant right ventricular and atrial dilatation, and a prominent jet of TR.

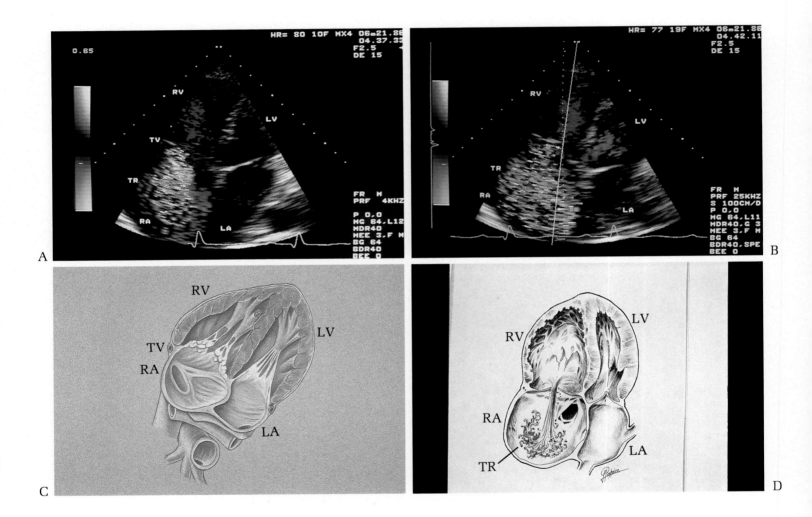

SECTION 5   TRICUSPID VALVE

Figure TV-8   **Tricuspid regurgitation.** Apical views (A on the right and B with 2D image turned off) in an adult patient with MV and TV disease show bluish-green signals on the ventricular aspect of the TV. These signals represent flow acceleration (FA) of tricuspid regurgitant jet. The jet is initially red in color, which implies aliasing. Then the jet becomes mosaic and, finally, blue in color farther in the RA as its velocity decreases. The color M-mode (A) on the left shows, during systole in the RA, bluish-green signals at the level of the TV, representing flow acceleration of the regurgitant jet and red signals just behind the TV representing aliasing (velocities have exceeded the Nyquist limit, first wraparound). The blue signals seen within the black area result from further aliasing, in which the velocities have twice exceeded the Nyquist limit (second wraparound). The black region represents flow signals with velocities very close to twice the Nyquist limit. During diastole, red signals of tricuspid inflow are observed at the periphery and prominent blue signals representing aliasing are seen in the center of these red signals. Small specks of red color located in the periphery of the blue signals represent secondary aliasing. These specks are expected to appear in the center of the blue signals, but, possibly because of both anteroposterior and "lateral" aliasing, they are confined to the periphery. TF = diastolic tricuspid inflow.

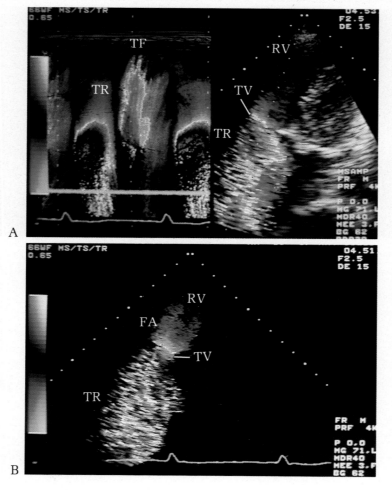

SECTION 5   TRICUSPID VALVE

Figure TV-9   **Calculation of pulmonary artery pressure in tricuspid regurgitation.** The continuous wave cursor is placed parallel to the mosaic signals of TR imaged in the short axis and the modified apical views as shown in A, B, and C. The velocity waveforms obtained in A, B, and C show peak velocities of 2.66, 2.89, and 3.5 m/sec, which translate into peak pressure gradients of 28, 33, and 49 mm Hg, respectively. Assuming a right atrial pressure of 10 mm Hg in these 3 patients, the calculated PA systolic pressure equals 38, 43, and 59 mm Hg for A, B, and C, respectively. Patient in D is a 58-year-old man referred for cardiac transplant evaluation, who demonstrates a peak TR velocity of 4.04 m/sec. This translates into a systolic PA pressure of 75 mm Hg.

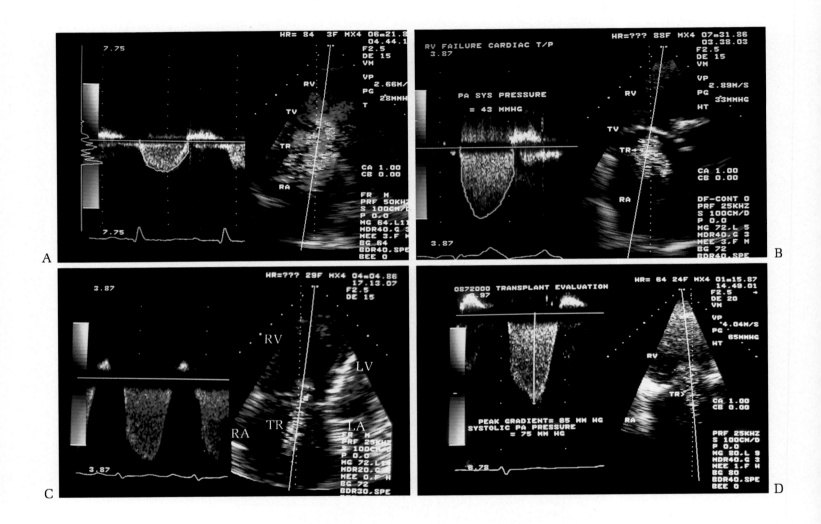

SECTION 5   TRICUSPID VALVE

Figure TV-10   Examination of the hepatic veins in tricuspid regurgitation. (A–E) Subcostal examination of the hepatic veins (HV) show these veins draining into the IVC. The blue signals during diastole (D) in A represent normal hepatic venous flow, and the faint red signals seen on the color M-mode during atrial systole indicate normal flow into these veins. Prominent red signals are seen in these veins during systole as shown in B and C. These signals represent retrograde or backward flow into them, which characterizes moderate to severe TR. The color M-mode examinations in C and D also show prominent red signals of retrograde flow (arrow) in the HVs during systole. Bluish-green signals within these red signals, as seen in C, result from aliasing (A), while blue signals as seen in C and D during diastole represent normal hepatic venous flow. The pulse Doppler sample volume (SV) placed within the systolic signals in a vertical HV as shown in E also displays systolic retrograde flow, represented by prominent Doppler shifts (F) above the baseline (B). L = liver.

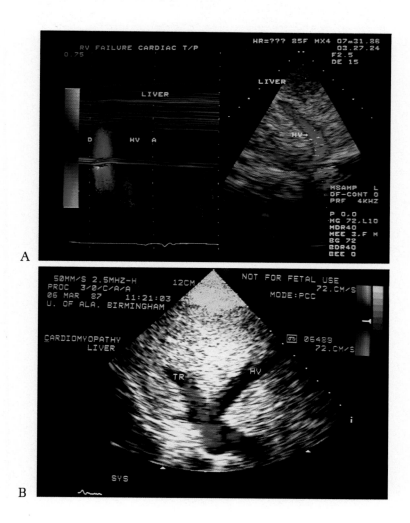

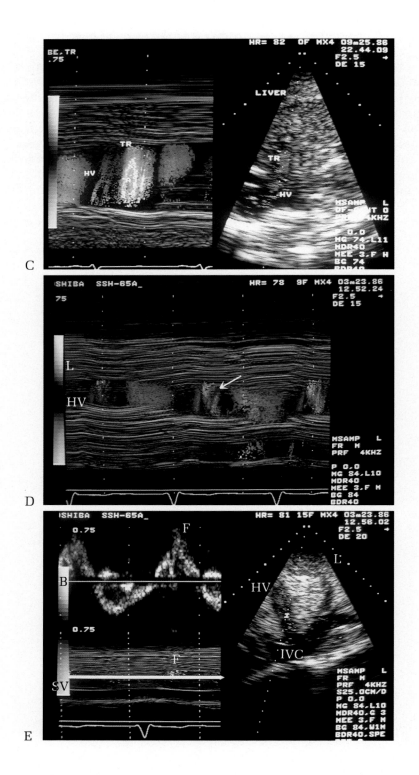

SECTION 5   TRICUSPID VALVE

Figure TV-11   **Tricuspid regurgitation visualized from right parasternal approach.** (A,B,C) Right parasternal views in a 59-year-old man show mosaic signals originating from the TV and moving anteriorly and superiorly into the RA. The coronary sinus (CS) flow is shown as a small area of red signals moving from the CS into the RA. The prominent blue signals represent the swirling of the tricuspid regurgitant flow as it strikes the back wall of the RA and then moves posteriorly. The TR and CS flow signals are shown in D with the 2D image turned off.

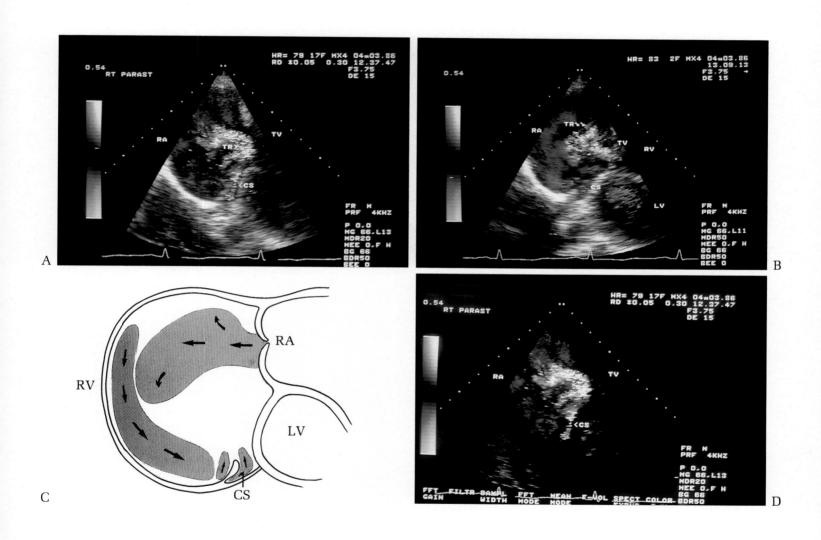

SECTION 5 TRICUSPID VALVE

Figure TV-12 **Tricuspid regurgitation visualized from right parasternal approach.** Right parasternal view in a 21-year-old man shows red signals of TR in the RA moving anteriorly and then turning blue as they turn posteriorly toward the back wall of the RA. The absence of aliasing in this frame could be caused by either a nonparallel orientation of the Doppler beam to the tricuspid regurgitant flow or a small gradient between the RV and RA systolic pressures. These cause low velocities below the Nyquist limit to be recorded for the tricuspid regurgitant jet. This phenomenon occurs in some cases of severe TR. The small area of red signals located near the AS may represent coronary sinus flow.

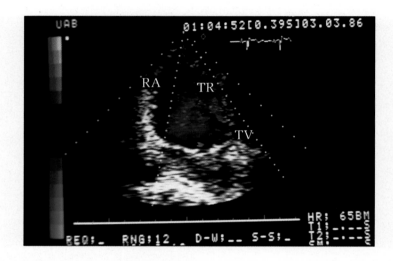

SECTION 5   TRICUSPID VALVE

Figure TV-13   **Two jets of tricuspid regurgitation.** The aortic short axis view in a 56-year-old man with scleroderma shows two distinct mosaic jets of TR. One of the jets originates from the septal leaflet and the other from the anterior leaflet. These two jets merge farther in the RA.

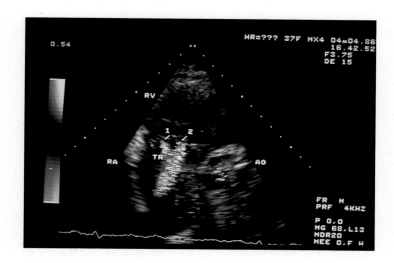

SECTION 5 TRICUSPID VALVE

Figure TV-14 **Tricuspid regurgitation.** Aortic short axis view in a 101-year-old man shows a jet of bluish-green signals of moderate TR in the RA, bifurcating farther in the cavity. This jet does not appear to originate from the TV. The apparent discontinuity in these flow signals at the origin of the TV results from transducer angulation. Careful manipulation of the transducer can help to define clearly the origin of these flow signals from the TV.

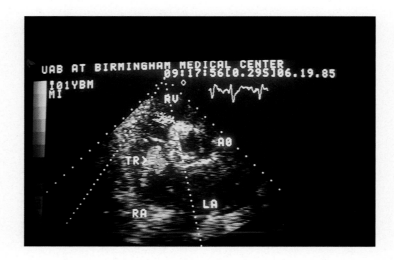

SECTION 5   TRICUSPID VALVE

Figure TV-15   **Tricuspid regurgitation.** The aortic short axis view shows mosaic signals of TR originating from the TV and moving medially in the RA toward the AS. Farther in the RA, these mosaic signals turn blue because their velocity decreases below the Nyquist limit of 0.65 m/sec.

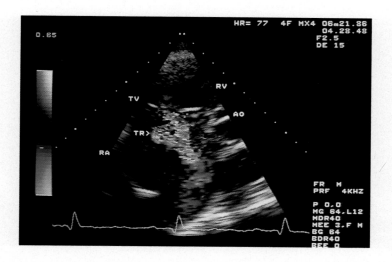

SECTION 5 TRICUSPID VALVE

Figure TV-16 **Tricuspid regurgitation.** (A, B, and C) The modified apical views using different color Doppler machines in different patients show mosaic signals of TR originating near the septal leaflet of the TV and moving toward the AS. Bluish-green and red signals on the ventricular aspect of the TV are more clearly seen in B and C. These signals represent flow acceleration of the tricuspid regurgitant jet and help define the site of the defect in the TV. Tricuspid regurgitant signals move along the AS in B and C and turn deep blue as the velocity of the jet decreases below the Nyquist limit. The pacemaker lead in the patient in C could have contributed to the eccentric direction of the tricuspid regurgitant jet. The schematic (D) illustrates a dilated RV and RA, the eccentrically directed TR jet, and the bulging of the AS toward the LA.

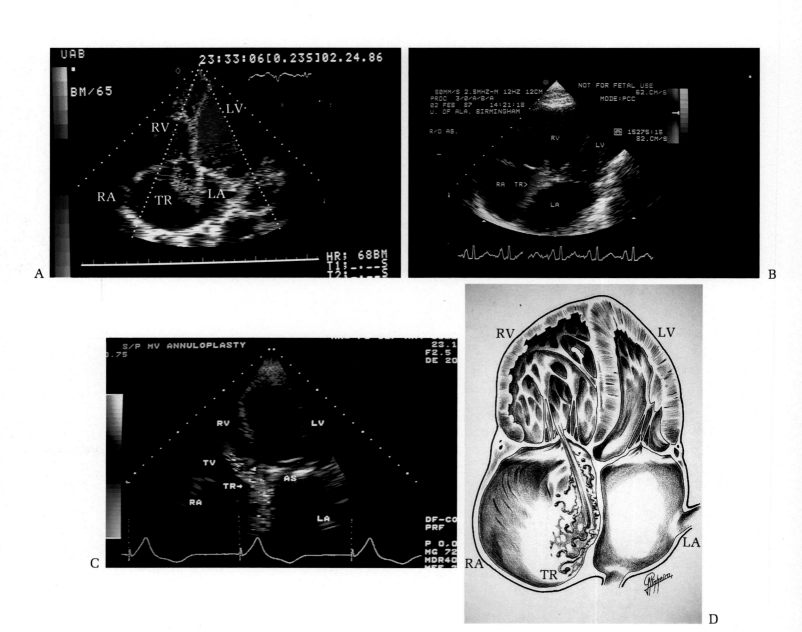

SECTION 5   TRICUSPID VALVE

Figure TV-17   **Severe tricuspid regurgitation.** Apical 4-chamber view in a 33-year-old man who has had AV replacement shows a large band of mosaic signals of TR in the RA. The adjacent red signals represent a swirling of the tricuspid regurgitant flow that occurs when the jet moves back toward the TV after impacting the back wall of the RA. This swirling effect is commonly seen in patients with severe TR.

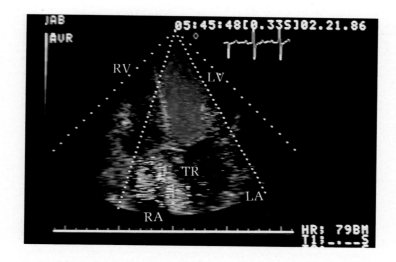

SECTION 5 TRICUSPID VALVE

Figure TV-18 **Tricuspid regurgitation.** (A) Right ventricular inflow view in a 38-year-old woman with complex cyanotic heart disease displays a red jet of TR in the RA during systole. The blue signals within this red jet represent aliasing. The color M-mode examinations (A and B) show this jet to be present throughout systole. In B, the regurgitant jet is mosaic in early systole and red in middle to late systole. The red signals during diastole represent tricuspid inflow moving from the RA to the RV, and a vertical band of blue signals seen at the closure point of the TV represents a ghosting artifact corresponding to the linear high amplitude and high-frequency signals on a pulse Doppler examination.

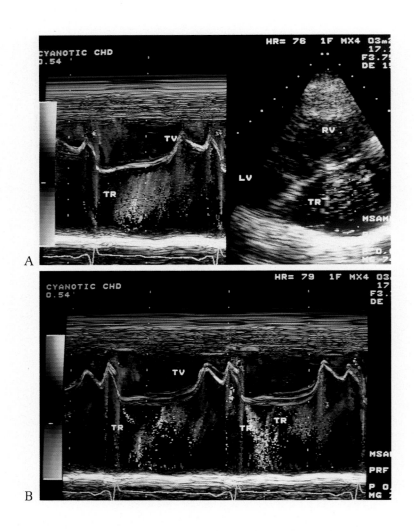

SECTION 5   TRICUSPID VALVE

Figure TV-19   **Tricuspid regurgitation from bacterial endocarditis.** (A) Autopsy specimen shows large vegetations (VEG) which have destroyed one of the TV leaflets. (B and C) Aortic short axis views in a 24-year-old woman with vegetations on her TV show flow signals of severe TR occupying the entire right atrial cavity. When the PRF is increased from 4 kHz in B to 6 kHz in C, the Nyquist limit increases from 0.75 to 1.13 m/sec, thus causing the tricuspid regurgitant signals to change from mosaic to blue in color. Velocities in this range are relatively low for TR, but can occur in severe regurgitation when a small systolic gradient exists between the RA and the RV. Color M-mode examination (D) shows prominent blue signals in the RA behind the TV during systole. The low-velocity signals below the baseline during systole on pulse Doppler examinations (E and F) correspond to the blue signals seen on color M-mode below. Because no aliasing is present on the spectral trace, a confident diagnosis of significant TR by conventional Doppler can be difficult. Diastolic frame (G) shows red signals of prominent right ventricular inflow.

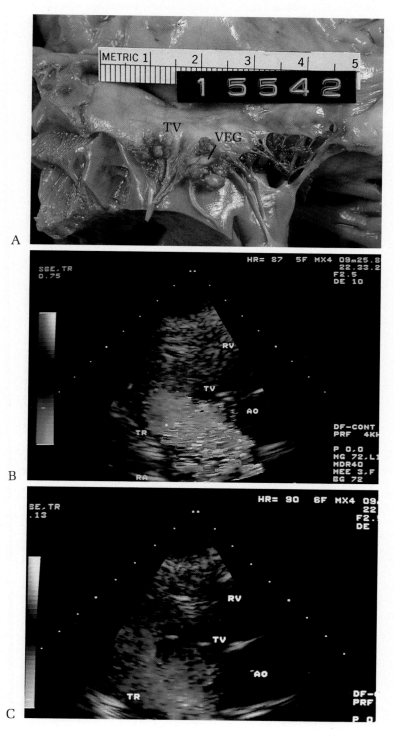

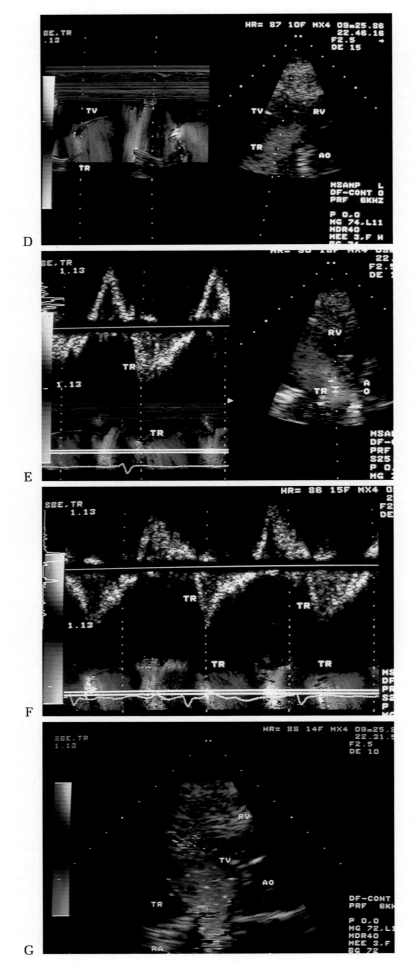

214

Figure TV-20   **Tricuspid regurgitation from bacterial endocarditis.** Apical 4-chamber view in a 54-year-old man with TV endocarditis shows mosaic signals of severe TR in the RA. The vegetation (VEG) on the TV is clearly seen.

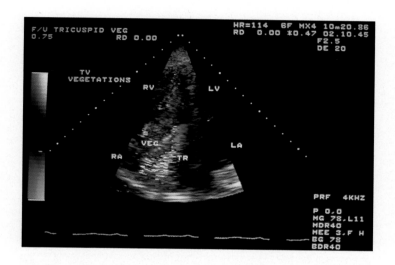

SECTION 5 TRICUSPID VALVE

Figure TV-21 **Severe tricuspid regurgitation.** (A) 2D echocardiogram in a 41-year-old woman with congestive heart failure shows a dilated RA and RV. (B) Color examination shows low-velocity blue signals filling a large portion of the RA with small areas of red and green signals that indicate aliasing and turbulence. In this patient, because most of the tricuspid regurgitant signals have low velocities, a confident diagnosis of severe TR by conventional Doppler can be difficult.

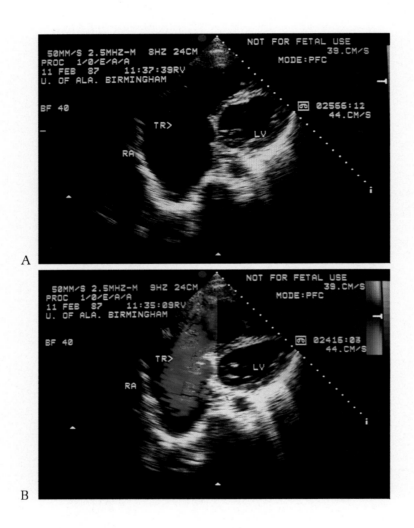

SECTION 5   TRICUSPID VALVE

Figure TV-22   **Tricuspid regurgitation due to RV papillary muscle dysfunction.** Aortic short axis view in an elderly patient with ischemic heart disease shows mosaic signals of moderate TR in the RA. The coaptation point of the TV is displaced inferiorly below the annulus, suggesting papillary muscle dysfunction. Further in the RA, the mosaic signals turn blue because of reduced velocity.

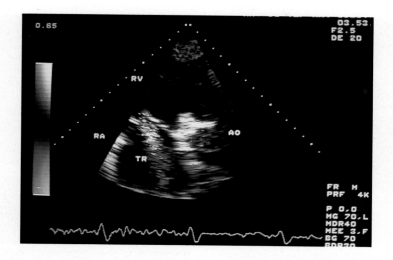

SECTION 5 TRICUSPID VALVE

Figure TV-23 **Traumatic tricuspid regurgitation.** (A) 2D echocardiogram performed from the right parasternal approach in a 23-year-old woman who was involved in a car accident shows the presence of a flail septal tricuspid leaflet (STV) in the dilated RA during systole. (B) Color flow examination shows mosaic signals of severe TR originating from the flail leaflet. These mosaic signals become red farther in the RA because of the anteriorly directed TR jet. (C) Pulse Doppler examination confirms the direction of the jet by displaying the spectral waveform above the baseline. The large area obtained by planimetry (D) of regurgitant mosaic and red signals substantiates the presence of severe regurgitation. Exclusion of the red signals in the planimetry would result in gross underestimation of the severity of the regurgitation. (ATV = Anterior tricuspid leaflet and CS = coronary sinus.)

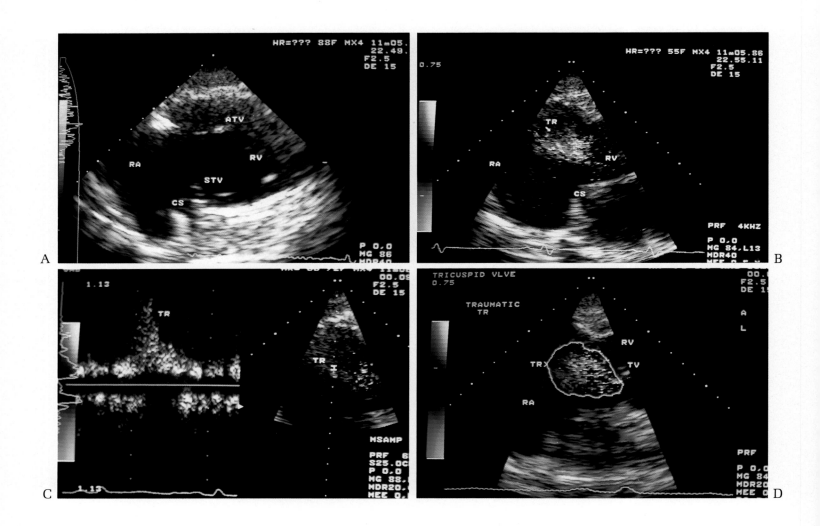

SECTION 5 TRICUSPID VALVE

Figure TV-24 **Tricuspid regurgitation associated with carcinoid syndrome.** Aortic short axis view in a 71-year-old woman with carcinoid syndrome shows mosaic signals of severe TR occupying a large part of the RA.

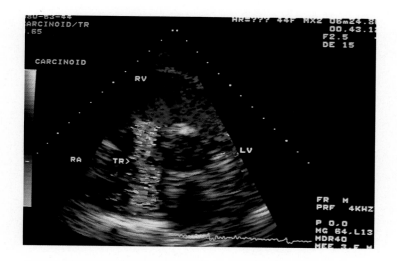

SECTION 5   TRICUSPID VALVE

Figure TV-25   **Tricuspid regurgitation due to acute rheumatic fever.** RV inflow plane in a 15-year-old boy with acute rheumatic fever shows bluish-green signals of moderate TR in the RA.

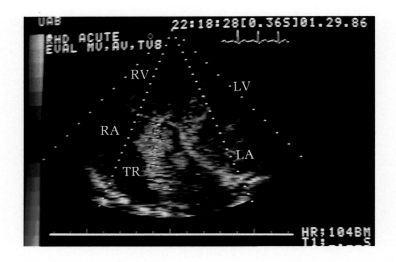

SECTION 5 TRICUSPID VALVE

Figure TV-26 **Severe tricuspid regurgitation.** (A) Systolic frame of the RV inflow view in a 93-year-old woman with congestive heart failure shows blue and red signals of FA (arrow) on the ventricular side of the TV and mosaic signals of severe TR occupying a large portion of a dilated RA. Diastolic frame (B) shows aliased flow in the RV because of increased tricuspid inflow. The pulse Doppler sample volume (C) placed in the systolic mosaic signals in the RA gives a spectral waveform showing aliasing. Apical 4-chamber views (D–G) using different color Doppler machines in the same patient also show the same signals as the systolic RV inflow view in (A). In addition, the mosaic signals in the RA are observed to strike the back wall and turn back as red signals toward the TV (E–G). This swirling pattern is commonly seen with severe TR. Color M-mode examinations (H and I) show mosaic signals of TR during systole and red signals of tricuspid inflow (TF) during diastole. The blue color within the red signals results from aliasing. The blue signals in the RA during middle to late diastole result from swirling. The apical views (J and K) show a markedly dilated CS resulting from this regurgitation. The regurgitant signals move toward the CS as shown by the color flow (K). Subcostal examination (L) confirms the swirling pattern in the RA. 2D examination performed from the right parasternal view (M) shows a dilated IVC and a prominent Eustachian valve (EV). Additional right parasternal color flow examinations (N–P) show mosaic signals of severe TR in the RA, turning red and blue as they move anteriorly and posteriorly, respectively. Other color flow examinations from this approach (Q–T) with three different color Doppler machines show the swirling pattern in the RA and red systolic retrograde signals in the IVC. The subcostal systolic frame (U) also shows these retrograde signals in the hepatic veins. Color M-mode (V) of the SVC (right supraclavicular approach) shows blue signals during diastole due to antegrade flow from the SVC to the RA. The red signals in systole represent retrograde flow in the SVC. This flow is also seen on the pulse Doppler examination (W). The presence of systolic retrograde flow into the SVC is rare and indicates very severe TR. X represents aortic short axis view in another patient (66-year-old man with congestive cardiomyopathy and pulmonary hypertension) showing a swirling effect in the RA from severe TR.

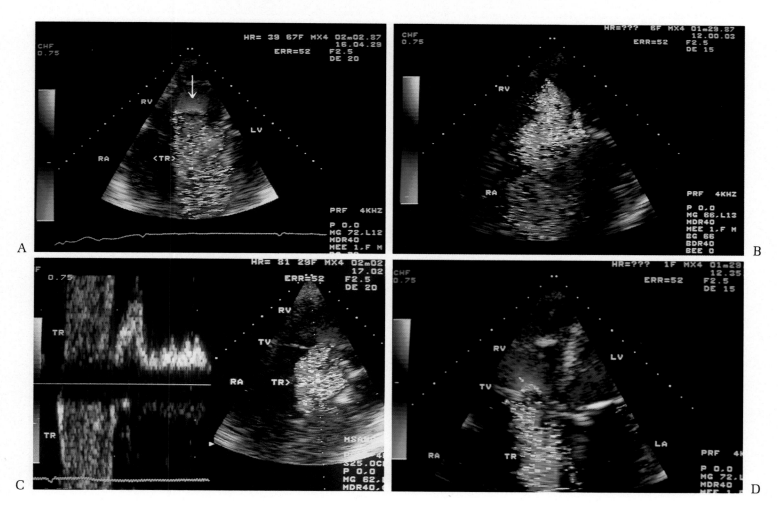

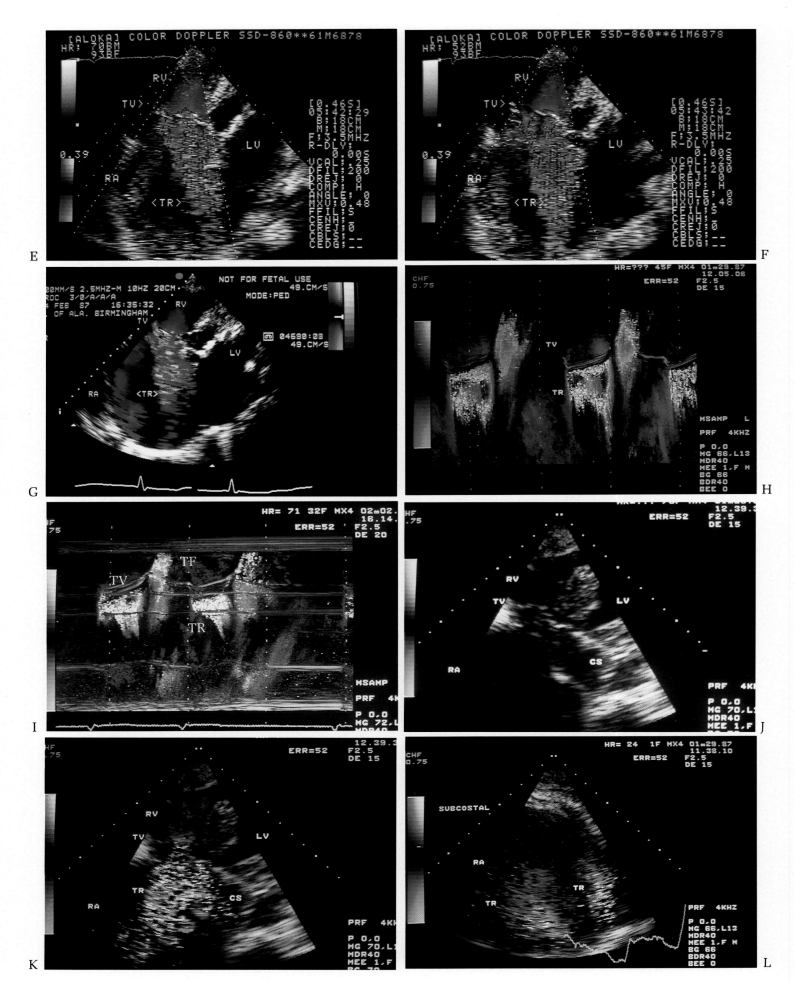

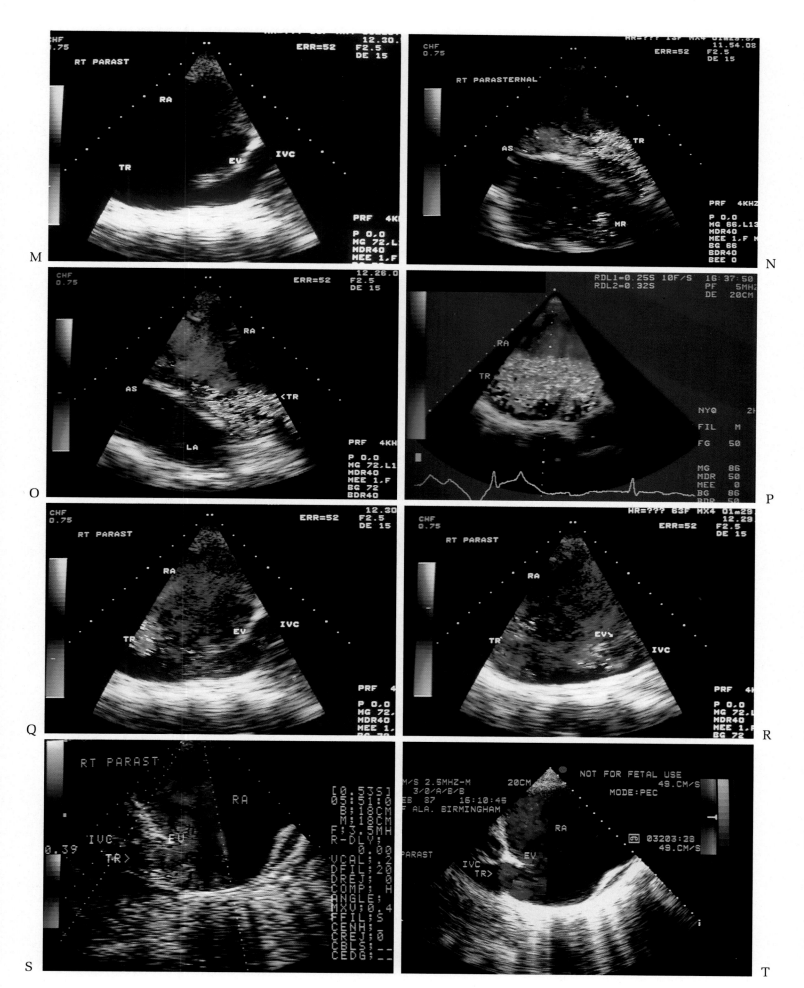

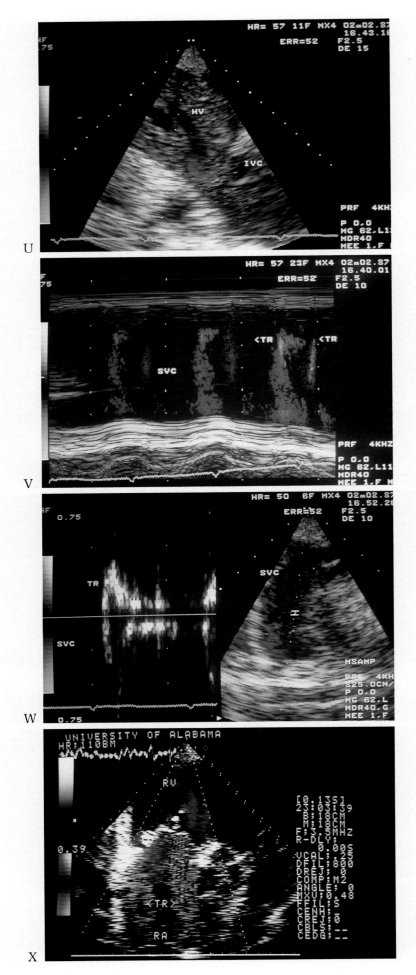

SECTION 5   TRICUSPID VALVE

Figure TV-27   **Tricuspid regurgitation associated with mitral regurgitation.** (A) Aortic short axis view in a 59-year-old woman with MV and TV prolapse shows a small jet of TR originating from the TV and a much larger jet of MR. Apical 4-chamber views (B and C) in another patient, using different color maps, show a relatively large area of bluish-green signals of TR in the RA and a smaller area of bluish-green signals of MR in the LA. The color map used in B has additional green color added to indicate the presence of turbulence.

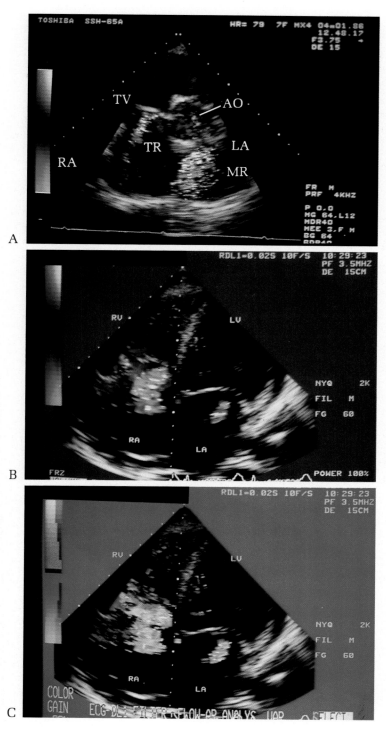

SECTION 5   TRICUSPID VALVE

Figure TV-28   **Residual tricuspid regurgitation following tricuspid annuloplasty.** (A) Apical view in a 24-year-old woman who has undergone MV replacement and tricuspid annuloplasty shows small areas of mosaic signals in the RA resulting from mild TR. The mosaic signals on the ventricular aspect of the TV result from flow acceleration (FA, arrow). Diastolic frame (B) shows the red tricuspid inflow in the RV.

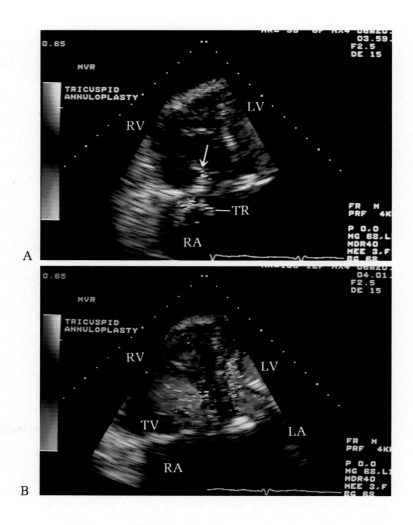

SECTION 5   TRICUSPID VALVE

Figure TV-29   **Tricuspid stenosis.** (A) Apical 4-chamber view at the level of the TV in a 50-year-old woman who had AV and MV replacement in 1973 shows mosaic signals of TS in the RV during diastole originating from the TV. These signals are very narrow at the origin, implying severe stenosis, and widen considerably farther in the RV because of a large diastolic pressure gradient between the RA and the RV. Red signals of flow acceleration are seen on the atrial aspect of the TV. In B, the PRF is increased from 4 to 6 kHz, and thus the Nyquist limit is changed from 0.54 to 0.81 m/sec. This PRF increase causes the mosaic signals to turn predominantly red with blue specks; thus some aliasing is still observed despite a PRF increase. C is a schematic. AP = aortic prosthesis.

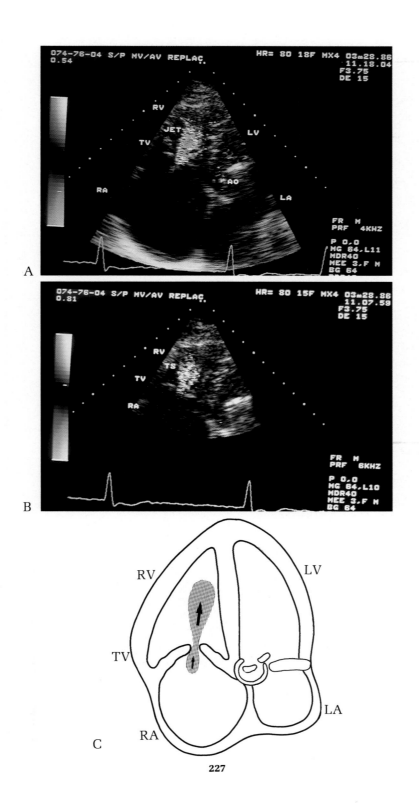

SECTION 5   TRICUSPID VALVE

Figure TV-30   **Tricuspid valve stenosis.** (A) RV inflow view in a 30-year-old woman with rheumatic heart disease shows a narrow aliased jet in the RV originating from the TV during diastole, implying severe TS. The pulse Doppler sample volume placed in the red signals in a hepatic vein (HV,B) shows a large A wave on the spectral waveform (arrow), implying a retrograde flow into the HV during atrial systole from severe TS. This is further substantiated by the concurrent red signals on the color M-mode (arrow). The prominent corresponding P wave on the electrocardiogram indicates RA enlargement. L = liver.

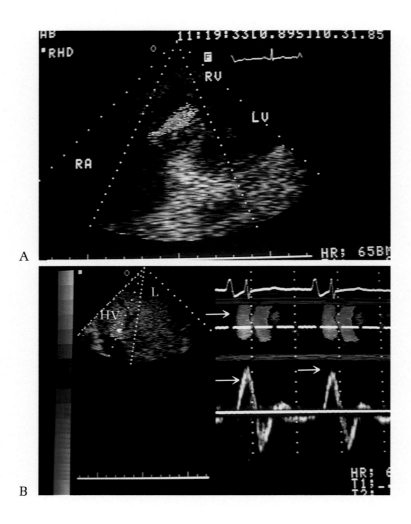

Section 6

PULMONARY VALVE

PULMONARY REGURGITATION

Color Doppler is superior to pulsed Doppler in the examination of pulmonary valve (PV) regurgitation. The width and depth of the regurgitant signals can be delineated rapidly and accurately with color Doppler. With pulsed Doppler, however, much time is required to assess these parameters, making these measurements tedious for the examiner and inconvenient for the patient.

The presence of PV regurgitation is indicated by color Doppler when retrograde signals are displayed originating from the PV and moving into the RVOT during diastole. These retrograde signals are usually mosaic in color because of turbulent flow. Non-turbulent red signals may, however, occasionally result from lower velocity flows when a small pressure gradient exists across the PV during diastole or when the Doppler ultrasonic beam is not oriented parallel to the flow. These signals are best visualized using the aortic and mitral-pulmonic short axis and left ventricular-pulmonic imaging planes. In some patients, PV regurgitation may also be well delineated using the subcostal right ventricular inflow-apical outflow imaging plane.

The severity of PV regurgitation is assessed by considering both the length and width of the regurgitant jet. If the proximal width of the pulmonary regurgitant jet at its origin from the PV is less than 50% of the RVOT width at the same location, the severity of the regurgitation is classified as mild or moderate. If this jet width is wide and greater than 50% of the RVOT width, the severity of the pulmonary valve regurgitation is classified as moderately severe to severe. In patients with severe PV regurgitation, the proximal RVOT width may be completely filled with diastolic mosaic signals and prominent antegrade signals may be seen moving into the pulmonary artery during systole because of the combined flow resulting from the pulmonic regurgitant flow and the normal flows occurring in the right heart. Severe PV regurgitation is also indicated when the re-

gurgitant jet extends the entire distance to the level of the TV. When the pulmonic regurgitant jet in an adult extends more than and less than four cm into the RVOT, moderate and mild pulmonary valve regurgitations are present, respectively. To ensure that the maximum width and length of the regurgitant jet are measured, a complete 3-dimensional view of the jet must be obtained by angling and rotating the transducer in multiple directions. In addition, the mosaic regurgitant jet may lose its mosaic color farther downstream in the RVOT because the velocity of the jet decreases below the Nyquist limit and the flow becomes laminar. This must be considered when noting the length of the regurgitant jet.

Occasionally, in patients with infundibular stenosis and severe pulmonary regurgitation, pulmonic regurgitant jet may appear narrow because of the narrowing of the RVOT. Observation of this jet extending downstream into the RV up to the level of the TV, however, allows a definite conclusion to be made that this PV regurgitation is severe. In these cases, an examination of the TV inflow region is very useful because this allows the extension of the pulmonary regurgitant jet to be observed.

In many patients with PV regurgitation, flow acceleration may be seen on the pulmonary artery side of the PV. These signals may pinpoint the exact location of an anatomical defect in the PV leaflets and, by noting their width near the PV, may provide an estimate of the size of this anatomical defect.

A narrow band of diastolic flow signals, occurring usually at the coaptation point of the PV leaflets and extending only a short distance into the RVOT, consistent with minimal or mild PR, may occur in a significant number of apparently healthy individuals, and thus its presence may not indicate any pathologic abnormality of the pulmonary valve or annulus. The presence of a wide jet originating from the PV and extending deep into the RVOT, however, indicates significant PV regurgitation and is always abnormal. Multiple jets of PR originating from either one leaflet or two different leaflets of the PV may also be seen in some patients. A pulmonic regurgitant jet originating from the PV as a single jet and bifurcating into two jets farther downstream in the RVOT or two pulmonic regurgitant jets occurring separately during early diastole and mid diastole may also sometimes be observed.

The pulmonic regurgitant jet signals may be oriented centrally, medially, or laterally. Occasionally, instead of being centrally located, the jet may be directed posteriorly in the RV until it hits the VS and turns anteriorly, taking on a "J"-shaped appearance. In some patients, the pulmonic regurgitant jet may be directed anteriorly until it strikes the anterior right ventricular wall and turns posteriorly. The flow pattern for this jet is thus displayed as an inverted "U" shape. The pulmonic regurgitant jet may also swirl in the RV after impacting the wall of the RVOT. Some of this flow may then turn back toward the PV during late diastole.

As mentioned previously, in patients with severe PR, the regurgitant jet may extend all the way down to the TV level and its impingement on the TV may cause it to flutter in diastole. In some patients, severe PR may cause late diastolic TV regurgitation. This can be confirmed by color M-mode examination, which clearly shows reversed flow signals in late diastole in the RA orginating from the TV and reversed diastolic flow signals in the RV impinging on the TV. This diastolic TR results from transient reversal of the pressure gradient across a partially closed TV in late diastole due to marked increase in right ventricular diastolic pressure from severe PR. It is important to emphasize that late diastolic TR may also be noted in patients with a prolonged PR interval who have no evidence of PR. Thus, in patients with severe PR, it is important to exclude first-degree atrio-ventricular block or complete heart block before attributing the late diastolic TR to marked increase in right ventricular diastolic pressure.

Color Doppler can diagnose the presence of PR even in patients with tricuspid prostheses. In these patients, the inflow originating from the prosthesis and the PV regurgitation are displayed by mosaic signals. The origin of these two different sets of signals can be easily delineated, allowing their classification, but farther downstream in the RV, these signals from PR and tricuspid inflow through the prosthesis tend to merge, making their delineation difficult. In these patients, only the width of the PR signals at their origin from the pulmonic valve can be used to estimate the severity of regurgitation. Color-guided continuous wave Doppler can also be used in the evaluation of patients with pulmonic regurgitation. A continuous wave Doppler cursor passed through the pulmonic regurgitant jet signals obtains a reliable diastolic pressure gradient across the PV. In the absence of right heart failure, a high peak pressure gradient between the PA and RV indicates an increased diastolic gradient which occurs with significant pulmo-

nary hypertension, while a low-pressure gradient across the pulmonary valve indicates normal PA pressure. This low-pressure gradient is often noted in an apparently healthy individual with minimal PV regurgitation. A rapid deceleration in the spectral trace of the pulmonary diastolic waveform indicates a rapid equalization of the PA and right ventricular diastolic pressures. This suggests that the right ventricular end-diastolic pressure may be elevated. Therefore, evaluation of the PV regurgitation may be useful in assessing the presence of pulmonary hypertension and providing an estimate of the right ventricular end-diastolic pressure.

A color M-mode examination is useful to assess the duration of the pulmonic regurgitant flow. Even in patients with mild PR, abnormal retrograde signals may be seen throughout diastole, indicating that the leakage is pandiastolic. Prominent color signals of very brief duration observed during PV closure should not be mistaken for PR because these signals simply represent a ghosting artifact resulting from the valve moving rapidly. These signals are similar to the linear high-frequency signals observed during conventional Doppler examination.

PULMONARY ARTERY DILATATION

Interesting flow patterns are seen in patients with PA dilatation from any cause. During early systole, normal antegrade flow is seen moving into the PA, but during mid to late systole, this flow is seen to swirl in the PA after it hits the wall of the artery and moves back toward the PV. This swirling effect may explain the partial pre-closure and systolic fluttering of the PV observed in these patients. Similar flow patterns are also observed in patients with PA aneurysms. PR is also often associated with PA dilatation.

REFERENCES

Pulmonary Regurgitation

1. Miyatake, K., Okamoto, M., Kinoshita, N., Matsuhisa, M., Nagata Beppu, S., Park, Y.D., Sakakibara, H., and Nimura, Y.: Pulmonary regurgitation studied with the ultrasonic pulsed Doppler technique. Circulation 65:969, 1982.
2. Patel, A., Rowe, G., Dhanasi, S., Kosolcharoen, P., Lyle, L.E.W., and Thompson, J.: Pulsed Doppler echocardiography in diagnosis of pulmonary regurgitation: Its value and limitations. Am. J. Cardiol. 49:1801, 1982.
3. Masuyama, T., Kodama, K., Kitabatake, A., Soto, H., Nanto, S., and Inoue, M.: Continuous-wave Doppler echocardiographic detection of pulmonary regurgitation and its application to noninvasive estimation of pulmonary artery pressure. Circulation 74:484, 1986.

Pulmonary Artery Dilation

1. Helmcke, F., Pinamonti, B., Colvin, E.C., Kan, M.N., Goyal, R., Moss, S., and Nanda, N.C.: Color Doppler detection of abnormal pulmonary flow patterns and their significance (Abstract). Clin. Res. 35:286A, 1987.

SECTION 6   PULMONARY VALVE

This section mainly covers color Doppler assessment of pulmonary regurgitation and illustrates some of the pitfalls to be avoided when assessing its severity.

Figure PV-1   **Pulmonary valve regurgitation.** Schematic illustrates some of the possible etiologies of PR. In this short axis view, the thickened PV leaflets with incomplete coaptation during diastole are clearly shown. This incomplete coaptation results from dilatation of the MPA and the RVOT. In addition, a hole (arrow) as shown in the pulmonary leaflet represents a fenestrated PV.

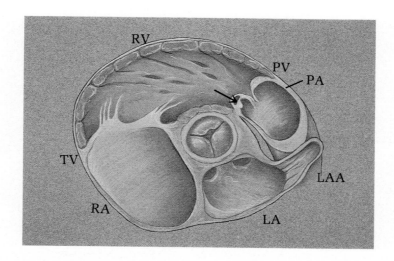

SECTION 6   PULMONARY VALVE

Figure PV-2   Mild pulmonary valve regurgitation. (A–D) Short axis views in these patients display small, narrow bands of red signals in the RVOT originating from the PV in diastole. The presence of these red signals indicates PR, and their narrow width and small length imply mild regurgitation. Such regurgitation signals can occur in a significant proportion of apparently healthy subjects and thus may not indicate abnormal hemodynamics. The bluish-green signals in the LVOT during diastole in D (right) result from associated mild AR. Color M-mode examination as shown in D (left) shows red signals throughout diastole, indicating that even mild PR is pandiastolic. The blue systolic signals in the RVOT, as shown in D, represent normal flow in the PA.

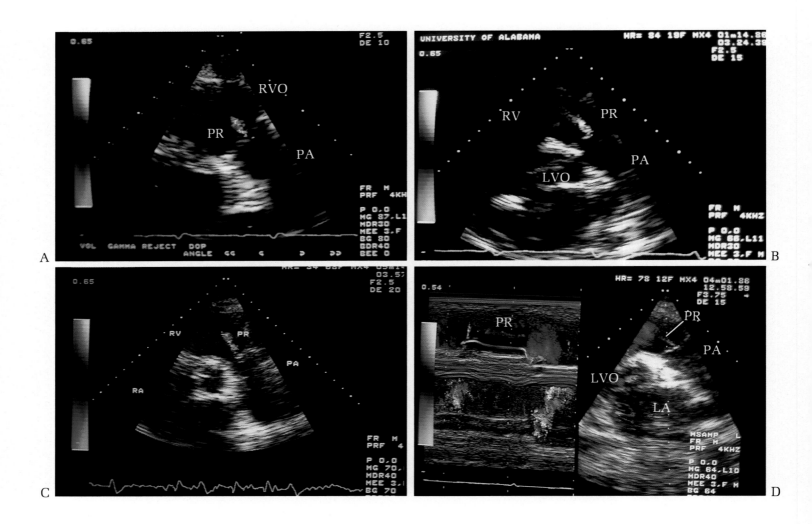

SECTION 6 PULMONARY VALVE

Figure PV-3   **Mild pulmonary valve regurgitation.** (A) Aortic short axis view in a 27-year-old man shows a small narrow band of mosaic signals originating, during diastole, from the PV, indicating mild PR. A pulse Doppler sample volume (SV) is placed in these signals (B) and the color M-mode and the spectral waveform obtained on the right show pandiastolic PR. The blue signals during systole in B represent normal flow through the PV, while the red signals within them represent aliasing. B = Doppler baseline.

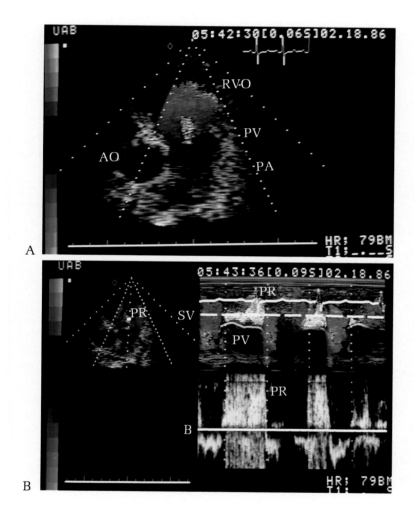

SECTION 6   PULMONARY VALVE

Figure PV-4   **Mild pulmonary valve regurgitation.** Subcostal short axis view in an 82-year-old man shows a small narrow band of yellow signals in the RVOT during diastole, indicating mild PV regurgitation.

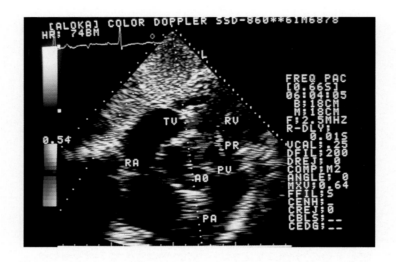

SECTION 6 PULMONARY VALVE

Figure PV-5 **Moderate pulmonary valve regurgitation.** (A and B) Aortic short axis views in these patients show a relatively wide band of mosaic signals originating from the PV, indicating moderate PR. These signals turn red as the velocity of the jet decreases below the Nyquist limit in the RV. Color M-mode examinations (B and C) show the mosaic signals along the entire diastolic period of the PV echoes. The blue signals during systole represent normal flow into the PA, and the red and yellow signals within them result from aliasing.

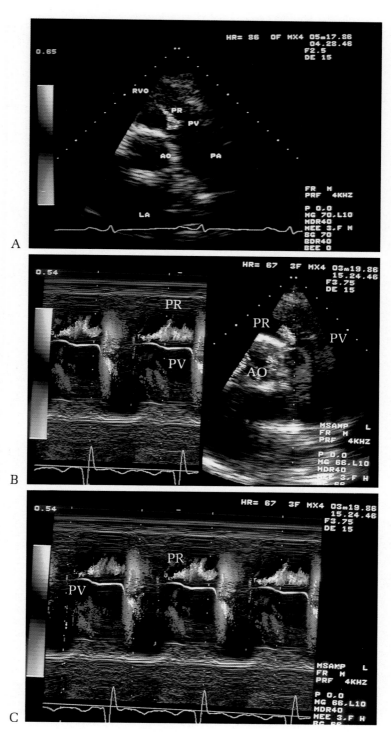

Figure PV-6   **Moderate pulmonary valve regurgitation.** Both the short axis view (A) and the modified long axis view (B) obtained from two different patients show long, narrow bands of red signals originating from the PV. These signals extend approximately 4 cm into the RVOT, indicating the presence of moderate PV regurgitation. Therefore, in assessing the severity of PR, both the length and the width of the regurgitant signals must be considered.

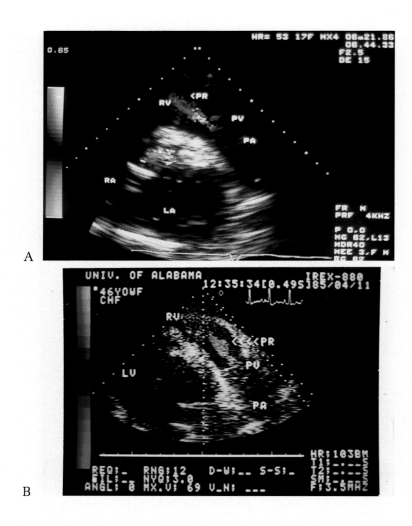

SECTION 6 PULMONARY VALVE

Figure PV-7 **Color M-Mode examination in pulmonic regurgitation.** Color M-mode examination in this patient shows reddish-brown signals during diastole in front of the PV echoes, indicating PR. The regurgitant jet appears to be divided into multiple bands because of fluctuations in the alignment of the Doppler beam with the regurgitation flow. These fluctuations result from cardiac and respiratory motion. The blue signals during diastole result from the swirling of these regurgitant signals. The blue signals in systole represent normal systolic flow into the PA, and the red signals within them represent aliasing. The red signals observed during PV closure represent a ghosting artifact resulting from rapid valve motion similar to the linear high frequency signal observed during conventional Doppler examination.

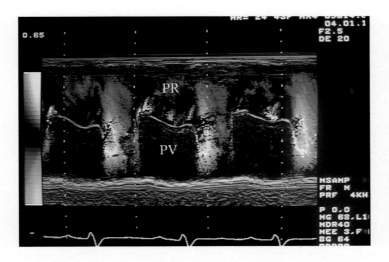

SECTION 6   PULMONARY VALVE

Figure PV-8   **Severe pulmonary valve regurgitation.** 46-year-old man had replacement of his AV and MV in 1974 and his TV in 1985. (A, B, and C) Three short axis views in this patient demonstrate that minimal successive angulations of the transducer cause both the width and length of the mosaic pulmonic regurgitant signals to increase considerably, indicating severe PR. Therefore, in assessing the severity of PR, the maximum width and length obtained for the regurgitant signals must be considered. The blue signals in the RVOT represent swirling pulmonic regurgitant flow. Blue signals are also seen when the mosaic signals of PR change direction and move toward the right ventricular inflow. These blue signals then merge with the red tricuspid prosthetic (TP) inflow signals as shown in C. The modified long axis view (D) shows, in addition, the third dimension of the mosaic pulmonic regurgitant jet. Red signals in the LV, as shown in D, represent the mitral prosthetic (MP) inflow, while mosaic signals in the LVOT, as shown in A and B, represent AR from the aortic prosthesis (AP).

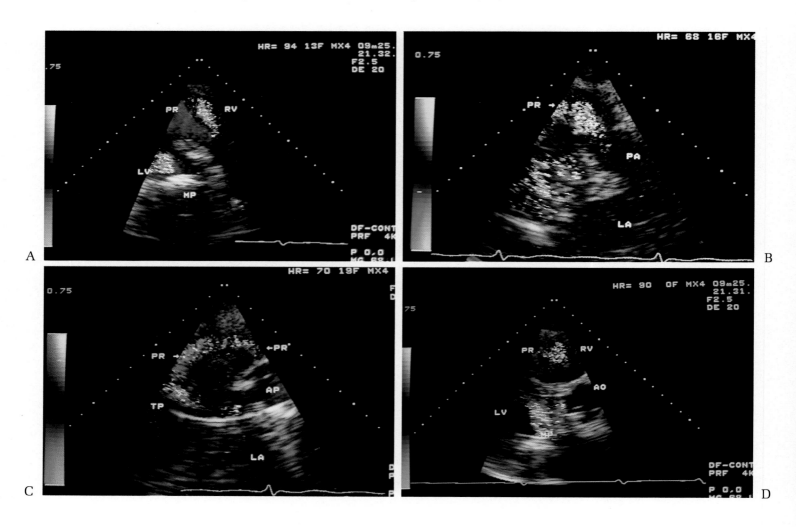

SECTION 6 PULMONARY VALVE

Figure PV-9   **Severe pulmonary valve regurgitation.** (A, B, and C) Left ventricular short axis views in a 66-year-old man with pulmonary hypertension due to cardiomyopathy demonstrate that minimal successive angulations of the transducer cause the size of the mosaic pulmonic regurgitant signals to increase significantly, indicating severe PR. These mosaic pulmonic regurgitant signals turn red farther in the RV because of the velocity decrease shown in B. The red signals on the PA side of the PV represent flow acceleration (arrow). The blue signals in the RVOT in C result from the pulmonary regurgitant flow swirling in the RVO.

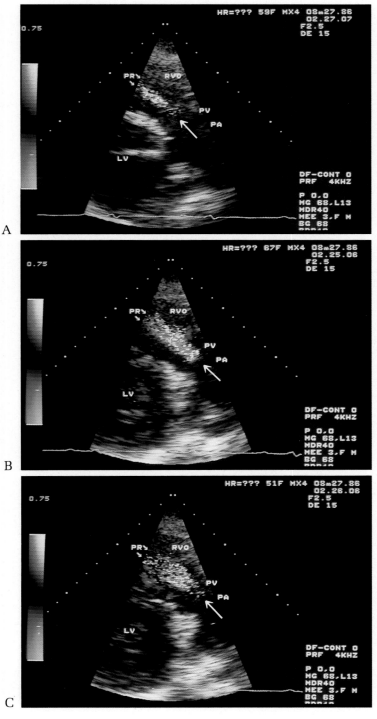

SECTION 6 PULMONARY VALVE

Figure PV-10 **Severe pulmonary valve regurgitation.** (A and B) Aortic short axis views in two women with congestive heart failure show wide bands of mosaic signals in the RVOT during diastole, implying severe PR. C is an aortic short axis view in another woman with severe PR in whom mosaic-colored signals almost completely fill the entire extent of the RVO during diastole.

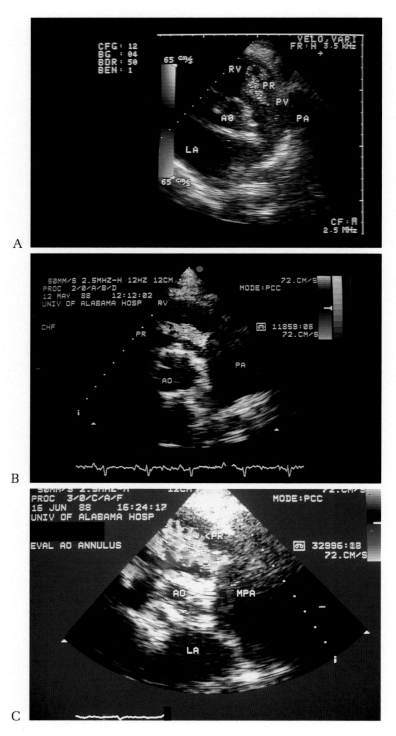

SECTION 6   PULMONARY VALVE

Figure PV-11   **Severe pulmonary valve regurgitation.** Late diastolic frame of an aortic short axis view in a 51-year-old man with right ventricular failure displays prominent blue signals of severe PR extending from the RVOT to the level of the TV. The red signals in the dilated RA represent tricuspid inflow.

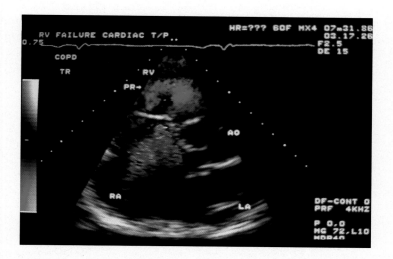

Figure PV-12 **Severe pulmonary valve regurgitation.** (A) 2D echocardiogram in a 20-year-old man who underwent valvotomy in childhood for PV stenosis shows a thick PV and a dilated RVOT. (B and C) Color Doppler examinations show diastolic mosaic signals filling the entire RVOT and extending to the TV, and red signals in the PA (B) represent diastolic backflow. Both of these signals result from severe PR. The observed mosaic signals turn predominantly blue as the pulmonary regurgitant jet moves away from the transducer toward the RV inflow. (D, E, and F) Color M-mode examinations show mosaic signals of PR impinging on the TV, causing it to flutter in diastole. The systolic red signals in these examinations represent RV flow moving toward the PA, while the diastolic red signals represent tricuspid inflow. The right ventricular inflow view (G) reveals blue signals in the RA (REG), originating from the TV during diastole. Color M-mode examination (H) at this level clearly shows these blue signals just before the TV closing, indicating late diastolic TR (REG). Blue signals of TR are also present during systole. The pulse Doppler sample volume placed in the diastolic blue signals (I) also displays a spectral waveform below the baseline during late diastole. Diastolic TR resulting from the pulmonic regurgitant flow moving through the partially open TV into the RA is clearly illustrated in the schematic (J). Diastolic TR results from transient reversal of the pressure gradient across a partially closed TV in late diastole due to marked increase in RV diastolic pressure from severe PR.

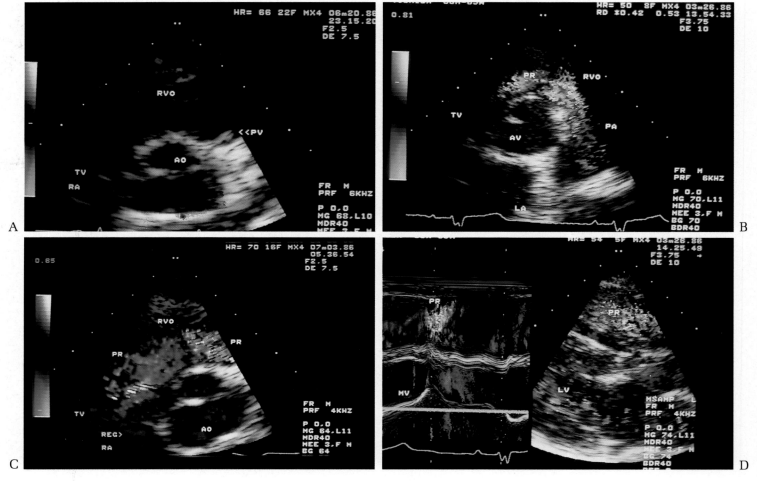

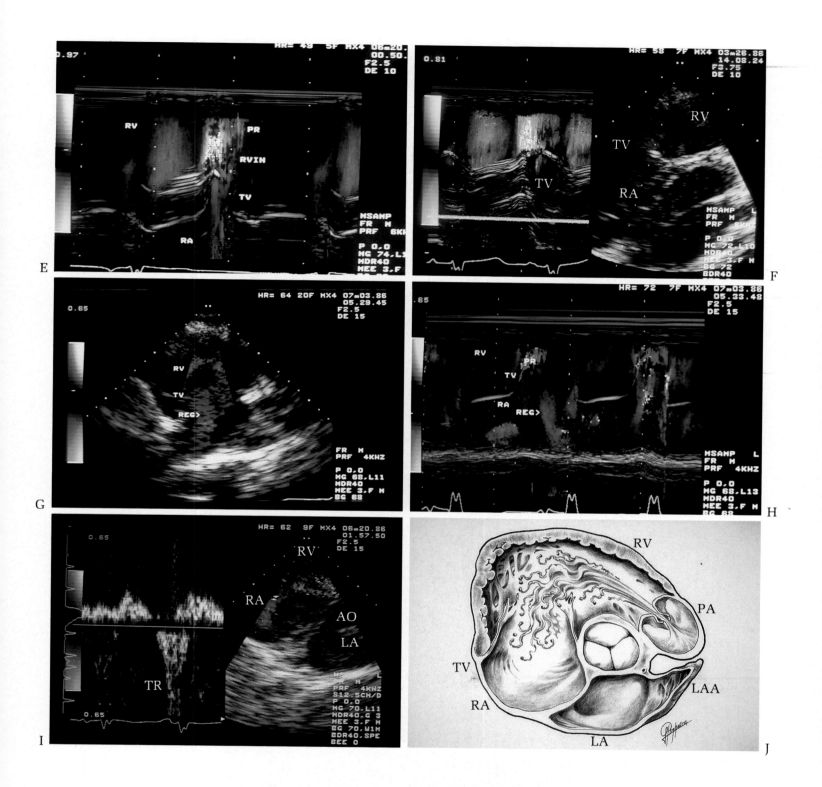

SECTION 6   PULMONARY VALVE

Figure PV-13   **"Inverted U" shaped jet of pulmonic regurgitation.** (A) Short axis view in a 27-year-old woman who had a PV replacement in 1974 shows a narrow jet of red signals originating from the prosthetic pulmonary valve (PVR) and directed anteriorly toward the right ventricular wall. After striking the RV wall, the pulmonary regurgitant jet moves posteriorly until it strikes the interventricular septum, thus creating an "inverted U." The schematic (B) clearly illustrates the formation of this "inverted U"-shaped jet of mild PR. The continuous wave Doppler cursor (C) placed in the posteriorly directed portion of the jet as shown by the arrows records a spectral waveform of PR below the baseline.

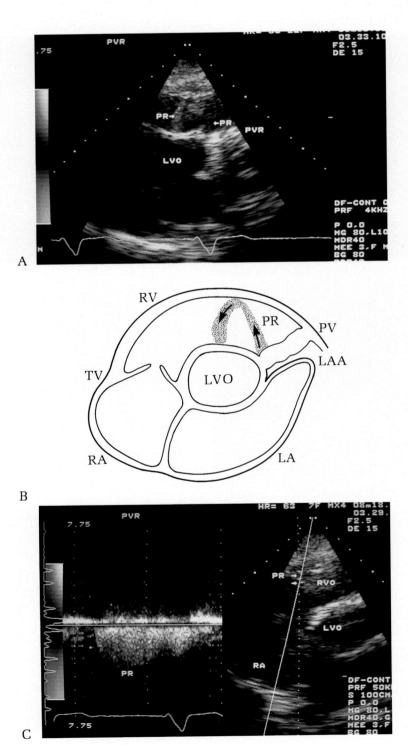

SECTION 6 PULMONARY VALVE

Figure PV-14   **Severe pulmonary valve regurgitation.** Aortic short axis view in a 14-year-old boy who had a valvotomy for PS and a TV replacement in early childhood shows red signals of the pulmonic regurgitant jet extending from the high RVOT to the level of the tricuspid prosthesis (TP). This jet is easily distinguished from the mosaic tricuspid inflow jet.

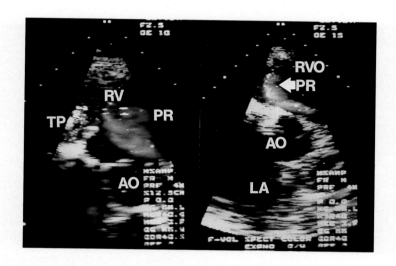

SECTION 6 PULMONARY VALVE

Figure PV-15 **Multiple pulmonic regurgitant jets.** (A) Short axis view in a 21-year-old man with a dilated cardiomyopathy and first-degree A-V block shows a red jet of PR originating from the lateral aspect of the PV. When the transducer is slightly angulated (B), central, medial, and lateral jets are visualized, as schematically illustrated in C. Color M-mode examinations (D and E) of the pulmonary regurgitant jet show at least two distinct bands of red signals anterior to the PV echoes. One band originates just before atrial systole (the patient has first-degree heart block) and the other originates during late diastole. The blue color in the red signals represents aliasing, while the systolic blue color represents systolic flow into the PA.

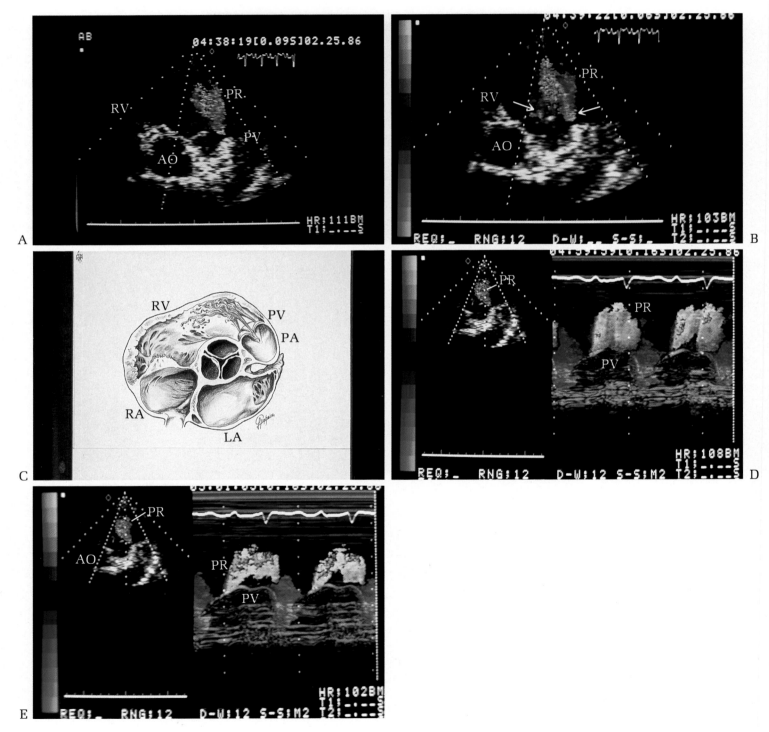

Figure PV-16   **Multiple pulmonic regurgitant jets.** (A and B) Aortic short axis views in two men clearly show multiple mosaic jets of PR. In A, the two distinct jets merge together in the RVOT, while in B, three distinct jets as indicated by arrowheads are visualized.

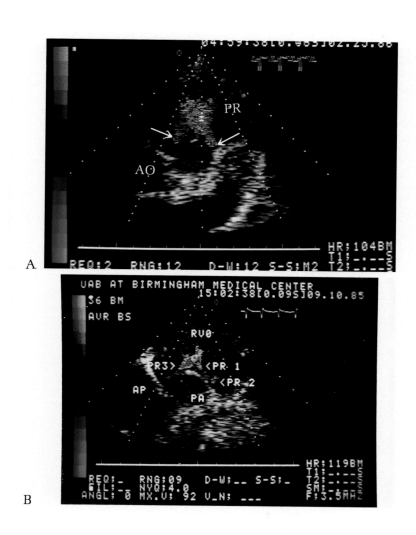

SECTION 6 PULMONARY VALVE

Figure PV-17 **Pulmonary valve regurgitation.** Aortic short axis view in a 51-year-old man with right ventricular failure displays mosaic signals of PR starting as a single jet from the PV and appearing to bifurcate into two jets farther in the RVOT. These two jets then merge in the distal RVOT.

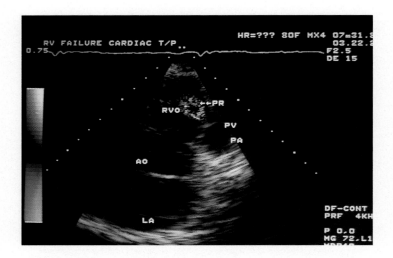

SECTION 6 PULMONARY VALVE

Figure PV-18   **Continuous wave Doppler examination of pulmonary valve regurgitation.** In a continuous wave Doppler examination of a 63-year-old man with pulmonary hypertension, the cursor is placed in the pulmonic regurgitant signals to obtain a peak velocity of 2.14 m/sec on the spectral display. This translates into a peak pressure gradient of 18 mm Hg between the PA and the RV during diastole, thus indicating significant pulmonary hypertension.

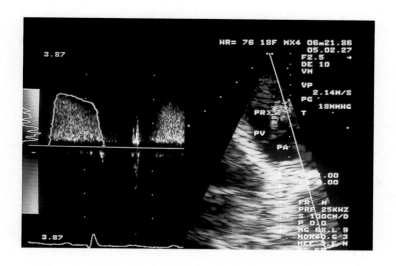

Figure PV-19 **Continuous wave Doppler examination of pulmonary valve regurgitation.** In a continuous wave Doppler examination of a 66-year-old man with pulmonary hypertension due to cardiomyopathy, the cursor is placed in the mosaic PR signals to obtain a relatively high peak velocity in early diastole of 2.0 m/sec on the spectral trace. Later in diastole, the peak velocity drops sharply until atrial systole, when the velocity again increases, thus forming an M-shaped pattern on the spectral trace.

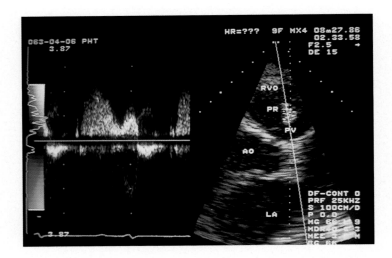

Figure PV-20   **Continuous wave Doppler examination of pulmonary valve regurgitation.** In a continuous wave Doppler examination of a 31-year-old man who has undergone a repair of an ASD and a valvotomy of the PV, the cursor is placed through the pulmonic regurgitant jet. The spectral trace obtained shows a relatively high peak velocity of 1.8 m/sec in early diastole, but this velocity drops sharply in mid to late diastole, indicating a relatively rapid equalization of the PA and the right ventricular diastolic pressures. This suggests that the RV end-diastolic pressure is elevated; this finding was confirmed by cardiac catheterization.

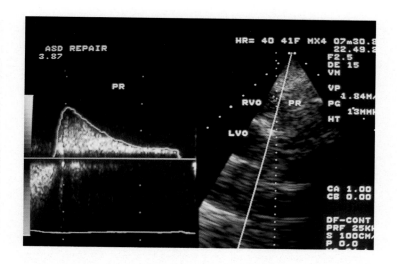

SECTION 6   PULMONARY VALVE

Figure PV-21   **Pulmonary valve regurgitation following pulmonary valvotomy.** (A) Modified long axis view in a 45-year-old woman who had total correction of tetralogy of Fallot shows two small jets of red signals in the narrow RVOT originating from the thickened PV. This indicates significant PR following pulmonary valvotomy. A continuous wave cursor (B) is placed parallel to the systolic flow signals in the PA, and a peak pressure gradient of 54 mm Hg is obtained across the RVOT, implying significant residual obstruction. The diastolic signals above the baseline in the spectral tracing result from PR.

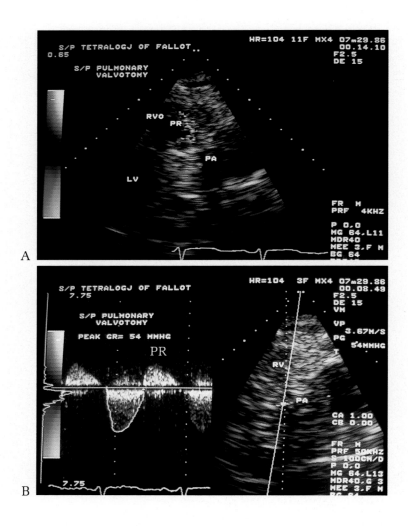

SECTION 6 PULMONARY VALVE

Figure PV-22 **Pulmonary valve regurgitation following pulmonary valve replacement.** Aortic short axis view in a 33-year-old woman who has had a repair of tetralogy of Fallot and a PV replacement, shows red signals in the RVOT due to mild PR. The continuous wave Doppler cursor passed through the PV prosthesis records a peak velocity in systole of only 2.0 m/sec, implying the absence of a significant obstruction across the RVO and the pulmonary prosthesis. PP = prosthetic pulmonic valve, C = prosthetic valve closing signal, F = systolic flow signals.

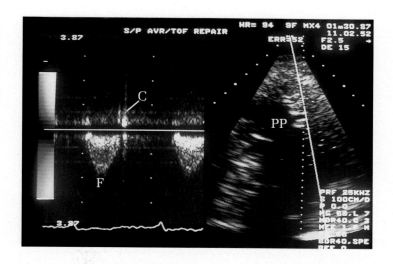

SECTION 6 PULMONARY VALVE

Figure PV-23 **Dilated pulmonary artery.** (A) Aortic short axis view in a patient with idiopathic dilatation of the PA shows, during systole, blue signals moving laterally into the PA. These signals contain small red flecks that represent aliasing. The predominantly blue signals then turn red as they swirl medially back toward the PV. This swirling effect is characteristic of a dilated PA from any cause. (B and C) Color M-mode examination shows the swirling by displaying blue signals moving into the PA in early systole and red signals moving from the PA toward the PV in mid to late systole. This swirling effect results in preclosure of the PV and systolic fluttering. The red signals seen in front of the PV in early diastole result from mild PR. The red signals contained within blue in systole in C are due to aliasing.

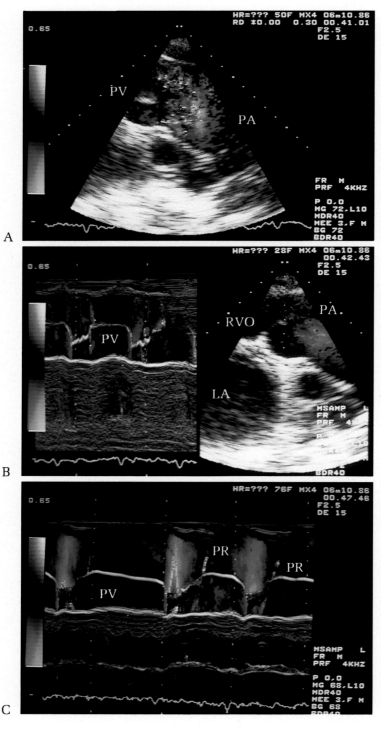

SECTION 6   PULMONARY VALVE

Figure PV-24   **Dilated pulmonary artery.** On the right, the modified short axis view (systole) in a patient who has had closure of a PDA shows a swirling effect by displaying blue signals that move laterally into the PA and then turn red as they flow medially back toward the PV. The color M-mode examination on the left shows blue signals moving into the PA in early systole, while in late systole red signals (BF) indicate a flow reversal, thus further demonstrating a swirling effect.

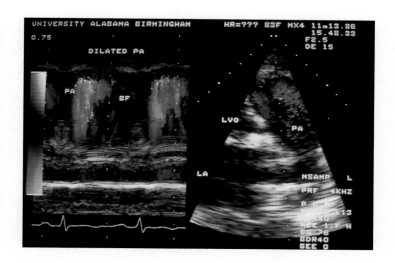

Figure PV-25   **Dilated pulmonary artery.** Aortic short axis view in a 20-year-old woman with lupus erythematosus was obtained by using a newer commerically available machine. Color M-mode examination on the left clearly displays flow reversal in late systole, shown by the red signals. The blue signals indicate antegrade flow in the MPA during early systole, and red signals within blue represent aliasing. Multiple distinct jets of PR are clearly seen in front of the diastolic tracing of the PV. S = systole.

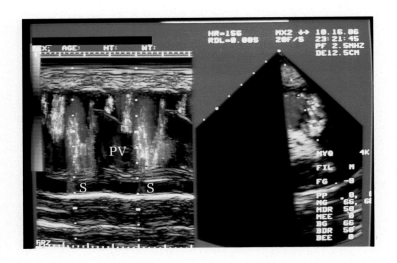

SECTION 6 PULMONARY VALVE

Figure PV-26 **Pulmonary artery aneurysm.** A 60-year-old woman with PS had a balloon valvoplasty of the PV in 1986. Aortic short axis view in this patient shows prominent poststenotic dilatation of the PA and swirling of blood flow in late systole. The blue signals represent forward flow (FF), and the red signals result from flow reversal (BF).

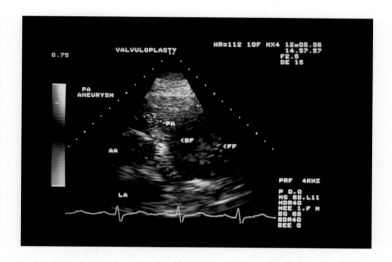

SECTION 6   PULMONARY VALVE

Figure PV-27   **Dilated pulmonary arteries in sarcoidosis.** (A) Aortic short axis view in a 33-year-old woman with sarcoidosis shows dilatation of the MPA and the proximal right (RPA) and left (LPA) branches. (B and C) Color flow examinations show prominent blue signals representing antegrade systolic blood flow in the main and proximal right and left PA. The swirling effect is not seen in this frame.

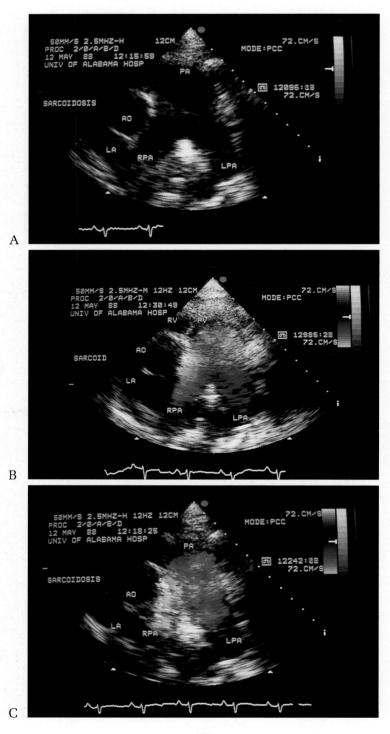

SECTION 7

PROSTHESES

MECHANICAL MITRAL PROSTHESES

In our experience, color Doppler has been useful in the evaluation of mechanical mitral prosthetic valves. It supplements 2D and conventional Doppler echocardiography in the assessment of prosthetic valve function. Color Doppler examination of one mechanical mitral prosthesis (Starr-Edwards) often shows two flow jets located on each side of the prosthesis during diastole as the flow moves around the ball from the LA into the LV. A small central jet representing the flow displaced by the poppet moving into the open position at the apex of the cage may also be seen. This central jet seen in the apical 4-chamber view may also denote the flow entering the LV along the side of the poppet because the cage and the poppet are 3-dimensional structures and the central jet may represent the flow moving around the poppet in the third dimension, or moving from the anterior or posterior aspect of the poppet. Visualization of these flow patterns facilitates parallel positioning of a pulsed Doppler sample volume or a continuous wave Doppler cursor in the flow to obtain reliable velocities from which the pressure gradient across the prosthetic valve can be calculated using the modified Bernoulli equation. The sample volume or cursor does not have to be placed in all three flow jets; placement in any of them provides reliable velocities because the velocities in all three jets are assumed to be equal. Color Doppler examination of another mechanical prosthesis (Bjork-Shiley) often shows two jets originating on either side of the prosthetic valve and merging farther downstream in the LV. Color Doppler examination of the St. Jude mitral prosthesis using the apical 4-chamber imaging plane generally shows two inflow jets moving through the prosthesis into the LV during diastole. In vitro studies conducted with color Doppler frequently show three jets originating from this mitral prosthesis, with two originating from the leaflets and one from the central area. This flow pattern, however, is not commonly seen in in vivo studies.

We have noticed fairly high pressure gradients in apparently normally functioning prosthetic valves and in such valves soon after their implantation, even without 2D echocardiographic and clinical evidence of obvious dysfunction. A relatively high pressure gradient obtained at a baseline examination simply indicates that prosthetic valves are not an ideal replacement for natural valves because they are inherently mildly stenotic. Patients must therefore be examined in the immediate postoperative period so that they can be followed serially to see if there is any significant increase in their pressure gradients or, in other words, if the prosthesis has become obstructed. In a patient with catheterization or surgically documented prosthetic valve stenosis, both the peak and mean pressure gradients across the prosthetic valve are high. Two-dimensional and M-mode echocardiography may also help to diagnose an obstructed prosthesis by showing the presence of an echo density, indicating a thrombus on the prosthesis and restricted motion of the poppet or disc.

Two-dimensional echo imaging of prosthetic valves produces numerous reverberations and artifacts. These cause significant problems in the parallel positioning of the pulsed Doppler sample volume or continuous wave Doppler cursor to the direction of flow across the prosthesis. Color Doppler alleviates this problem by helping to distinguish between the artifacts and reverberations and the actual flow signals. In general, color reverberations can be distinguished from actual flow signals by their short durations and their overlapping of adjacent stuctures.

Regurgitation in patients with mechanical mitral prostheses may be diagnosed by noting reversed flow signals in the LA originating from the prosthetic valve during systole. The MR in these patients may not be well visualized using the long and short axis parasternal and apical 4-chamber imaging planes because the extensive reverberations often clutter the LA, making the regurgitant flow signals difficult to visualize. In addition, the area immediately behind the mechanical prosthesis is acoustically silent because the metal in the prosthesis impedes the transmission of ultrasound waves. This frequently results in failure to adequately detect the regurgitant flow signals. Therefore, prosthetic MR may not be detected, or if it is, its severity may be grossly underestimated. To eliminate this problem, it is important for the examiner to use multiple imaging planes and transducer angulations to attempt to interrogate as much of the LA as possible. For example, prosthetic reverberations in the LA may not be displayed using the right parasternal approach with the patient in the right lateral decubitus position, thus allowing a larger segment of the left atrium to be interrogated successfully by color Doppler. We have been able to correctly diagnose severe prosthetic MR in some patients using this view when the apical, parasternal long axis, and short axis views suggested the absence of significant regurgitation.

The severity of the MR present is graded using the same method as is used to assess the severity of the regurgitant native valve. The proportion of the LA occupied by the regurgitant flow signals determines the grade of MR present. The MR is classified as mild or Grade 1, moderate or Grade 2, and severe or Grade 3 when the regurgitant jet occupies less than 20%, between 20 and 40%, and more than 40% of the LA, respectively.

The origin of the mitral regurgitant jet observed using color Doppler often determines the classification of the regurgitation present. For example, valvular and paravalvular regurgitation are suspected if the regurgitant signals originate from the central portion and the side of the prosthesis respectively. In cases of paravalvular regurgitation, the origin of the jet points to the site of the dehiscence of the suture line and determines whether the dehiscence is present medially or laterally in the apical 4-chamber view and anteriorly or posteriorly using the long axis and apical 2-chamber views. In some patients we have found systolic mosaic signals of MR moving into the LA between the mechanical mitral prosthesis and the atrial septum (AS) in the apical 4-chamber or right parasternal view, demonstrating the presence of paravalvular regurgitation.

The diagnosis of the type of prosthetic regurgitation may also be aided by observing a localized area of flow acceleration on the ventricular side of the mitral prosthesis and directly opposite the origin of the prosthetic mitral regurgitant jet. If the flow acceleration is seen beyond or between the stents, paravalvular or valvular regurgitation, respectively, is diagnosed.

PORCINE MITRAL PROSTHESES

In general, the function of a porcine mitral prosthesis is easier to assess than the function of a mechanical mitral prosthesis. With 2D echo imaging, all three stents of a porcine MV can be seen. The leaflets of a normal porcine mitral prosthesis are observed to be thin and freely mobile during diastole. If the valve leaflets are displayed as thickened or with restricted mobility, porcine MV dysfunction is suspected, and Doppler must then be used to assess the degree of dysfunction and stenosis.

Color Doppler, rather than conventional Doppler, provides the best approach for the assessment of valve function because it facilitates parallel placement of the continuous wave Doppler cursor to the flow moving across the prosthesis and thus provides more reliable pressure gradient measurements. Sometimes high pressure gradients may be recorded across a nonobstructed but leaking prosthesis, but the presence of a rapid diastolic deceleration and a relatively low mean pressure gradient indicate that the prosthesis is nonobstructed. In a patient with a relatively small LV, the protruding bioprosthetic MV may obstruct the outflow, creating turbulence, which is clearly displayed by color Doppler. In such patients, color Doppler also facilitates the placement of the continuous wave Doppler parallel to the turbulent flow and provides an accurate assessment of the severity of outflow obstruction produced by the prosthesis. The effective MV orifice area in a patient with a bioprosthetic MV prostheses can be accurately calculated using the pressure half-time method.

In general, a color Doppler examination of an unobstructed porcine prosthesis shows flow signals filling the entire space between the stents of the prosthesis. Flow signals seen consistently occupying only a portion of the area between the stents indicate that the prosthetic valve is obstructed. The presence of an obstructing clot, however, may be difficult to visualize unless the clot is large and protrudes into the LV. The width of the prosthetic inflow signals originating from the prosthetic valve is also useful in assessing its function. A markedly narrow jet implies significant obstruction, while a wide jet indicates no obstruction. The width of the jet must be assessed at its origin from the prosthetic valve because farther downstream the jet widens significantly.

Associated AR in patients with mitral prosthetic valves is difficult to diagnose, especially if the prosthesis is directed anteriorly. In these patients, mosaic turbulent signals due to prosthetic inflow are observed in the LVOT proximal to the origin of the AV. It is difficult to distinguish between these signals and the aortic regurgitant signals, especially in the parasternal long axis plane. Only careful frame-by-frame analysis reveals that these signals originate from the mitral prosthesis and not from the AV. Also, these mosaic signals are not seen during early diastole, unlike the aortic regurgitant signals. Continuous wave Doppler examination can be used to assess the presence and severity of associated AR, because if any AR is present, high-velocity signals are recorded in the LVOT. A comprehensive examination conducted using multiple imaging planes also resolves any confusion regarding the presence and severity of associated AR.

The regurgitant signals from a porcine mitral prosthesis are more easily visualized and more reliably differentiated into both valvular and paravalvular regurgitation than those from a mechanical mitral prosthesis. In valvular regurgitation, blood leaks through the valve, and in paravalvular regurgitation, the leak occurs at the attachment point of the prosthesis. Color Doppler shows valvular and paravalvular regurgitation by displaying mitral regurgitant signals occurring between the stents and at or beyond the stents, respectively.

As in the mechanical prosthesis, a localized area of flow acceleration may be seen on the ventricular aspect of the bioprosthetic valve directly opposite the origin of the mitral regurgitant signals. The site of this flow acceleration can be used to help differentiate valvular from paravalvular regurgitation. In some patients, both valvular and paravalvular regurgitation may be present.

The severity of bioprosthetic MR is graded by comparing the maximum area of the regurgitant signals to the area of the LA and is similar to grading regurgitation in the native MV. Color Doppler may underestimate the severity of regurgitation in some patients because of the difficulty in fully interrogating the LA due to interference produced by reverberations and to acoustically silent areas produced by the metallic components of the prosthesis. This problem is not as significant for the porcine prosthesis as for the mechanical prosthesis because in the porcine prosthesis only the ring is made of metal. In some patients with porcine prosthetic valves, two separate jets of MR may be detected. The severity of the regurgitation in these patients is estimated by adding the regurgitant areas of the two jets.

MITRAL ANNULOPLASTY

Color Doppler is also useful in examining patients who have undergone Carpentier mitral ring annuloplasty for severe MR. Color Doppler clearly displays the Carpentier ring and prominent inflow signals moving through the ring and the leaflets during diastole. Often these flow signals are anteriorly directed, and as they move through the mitral leaflets, they become posteriorly oriented. Occasionally, two inflow jets may be seen, with one jet anteriorly directed toward the VS and the other posteriorly directed toward the left ventricular posterior wall. During systole, the LA can be interrogated for the presence of residual MR. In some patients, MR can be seen originating beyond the level of the ring ("para-ring" mitral regurgitation). Regurgitant signals originating within the confines of the ring elements represent "ring" regurgitation. A color-guided continuous wave Doppler examination can also be used to exclude the presence of obstruction produced by ring annuloplasty by positioning the cursor parallel to the direction of the inflow jet and obtaining the pressure gradients across the ring.

MECHANICAL AORTIC PROSTHESES

Color Doppler examination of a normally functioning mechanical aortic prosthesis shows mosaic signals moving through the prothesis into the aortic root during systole. These findings have been seen with the Starr-Edwards, St. Jude, and Bjork-Shiley prostheses. As previously discussed, color Doppler provides an easier method of positioning the continuous wave Doppler cursor parallel to the direction of the jet originating from the prosthesis. This, in turn, generates more reliable velocities and pressure gradients. Even though the continuous wave Doppler cursor may appear to be parallel to the flow signals in the color image of the prothesis, it may not actually be parallel to the central "core" of the jet where the velocity is maximum. Therefore, the transducer needs to be angled slightly in various directions to make the cursor parallel to the "core" of the 3-dimensional jet moving through the prosthesis.

As in the mitral prostheses, significant pressure gradients can be measured even in apparently normally functioning prosthetic valves. This results from the valve being inherently mildly stenotic and/or from the increased cardiac output caused by the relief of either the stenotic or the regurgitant lesion. These prostheses must be studied in the immediate postoperative period so that they can be followed serially to see if there is any significant increase in the pressure gradients that would indicate the development of prosthetic obstruction.

Mechanical aortic prosthetic regurgitation is diagnosed by noting the presence of mosaic signals originating from the prosthetic valve and moving into the LVOT during diastole. As with the mechanical mitral prostheses, the severity of AR may be underestimated in these patients. Minimal AR is always present with some aortic prosthetic valves like the Bjork-Shiley or St. Jude's prosthesis. It may not be detected, however, because of the interference caused by prosthetic reverberations that clutter the LVOT and the acoustically silent area behind the metallic components of the prosthesis. It is, therefore, important to examine these patients using multiple planes and multiple transducer angulations to interrogate the LVOT as completely as possible in all three dimensions.

Prosthetic AR is graded in the same way as native aortic valve regurgitation. With a mechanical aortic prosthesis, it is not always easy to differentiate valvular from paravalvular prosthetic regurgitation, but prosthetic regurgitation that appears to originate from the center of the valve is generally classified as valvular. When it appears to occur anteriorly at or near the junction of the anterior aortic wall with the VS or posteriorly at or near the junction of the posterior aortic wall with the anterior mitral leaflet, paravalvular regurgitation is suspected. The presence of paravalvular regurgitation is also indicated when regurgitant jet signals are seen moving into the LV through an area between the prosthesis and the anterior or posterior aortic wall or when diastolic regurgitant signals are located near the extreme anterior or posterior aspect of the prosthesis. In some patients, both valvular and paravalvular regurgitation may occur and be diagnosed by color Doppler.

PORCINE AORTIC PROSTHESES

Porcine aortic prostheses are easier to assess by color Doppler than mechanical aortic prostheses because the metallic component is smaller and confined to the ring, and this results in a smaller acoustically silent area during a color Doppler examination. Even though the thin leaflets of the aortic prosthesis appear to open well, color-guided continuous wave Doppler records significant pressure gradients in patients who have no evidence by auscultation or 2D echocardiography of any abnormality of the valve. This may reflect the inherent stenotic nature of some of these valves and also an increase in the cardiac output, which may occur with relief of stenosis or regurgitation. Therefore, in many patients, the high-velocity flow signals moving through the aortic prosthesis show a mosaic pattern due to variance and turbulence. As in the mitral porcine prosthesis, color flow signals filling the entire space between the stents of the bioprosthetic aortic valve indicate the presence of unobstructed flow, and flow signals not completely filling the area between the stents should alert the examiner to the presence of prosthetic obstruction. In our experience, prosthetic obstruction is best assessed by color-guided continuous wave Doppler using the suprasternal view or in the right parasternal imaging plane with the patient in the right lateral decubitus position. In some patients, the maximum velocity may be obtained using the apical approach. Although uncertainty exists about applying the continuity equation to flow through a mechanical prosthesis, we have used it successfully in calculating the effective orifice areas for porcine aortic prostheses.

AR in porcine prostheses is diagnosed in a similar manner to AR in mechanical aortic prostheses, by noting retrograde flow originating from the AV and moving into the LVOT during diastole. The severity of prosthetic AR is graded in a manner similar to that used to grade native aortic valve regurgitation, by measuring the maximum width of the regurgitant signals at their origin from the prosthetic valve and comparing it to the width of the LVOT width taken at the same point.

Because it is sometimes difficult to visualize the stents of the bioprosthetic aortic valve, differentiating between valvular and paravalvular regurgitation may be difficult. If the regurgitation appears to originate centrally from the prosthetic valve or occurs eccentrically from the extreme anterior or posterior aspect of the prosthesis, valvular or paravalvular regurgitation is present, respectively. Occasionally, flow signals may be seen moving into the LVOT through a gap between the prosthetic valve and the anterior aortic root. This indicates the presence of significant prosthetic dehiscence with considerable paravalvular aortic regurgitation. In some patients, the leaflets of the porcine aortic prosthesis may protrude markedly into the LVOT during diastole, indicating the presence of significant valvular regurgitation.

HOMOGRAFT AORTIC VALVE

We have limited experience in examining patients with homograft valve replacement. The examination is conducted in a manner similar to that used for examining a porcine aortic prosthesis.

TRICUSPID PROSTHESIS

Color Doppler examination of a tricuspid prosthesis shows flow patterns very similar to those seen in an examination of a mitral prosthesis. Porcine tricuspid prosthetic stenosis can be diagnosed by noting high pressure gradients obtained using color-guided continuous wave Doppler examination. A narrow jet originating from a tricuspid prosthetic valve is also a good indicator of significant prosthetic obstruction.

Tricuspid prosthetic regurgitation can be assessed by noting the presence of flow signals originating from the prosthesis and spreading into the RA during systole. The grading of this regurgitation is the same as the grading for prosthetic MR.

LEFT VENTRICULAR-AORTIC CONDUIT

A left ventricular-aortic conduit is placed in patients in whom the LVOT or the AV is significantly obstructed and surgical relief of obstruction technically difficult to accomplish. A color Doppler examination performed in a patient with a normally functioning conduit shows normal left ventricular inflow signals during diastole and prominent flow signals moving through the conduit during systole. No evidence of conduit valve regurgitation is seen. Conduit regurgitation is diagnosed when flow signals are observed moving into the LV from the conduit during diastole.

The severity of the conduit regurgitation is assessed by noting the proportion of the regurgitant signals filling the left ventricular cavity. We have found that conduit regurgitation is mild if the regurgitant signals occupied less than 10% of the left ventricular cavity and severe if the signals occupied more than 50% of the cavity. We recently had two patients with severe left ventricular-aortic conduit regurgitation. This regurgitation was alleviated in one patient by replacing the porcine conduit valve with a St. Jude prosthesis.

REFERENCES

1. Norwood, W.I., Freed, M.D., Rocchini, A.P., Bernhard, W.F., and Castaneda, A.R.: Experience with valved conduits for repair of congenital cardiac lesions. Ann. Thorac. Surg. 24:223, 1977.
2. Heck, H.A., Schieken, R.M., Laurer, R.M., and Doty, D.B. Conduit repair for complex congenital heart disease. Late follow-up. J. Thorac. Cardiovasc. Surg. 75:806, 1978.
3. Ciaravella, J.M. Jr., McGoon, D.C., Danielson, G.K., Wallace, R.B., Mair, D.D., and Ilstrup, D.M.: Experience with the extracardiac conduit. J. Thorac. Cardiovasc. Surg. 78:920, 1979.

4. Carpentier, A., Chauvaud, S., Fabiani, J.N., Deloche, A., Relland, J., Lessana, A., D'Allaines, C., Blondeau, P., Piwnica, A., and Dubost, P.: Reconstructive surgery of mitral valve incompetence. Ten year appraisal. J. Thorac. Cardiovasc. Surg. 79:338, 1980.

5. King, H., Csicsko, J., and Leshnower, A.: Intraoperative assessment of the mitral valve following reconstructive procedures. Ann. Thorac. Surg. 29:81, 1980.

6. Bonchek, L.I.: Correction of mitral valve disease without mitral valve replacement. Am. Heart J. 104:865, 1982.

7. Williams, G.A., and Labovitz, A.J.: Doppler hemodynamic evaluation of prosthetic (Starr-Edwards and Bjork-Shiley) and bioprosthetic (Hancock and Carpentier-Edwards) cardiac valves. Am. J. Cardiol. 56:325, 1985.

8. Switzer, D.F., Yoganathan, A.P., Nanda, N.C., Woo, Y.R., and Ridgway, A.J.: In vitro evaluation of prosthetic aortic regurgitation by color Doppler (Abstract). Circulation 72 (Supp.III);III-207, 1985.

9. Okumachi, F., Yoshikawa, J., Yoshida, K., Asaka, T., Takao, S., and Shiratori, K.: Diagnostic value and limitations of two-dimensional Doppler color flow mapping in the evaluation of prosthetic valve dysfunction (Abstract). Circulation 72(Supp.III):III-101, 1985.

10. Jones, S., McMillan, S.T., Eidbo, E.E., Woo, Y.-R., and Yoganathan, A.P.: Evaluation of prosthetic heart valves by Doppler flow imaging. Echocardiography 3:513, 1986.

11. Goyal, R.G., Kan, M.N., Soto, B., Hsiung, M.C., Helmcke, F., Moos, S., and Nanda, N.C.: Color Doppler assessment of prosthetic valve function and its limitations (Abstract). Circulation 74(Supp. IV):IV-389, 1986.

12. Shah, R.M., Roitman, D.I., and Nanda, N.C.: Color Doppler flow imaging in prosthetic valves (Abstract). J. Am. Coll. Cardiol. 7:188A, 1986.

13. Maurer, G., Czer, L., DeRobertis, M., Chaux, A., Kass, R., Lee, M., and Matloff, J.: Color Doppler flow mapping for intraoperative assessment of valvuloplasty and repair of congenital heart disease (Abstract). J. Am. Coll. Cardiol. 7:2A, 1986.

14. Goldman, M.E., Mora, F., Fuster, V., Guarino, T., and Mindich, B.P.: Is mitral valvuloplasty superior to mitral valve replacement for preservation of left ventricular function? An intraoperative two-dimensional echocardiographic study (Abstract). J. Am. Coll. Cardiol. 7:161A, 1986.

15. Goldman, M.E., Mora, F., Guarino, T., Fuster, V., Mindich, B.P.: Mitral valvuloplasty is superior to valve replacement for preservation of left ventricular function: an intraoperative two-dimensional echocardiographic study. J. Am. Coll. Cardiol. 10:568, 1987.

16. Yoganathan, A.P., McMillan, S., Sung, H.W., Nanda, N.C.: In vitro demonstration of regurgitant jets identified by color Doppler flow mapping in normally functioning mechanical valves (Abstract). Circulation 76 (Suppl. IV):IV-140, 1987.

17. Sprecher, D.L., Adamick, R., Adams, D., and Kisslo, J.: In vitro color flow, pulsed and continuous wave Doppler ultrasound masking of flow by prosthetic valves. J. Am. Coll. Cardiol. 9:1306, 1987.

18. Fan, P.H., Kapur, K.K., Aggarwal, K.K., Jain, S., Goyal, R., and Nanda, N.C.: Utility of color flow acceleration in differentiating valvar from paravalvar prosthetic mitral regurgitation (Abstract). Circulation 76(Supp.IV):IV-448, 1987.

19. Gupta, A., Helmcke, F., Pandey, B.J., Nanda, N.C., Aggarwal, K.K., and Yoganathan, A.P.: Color guided continuous wave Doppler assessment of effective prosthetic valve area (Abstract). J. Am. Coll. Cardiol. 11:177A, 1988.

SECTION 7 PROSTHESES

Normal and abnormal color Doppler flow patterns in various types of valvar prostheses, both mechanical and tissue, are presented in this section.

Figure PR-1 **Starr-Edwards mitral prosthesis.** (A) Prosthetic MV is shown in an autopsy specimen and schematically in (B) the closed position and (C) the open position. MP = Mitral prosthesis.

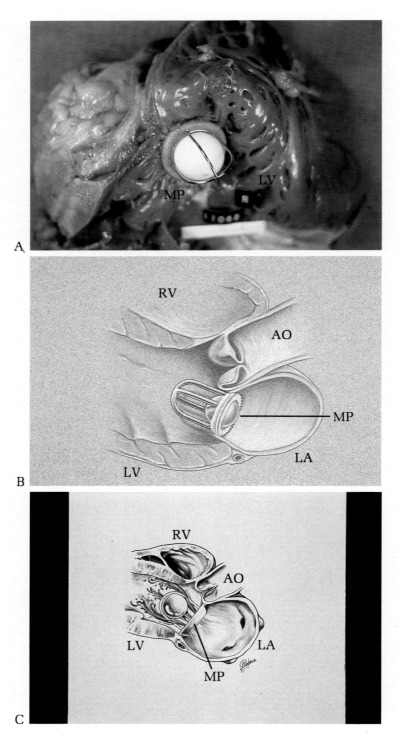

SECTION 7 PROSTHESES

Figure. PR-2 **Starr-Edwards mitral prosthesis (MP) visualized in apical 4-chamber view.**
(A) Two inflow jets (arrows) are present on each side of the prosthesis with distinct reverberations (RB). (B) Two inflow jets (arrows) are present on each side of the prosthesis. (C) Three inflow
jets (arrows) located on each side and through the center of the prosthesis are shown. (D) The
pulse Doppler sample volume (SV) is placed in the left inflow (FL) jet to characterize the velocity
waveform.

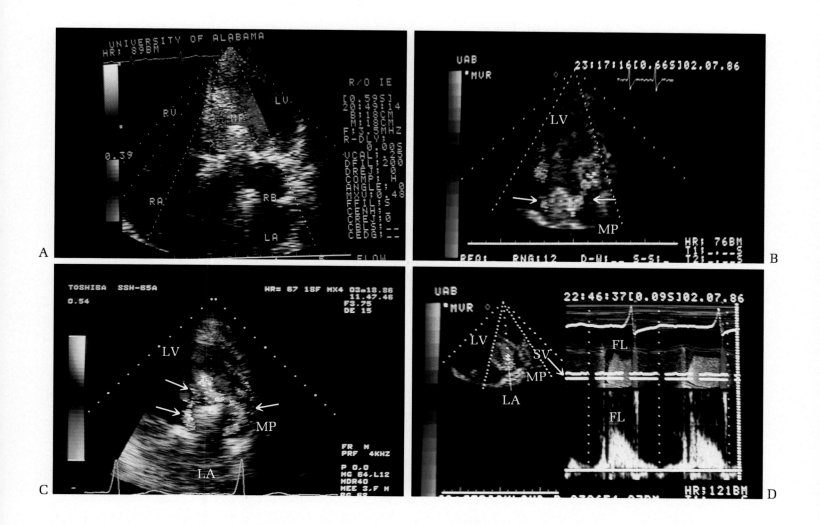

Figure PR-3 **Regurgitation from Starr-Edwards mitral prosthesis.** (A) Autopsy specimen shows a large gap (arrow) at the suture line, indicating dehiscence of the prosthesis. (B) Long axis view in a 36-year-old woman with a Starr Edwards MP shows a small area of blue signals in the LA originating from the side of the anterior stent, implying minimal paravalvular regurgitation. The small area of blue signals on the ventricular side represents flow acceleration (ACC), and its location beyond the anterior stent further supports the diagnosis of a paravalvular leak. The right parasternal view (C) shows these regurgitant signals more prominently and also shows a swirling pattern in the left atrial cavity, implying significant MR, which in this patient could not be well visualized from the long axis view because of extensive reverberations. In addition, the area immediately behind the metallic prosthesis is acoustically silent because the metal in the prosthesis impedes the transmission of ultrasound waves. This can result in failure to detect regurgitant flow signals. The continuous wave Doppler cursor (D) placed through the LA flow signals records a relatively high velocity of approximately 1.9 m/sec, implying that these signals result from MR and not pulmonary venous flow. E, F, and G represent long axis views in a 76-year-old man with a Starr-Edwards MP implanted 15 years ago who presented with recent onset of cardiac failure and severe hemolysis (HCT 20%). A prominent rounded mobile echo density (arrow) is seen originating from the medial aspect of the prosthesis (MP) and moving towards the aortic root in systole (F,G) consistent with a thrombus. Color-guided continuous wave Doppler examination revealed a peak diastolic pressure gradient of 22 mm Hg across the prosthesis, indicating obstruction. Mosaic-colored flow signals seen in the LA during the isovolumic contraction period (E) and appearing to originate directly opposite the echo density represent MR in this patient. These signals were more prominently seen in the apical 4-chamber and right parasternal views during systole, and we graded MR as 2/3. These findings were confirmed by cardiac catheterization and angiography. Autopsy specimen (H) from another patient shows a thrombus (TH) on the ventricular aspect of a Starr-Edwards MP. Damage to the LV wall produced by impaction of the prosthetic cage is also seen (arrows).

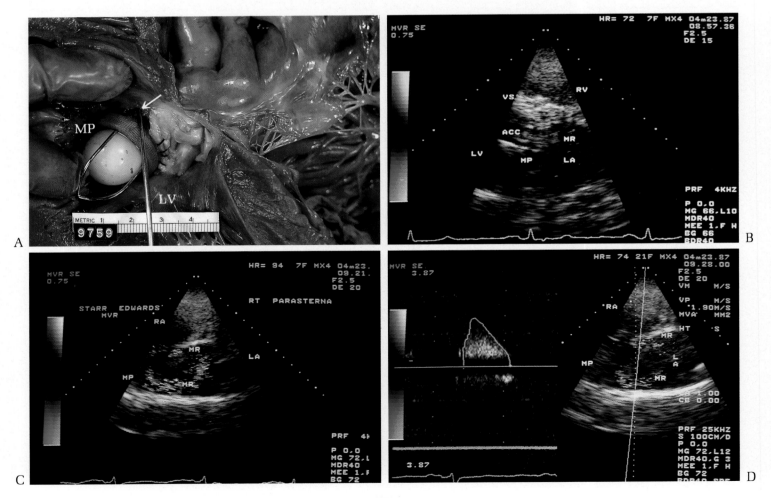

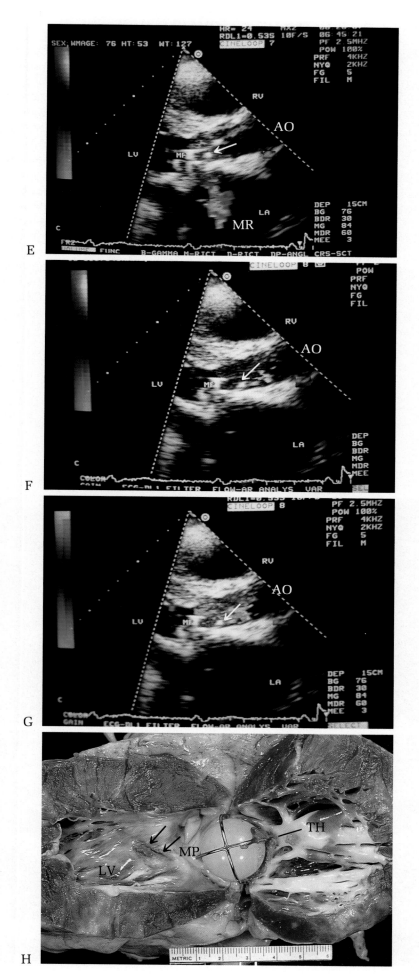

SECTION 7   PROSTHESES

Figure PR-4   Regurgitation from caged-ball mitral prosthesis. (A) Right parasternal view in a 65-year-old man who had a Starr-Edwards MV replacement in 1972 shows prominent mosaic signals originating from the prosthesis and moving into the LA, indicating significant MR, which in this patient could not be well visualized from the standard parasternal and apical views because of extensive reverberations and an acoustically silent area immediately behind the metallic prosthesis. (B) Right parasternal examination in another adult patient with a caged-ball prosthesis (Braunwald-Cutter) shows systolic blue signals in a markedly dilated LA, indicating significant MR. In this patient also, the regurgitant signals could not be detected from the conventional views. The mosaic signals in the RA indicate associated TR. C and D represent parasternal long axis views using 2 different flow maps in another patient (47-year-old woman) with a Starr-Edwards (SE) mitral prosthesis (MP) showing systolic bluish-white signals of MR in the LA adjacent to the LA posterior wall and separated from prosthetic echoes by an echolucent area (SA), probably related to incomplete penetration of the metallic prosthesis by the Doppler ultrasonic beam. Right parasternal examination (E) in the same patient shows the MR signals clearly originating from the prosthesis without encountering significant interference from its metallic components. Angulation of the transducer (F) so that a larger portion of the Doppler beam encounters the prosthesis produces artifactual color reverberations (RB), distinguished from MR signals by their very short duration ("lightning flashes") and overlapping of adjacent structures.

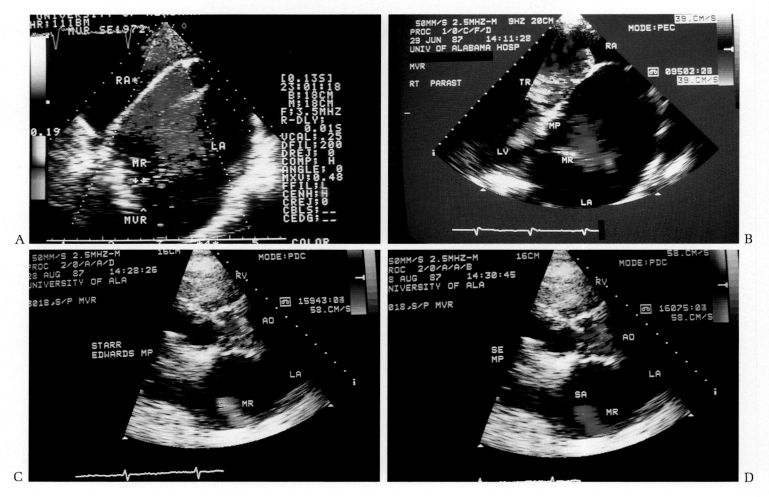

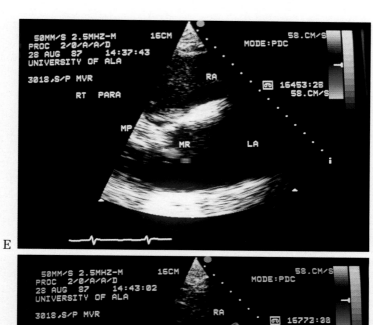

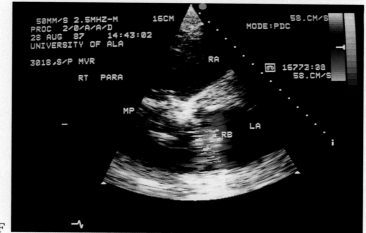

SECTION 7   PROSTHESES

Figure PR-5   **Bjork-Shiley prosthesis.** Prosthetic valve is shown in (A) mitral position and (B) both mitral and tricuspid positions in autopsy specimens. The apical views of patients with this prosthesis (C and D) show two jets (J1 and J2) originating from both sides of the prosthesis and merging farther downstream.

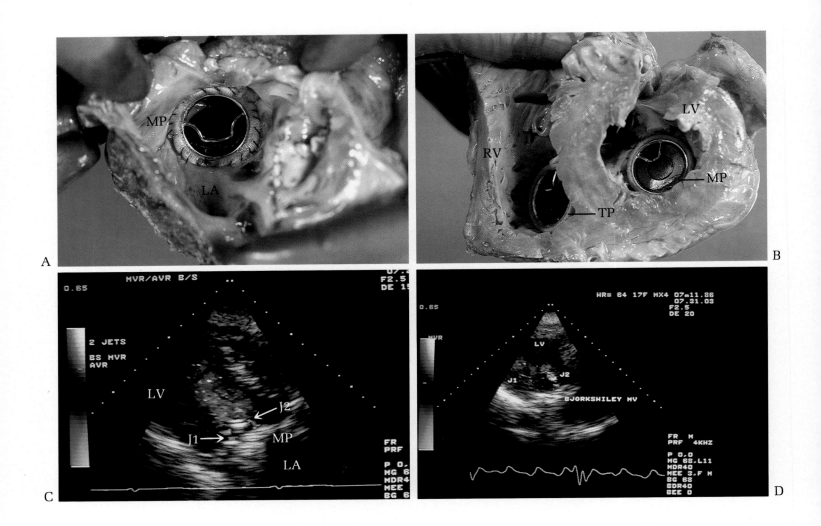

SECTION 7 PROSTHESES

Figure PR-6 **Regurgitation from Bjork-Shiley mitral prosthesis.** (A) Autopsy specimen shows a large gap (arrow) at the suture line indicating dehiscence of the prosthesis. (B) Apical view in a 54-year-old woman with a Bjork-Shiley MP displays mosaic signals in the LA along the atrial septum (AS). These signals appear to originate from the anterior side of the sewing ring, implying paravalvular regurgitation (PMR). (C) Right parasternal examination in a 30-year-old male shows systolic mosaic-colored signals moving into the LA between the Bjork-Shiley mitral prosthesis (BSP) and the AS, conclusively demonstrating paravalvular (PARA) regurgitation in this patient. With minimal transducer angulation (D), most of the LA is filled with mosaic and red signals, indicating severe MR. E shows MR in the apical 4-chamber view. FA = flow acceleration. The diastolic apical 4-chamber view (F) shows two inflow jets (J1 and J2) originating from both sides of the prosthesis. The blue signals within the red are due to aliasing. Color-guided continuous wave Doppler did not reveal significant prosthetic obstruction in this patient.

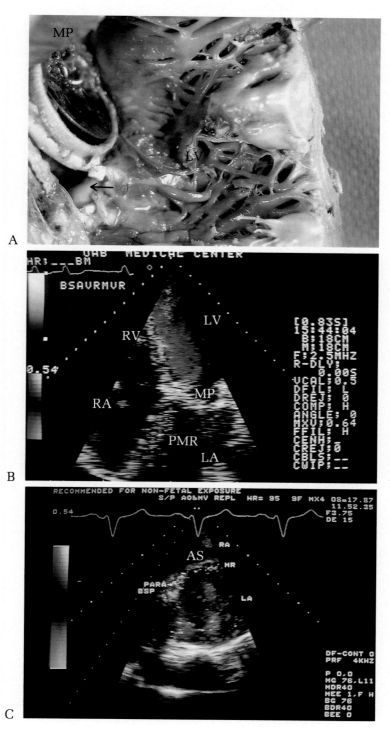

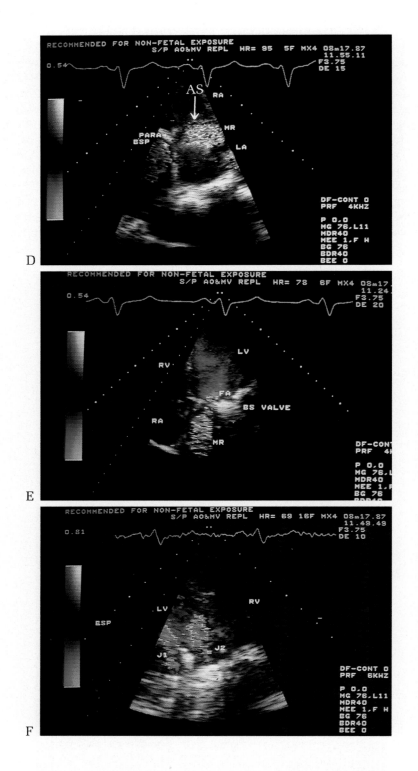

D

E

F

SECTION 7   PROSTHESES

Figure PR-7   **St. Jude mitral prosthesis.** (A) Prosthetic valve is shown schematically in the open position. (B) Apical 4-chamber view shows two jets (J1 and J2), displaying a mosaic pattern of colors indicating the presence of turbulence across the prosthesis. (C) Apical view shows an eccentric mosaic jet originating from the prosthesis and directed toward the VS.

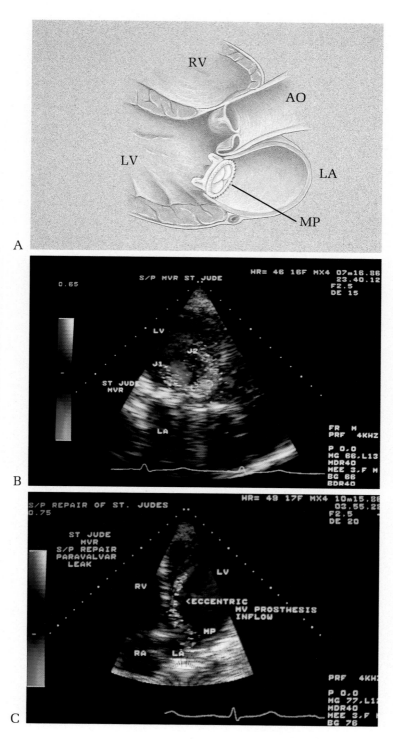

SECTION 7   PROSTHESES

Figure PR-8 **Regurgitation from St. Jude mitral prosthesis.** Aortic short axis view in a 26-year-old woman with a St. Jude prosthesis shows bluish-green signals of MR and a large LA. MR in this patient could not be well visualized from the long axis and apical views because of extensive reverberations. In addition, the area immediately behind the metallic prosthesis is acoustically silent because the metal in the prosthesis impedes the transmission of ultrasound waves. This can result in failure to detect regurgitant flow signals.

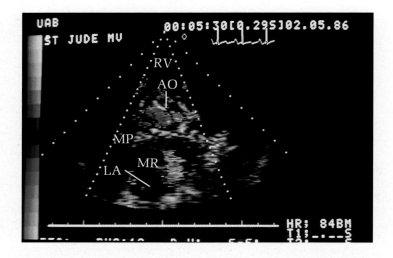

Figure PR-9 **Regurgitation from St. Jude prosthesis.** MR in an 18-year-old man with a St. Jude MP is best seen from a right parasternal view (A) as mosaic signals in the LA along the AS. These signals were recorded during the entire systolic period, as shown on color M-mode (B).

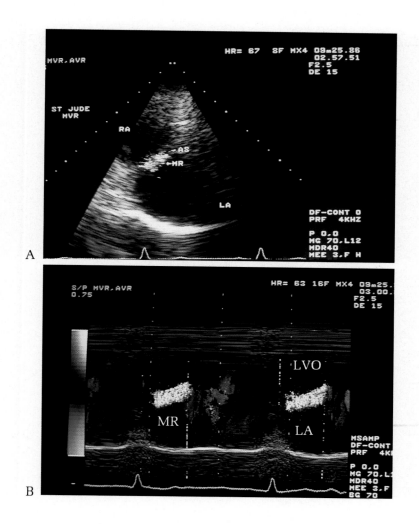

SECTION 7 PROSTHESES

Figure PR-10 **Porcine mitral prosthesis.** A specimen of the prosthetic valve as viewed from the atrial (A) and ventricular (B) sides is shown. The valve and the flow through it are shown in schematics (C and D). Long axis views (E, F, and G) in different patients visualize the color flow signals moving through normally functioning prosthetic valves toward the VS. The mosaic color in E and F represents turbulence, while the predominant blue color seen in G represents aliasing. The apical 4-chamber view (H) shows a red jet originating from the prosthesis and directed towards the VS. Blue color mixed in this red jet signifies the presence of aliasing. This 24-year old woman also had tricuspid annuloplasty for severe TR.

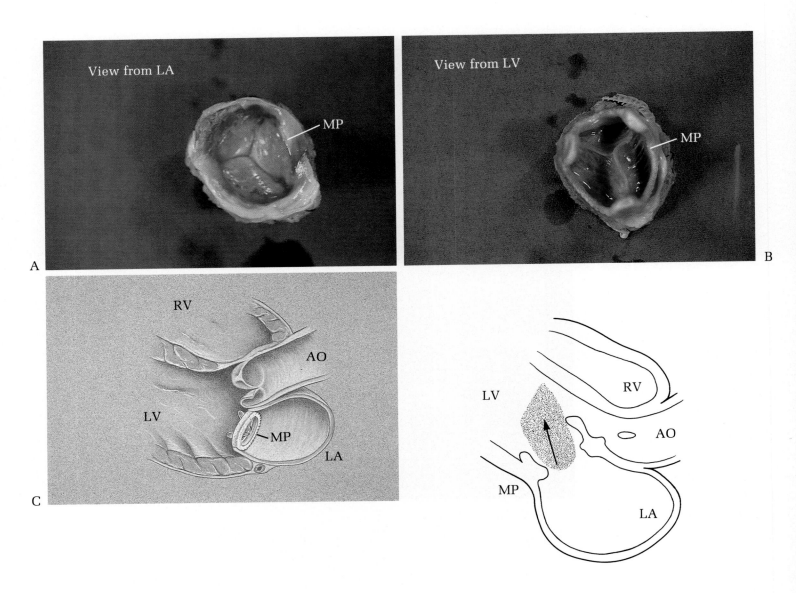

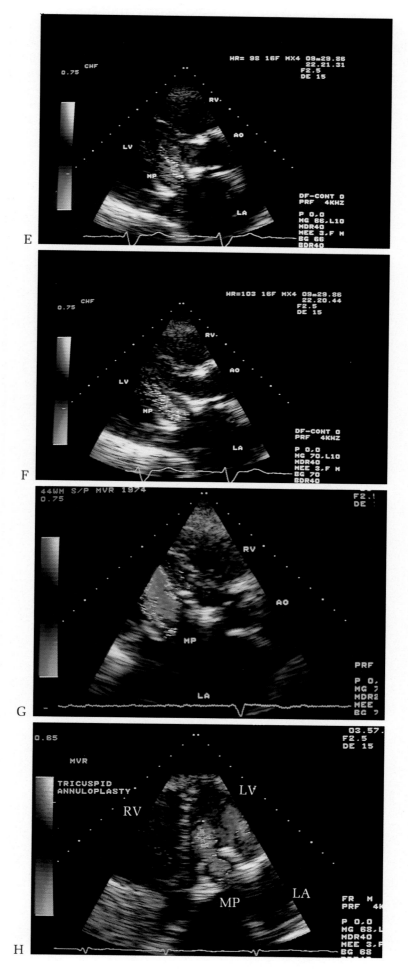

SECTION 7 PROSTHESES

Figure PR-11 **Porcine mitral prosthesis.** The continuous wave Doppler cursor is placed parallel to the mosaic-colored jet across the prosthesis shown in the apical 4-chamber view (right). The velocity waveform obtained as shown on the left shows a peak pressure gradient of only 8 mm Hg, indicating the absence of significant obstruction across the valve.

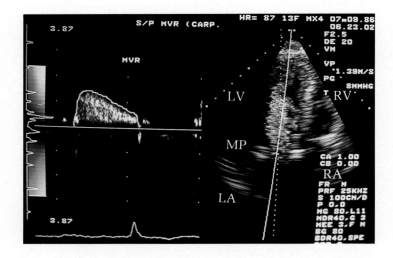

SECTION 7 PROSTHESES

Figure PR-12 **Porcine mitral prosthesis.** Apical 4-chamber view in a 52-year-old woman who had undergone porcine MV replacement in 1978 shows aliased flow signals originating from the MP during diastole. The continuous wave Doppler cursor placed parallel to this jet records a high peak pressure gradient of 18 mm Hg, but the diastolic deceleration is relatively rapid and the mean pressure gradient is only 8 mm Hg, implying no significant prosthetic obstruction. The high recorded peak gradient results from significant MR in this patient.

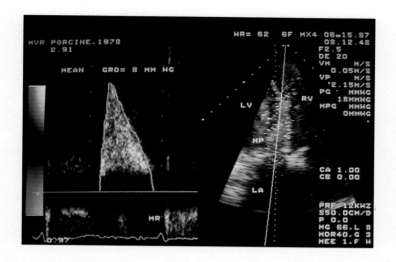

Figure PR-13 **Obstruction of porcine mitral prosthesis.** (A) Autopsy specimen of an obstructed porcine MP shows thickened leaflets and clots on the ventricular aspect (arrows). (B) Long axis view in a 23-year-old woman who had a porcine prosthesis replacement in 1981 shows the three stents of the prosthesis and a large LA. Long axis views (C and D) revealed a narrow band of mosaic signals originating from the MP, indicating significant stenosis and turbulence, while the red signals just below the valve represent flow acceleration. The mosaic signals broaden immediately downstream because of a high peak pressure gradient across the obstructed prosthesis. The continuous wave Doppler cursor in the apical view (E) is placed in the narrow jet to obtain a high peak pressure gradient of 22 mm Hg. The velocity waveform on the left shows a flat profile, also indicating the presence of severe stenosis. The MV area calculated from the pressure half time was 0.6 cm² in this patient. At surgery, the bio-prosthesis was replaced with a St. Jude valve.

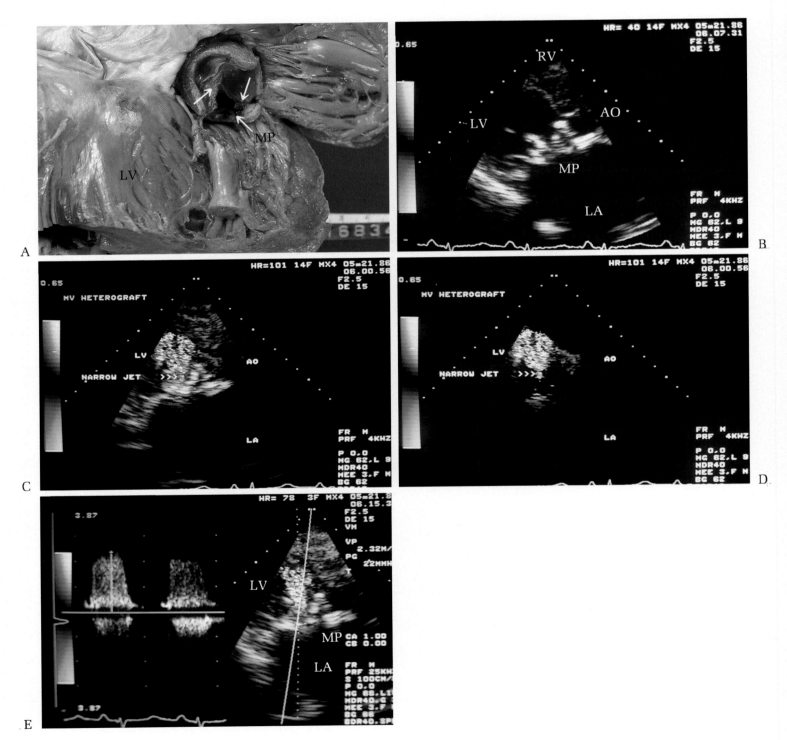

SECTION 7 PROSTHESES

Figure PR-14 **Obstruction of porcine mitral prosthesis.** (A) 2D examination from the long axis view in a 61-year-old man shows thickened leaflets (arrowhead) of the porcine prosthesis (MP), while color flow examination (B) shows a very narrow jet of mitral flow (MF) signals broadening downstream. The continuous wave cursor is positioned in the prosthetic inflow (C) to record a peak gradient of 32.6 mm Hg and the MV area of 0.72 cm². At surgery, the leaflets of the bio-prosthesis were replaced with a St. Jude valve.

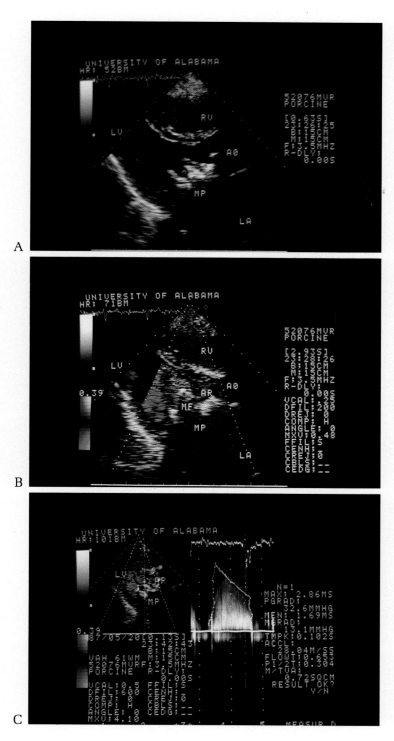

Figure PR-15 **LV outflow obstruction produced by mitral prosthesis.** (A) An indentation on the VS produced by a mitral bio-prosthesis (arrow) is shown in an autopsy specimen. (B) Schematic shows a mitral bio-prosthesis protruding into the LV and obstructing the outflow, which creates turbulence. (C) Long axis view in a 40-year-old woman shows mosaic signals from turbulence in the narrowed LVOT, while the continuous wave Doppler cursor positioned in the LVOT (D and E) records peak pressure gradients of 11 to 15 mm Hg across the LVO, indicating mild obstruction.

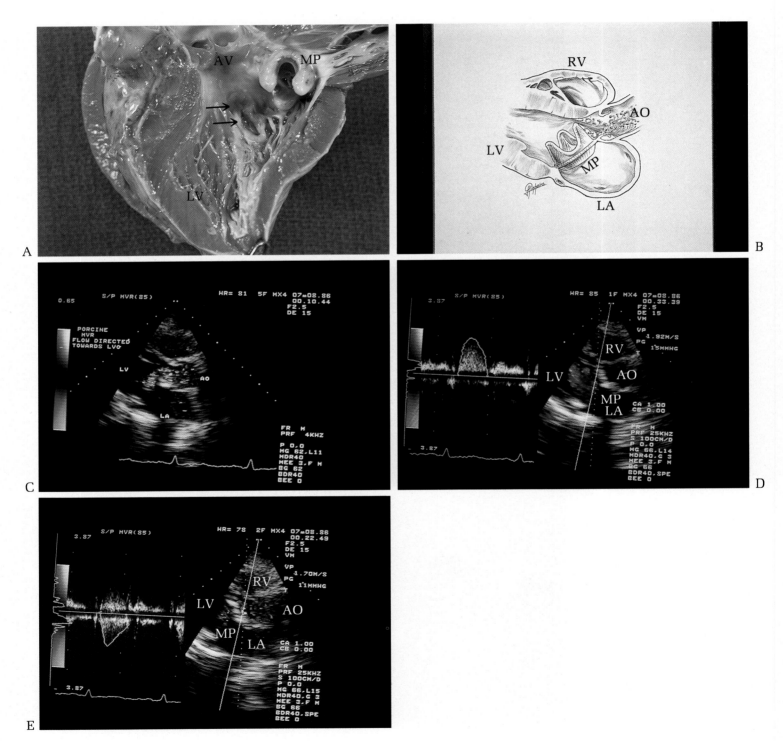

SECTION 7 PROSTHESES

Figure PR-16 **Mitral prosthetic inflow simulating aortic regurgitation.** Turbulence in the LVOT produced by mitral prosthetic inflow is shown schematically in A. Color Doppler examination of patients with mitral prosthesis (B—H) shows mosaic flow signals (arrow) in the LVOT in the vicinity of the AV, which could imply AR. Careful frame-by-frame analysis, however, reveals that these signals originate from the MP and not from the AV. Also, these signals were not seen in very early diastole, as would occur with AR.

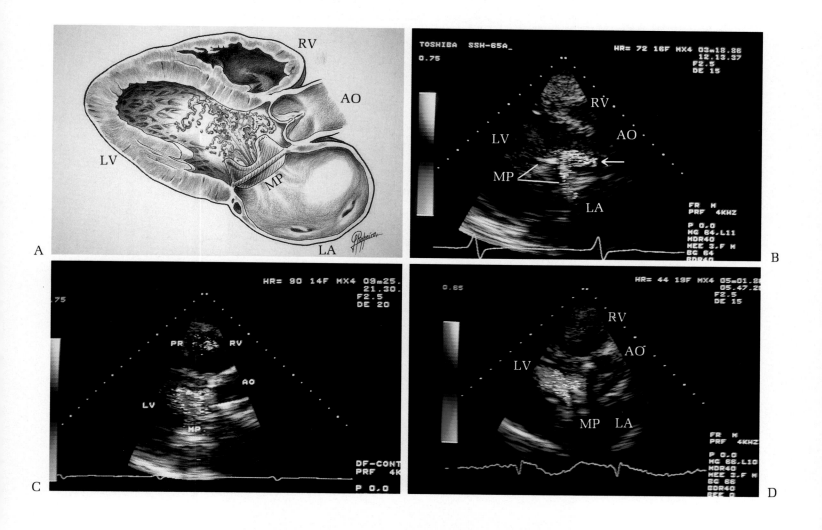

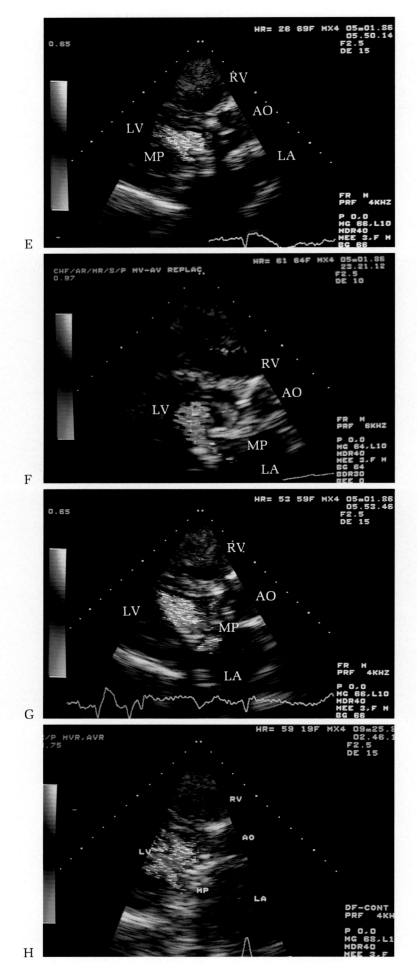

SECTION 7   PROSTHESES

Figure PR-17   Regurgitation from porcine mitral prosthesis. (A) Autopsy specimen shows marked degeneration of the leaflets of a Carpentier-Edwards porcine MP which resulted in severe regurgitation. The schematic (B) shows both valvular and paravalvular regurgitation from a MP. In valvular regurgitation, blood leaks through the valve, while in paravalvular regurgitation, the leak occurs at the attachment point of the prosthesis. Apical view (C) in a 59-year-old woman with a porcine heterograft reveals mosaic mitral regurgitant signals in the LA and bluish-green signals resulting from flow acceleration (FA) on the ventricular side of the prosthesis exactly opposite the origin of the regurgitant signals. The location of both the origin of the MR and the FA signals in an area between the stents categorizes this regurgitation as valvular. Slight angulation of the transducer (D and E) reveals the presence of a large area of mosaic signals that appear to originate from the side of the anterior stent, indicating the presence of additional paravalvular regurgitation. The red signals in E indicate the presence of anteriorly directed regurgitant signals after they have been deflected by the posterior wall of the LA. These signals also are clearly seen in the short axis view (F).

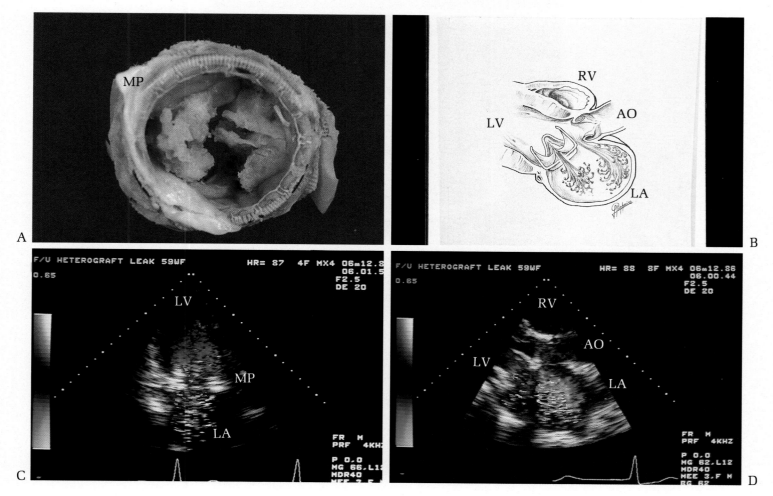

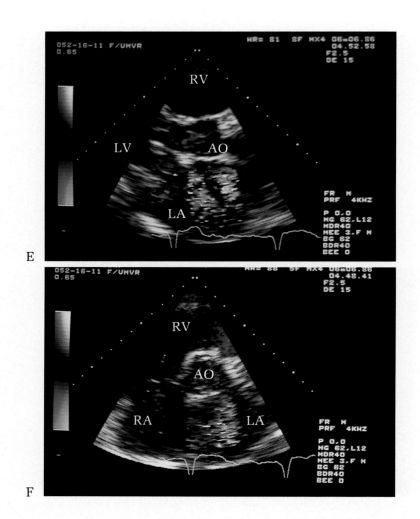

E

F

SECTION 7 PROSTHESES

Figure PR-18 **Regurgitation from porcine mitral prosthesis.** Apical views from 2D (A) and color Doppler (B) examinations of a 50-year-old man who had a porcine MV replacement in 1977 show prolapse of a thickened porcine leaflet into the LA. The mosaic signals in the LA during systole and originating from the prosthetic leaflets indicate valvular regurgitation in this patient. The green and red color signals on the left ventricular aspect of the leaflets represent flow acceleration (FA). The origin of the MR and the FA signals is not located beyond the prosthetic stents, indicating that the regurgitation is valvular and not paravalvular.

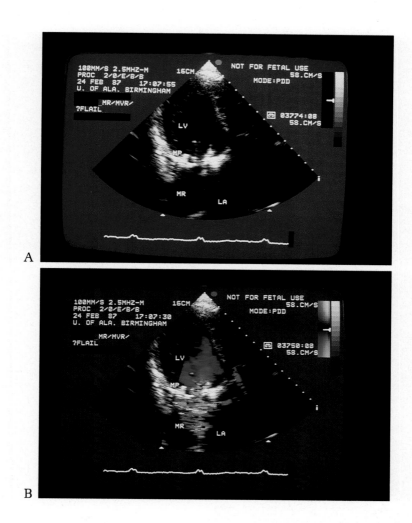

SECTION 7 PROSTHESES

Figure PR-19 **Regurgitation from porcine mitral prosthesis.** (A, B, and C) Apical views from a 78-year-old man with a Carpentier-Edwards MP show eccentrically directed mosaic signals originating from the side of the lateral stent. This implies the presence of paravalvular MR, which is displayed more prominently in B and C and represented schematically in D. The continuous wave Doppler cursor in the apical view on the right (E) is placed in the prosthetic inflow signals to record a peak pressure gradient of 20 mm Hg. The velocity waveform shown on the left shows a sharp downward slope from a high peak velocity, indicating that the high gradient obtained results from significant MR and not from prosthetic obstruction.

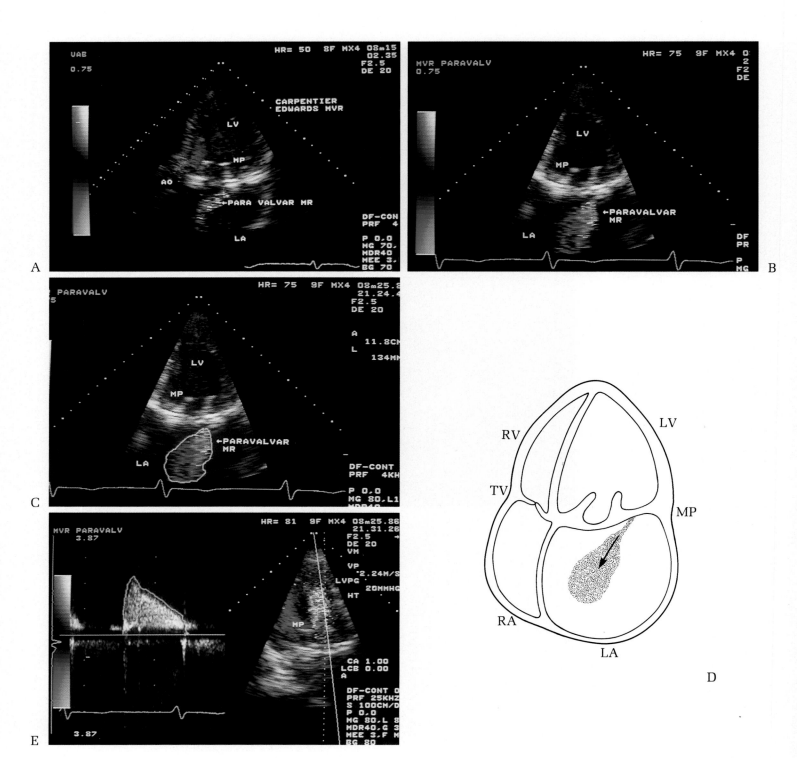

SECTION 7   PROSTHESES

Figure PR-20   **Regurgitation from porcine mitral prosthesis.** (A and B) Long axis view in a 30-year-old woman who had a porcine MV replacement in 1985 shows a narrow jet of mosaic signals in the LA during systole. These signals originate from the side of the anterior stent, implying paravalvular regurgitation. The small area of bluish-green signals on the ventricular side represents FA and its location beyond the anterior stent further supports the diagnosis of a paravalvular leak. The apical view (C) in this patient shows the blue signals of paravalvular regurgitation more prominently. The paravalvular leak in this patient was confirmed at surgery and repaired.

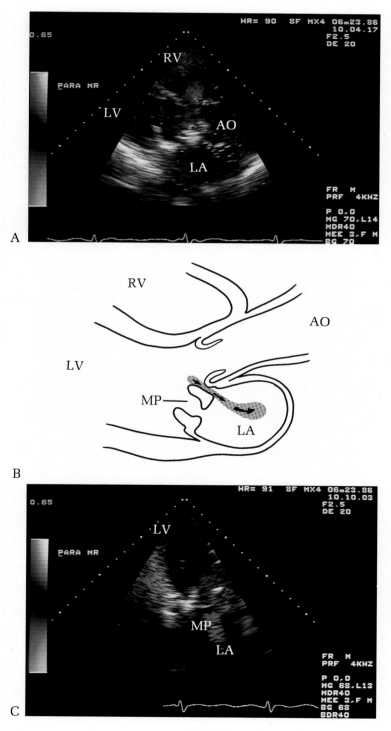

SECTION 7   PROSTHESES

Figure PR-21   **Regurgitation from porcine mitral prosthesis.** Long axis view in a 54-year-old man who has a Hancock MP reveals mosaic signals in the LA originating from the prosthesis. The green signals of FA (arrow) on the ventricular side of the prosthesis are located between the prosthetic stents, implying valvular regurgitation.

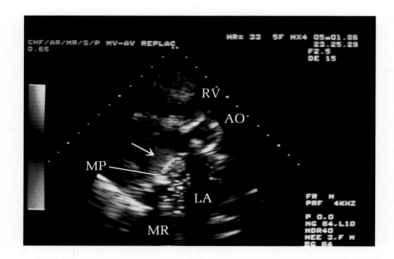

SECTION 7 PROSTHESES

Figure PR-22 **Regurgitation from porcine mitral prosthesis.** (A) Systolic frame of long axis view in a 61-year-old man who had a Carpentier-Edwards MV replacement shows mosaic signals of severe prosthetic regurgitation originating beyond the anterior stent. The tiny area of mosaic signals on the ventricular aspect of the MP represents flow acceleration (ACC), and its location beyond the stent confirms the presence of paravalvular regurgitation. (B) Apical view also shows MR signals and flow acceleration signals (ACC) beyond the anterior stent, further supporting the diagnosis of paravalvular MR from the anterior suture line. S = prosthetic stent.

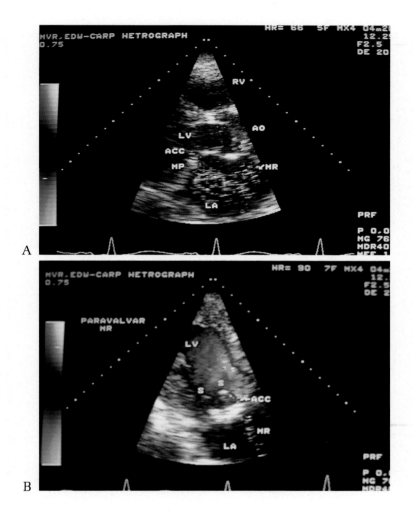

SECTION 7   PROSTHESES

Figure PR-23   **Regurgitation from porcine mitral prosthesis.** (A and B) Long axis views in a 52-year-old woman with a porcine MP shows blue signals of MR moving through the prosthesis into the LA, indicating valvular regurgitation. Minimal angulation of the transducer (C) reveals paravalvular MR from the side of the anterior stent. Further angulation of the transducer (D and E) reveals both valvular and paravalvular regurgitation. The valvular regurgitation is represented by mosaic signals moving within the stents, and the paravalvular regurgitation is represented by mosaic signals moving beyond the anterior stent. Note the presence of flow acceleration (A) in B, C, D, and E as a discrete linear band of mosaic-colored signals in the LVO along the outer margin of the anterior stent and directly opposite the paravalvar MR jet. Flow acceleration (A) is also noted in the LV within the confines of the stents and directly opposite the valvar MR jet in A, C, and D. The location of flow acceleration is useful in determining the type of prosthetic MR. In A, the flow signals have been turned off to show only the 2D image. (VMR = valvular regurgitation, PMR = paravalvular regurgitation, MP = mitral prosthesis.)

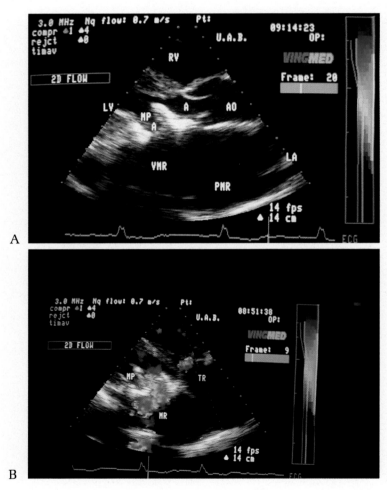

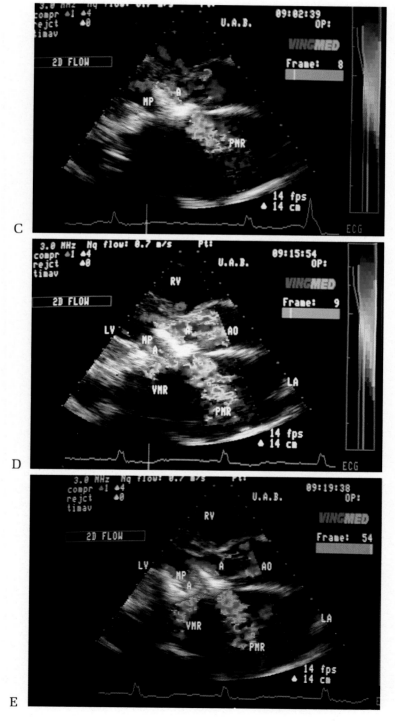

SECTION 7 PROSTHESES

Figure PR-24 **Regurgitation from porcine mitral prosthesis.** A 27-year-old man who had a recent porcine valve replacement had a fever of unknown etiology 2 weeks after surgery. The long axis view (A) in this patient at this time shows a small circular echolucent area between the MP and the aortic root, implying a possible abscess cavity. This area was constantly observed and did not appear to be an artifact. The systolic frame (B) shows mosaic signals originating from this echolucent area and moving into the LA, indicating significant paravalvular regurgitation PMR. Later, this patient was found to have bacterial endocarditis and underwent a reoperation. abs = abscess.

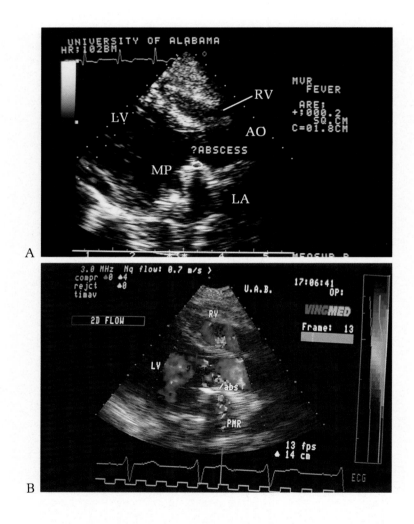

Figure PR-25 **Regurgitation from porcine mitral prosthesis.** Long axis view in a 72-year-old man who had a porcine MV replacement in 1978 shows two regurgitant jets during systole in the LA. These jets originate from within (vertical arrow) and beyond (horizontal arrow) the prosthetic stents, indicating both valvular and paravalvular regurgitation.

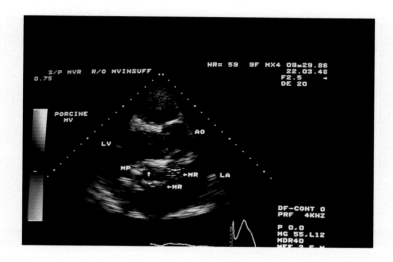

SECTION 7 PROSTHESES

Figure PR-26 **Regurgitation from porcine mitral prosthesis.** (A) Long axis view in a 46-year-old man who had a porcine MV valve replacement in 1974 shows a small area of mosaic signals in the LA during systole. These signals appear to originate beyond the posterior stent, implying PMR. The right parasternal views (B and C), however, disclose additional blue signals originating between the stents which suggests VMR. The mosaic PMR signals in these views become red after the jet strikes the left atrial posterior wall and moves anteriorly. Both the VMR and PMR regurgitant signals in a right parasternal view are well illustrated in the schematic (D). The malfunctioning porcine valve in this patient was replaced with a St. Jude prosthesis. S = stents.

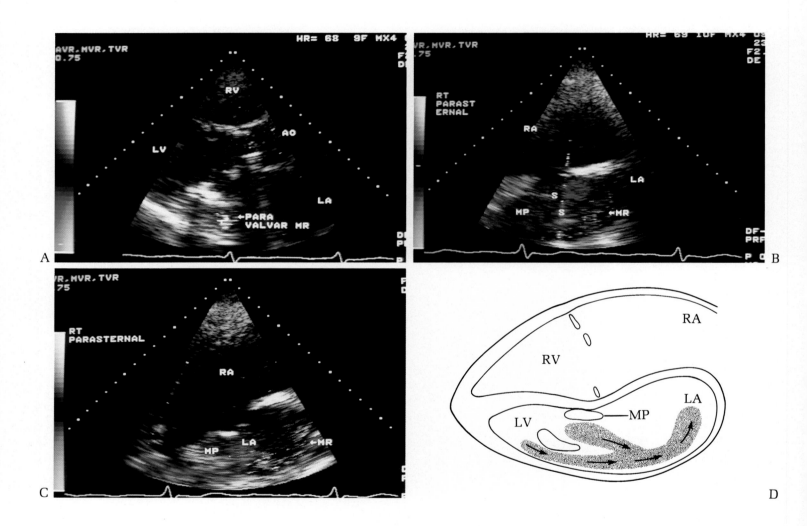

SECTION 7   PROSTHESES

Figure PR-27   **Regurgitation from porcine mitral prosthesis.** (A) Right parasternal view in a 65-year-old woman with a porcine MP shows blue signals moving from the LV into the LA through the prosthesis and the space between the atrial septum (AS) and the prosthesis. This flow pattern implies the presence of both VMR and PMR. The mosaic signals in the RA represent associated TR. Systolic frame (B) of a right parasternal view in another adult patient shows prominent blue signals filling a relatively large portion of the huge LA cavity. The origin of these signals is questionable, but because these signals fill the LA cavity only during systole, they are classified as mitral regurgitant signals. MR, confirmed subsequently at cardiac catheterization, could not be well visualized through the other conventional approaches.

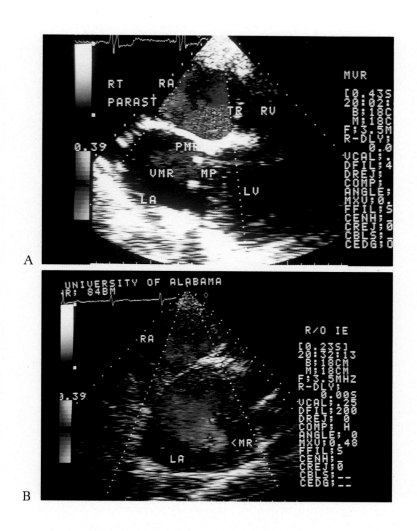

Figure PR-28 **Carpentier ring mitral annuloplasty.** (A) The Carpentier ring and thickened calcified leaflets (arrow) are observed in an autopsy specimen. Long axis views (B and C) in a 53-year-old man, who had a Carpentier ring inserted in 1986, display clearly the ring (R) and the mitral leaflets and show low-velocity flow signals moving from the LA to the LV through the ring. Red flow signals (B) are observed moving through the ring, but in the ventricle the flow signals become blue (C) as the flow moves posteriorly. Color M-mode examinations taken at the level of the ring (D) and through the leaflets (E) show red and blue flow signals, respectively, during diastole. The linear echoes observed posteriorly in D represent the reverberations from the ring (arrow). The continuous wave Doppler cursor in the long axis view (F) is placed parallel to the flow signals in the ring, and a peak pressure gradient of only 3 mm Hg is recorded, indicating no obstruction.

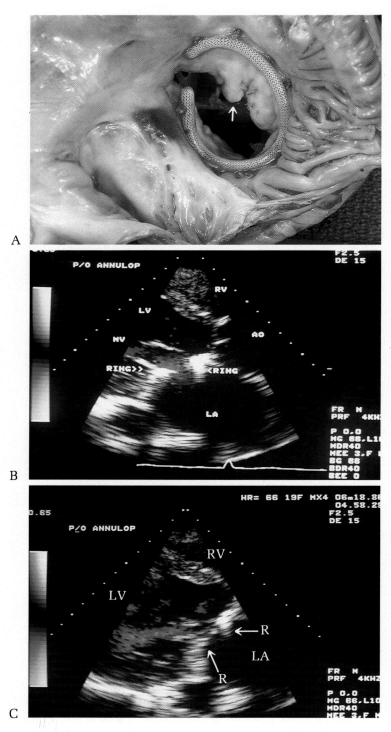

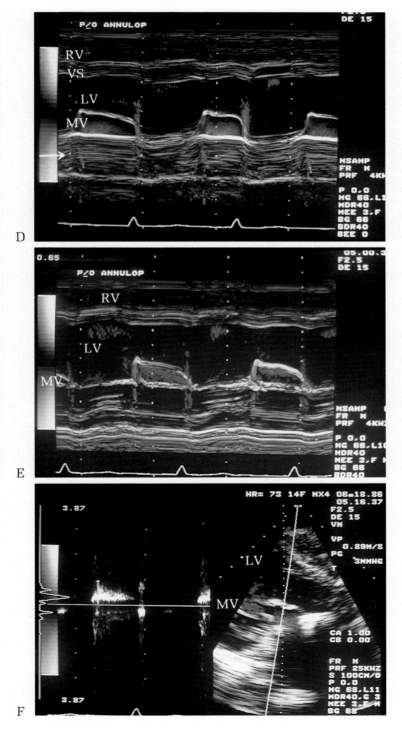

SECTION 7   PROSTHESES

Figure PR-29 **Carpentier ring annuloplasty.** (A) Apical 4-chamber view in a 28-year-old woman, who had a repair of an ostium primum ASD and a Carpentier ring inserted for significant MR, shows mosaic signals moving through the Carpentier ring into the LV. The continuous wave cursor (B) is placed parallel to the flow signals to obtain a peak pressure gradient of only 10 mm Hg. Therefore, the ring causes no obstruction. The arrows indicate parts of the Carpentier ring. Short axis view (C) shows a portion of the ring and red signals within the open mitral leaflets. Apical view (D) displays mosaic and blue signals in the LA, originating beyond the ring attachment or, in other words, "para-ring" MR, while E and F show blue signals originating through and beyond the ring, indicating the presence of additional regurgitation through the ring. The continuous wave cursor (G) passed through the "para-ring" regurgitant jet records the velocity waveform with a high peak velocity of 4.8 m/sec. Both types of regurgitation are represented schematically in H. R = Carpentier ring.

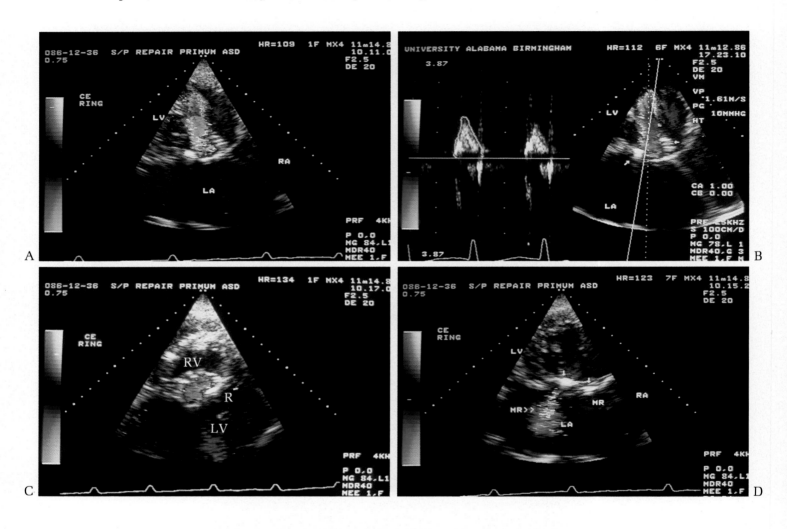

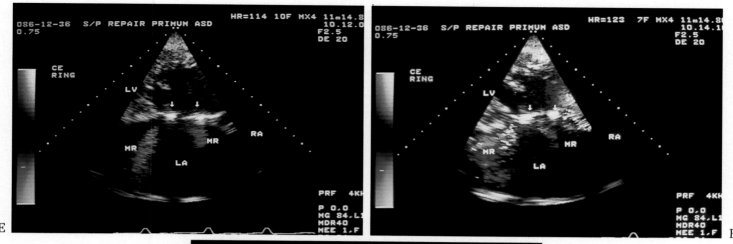

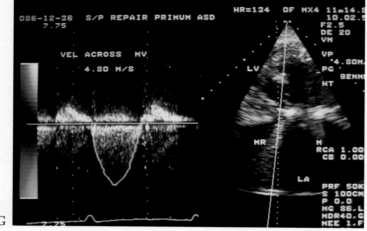

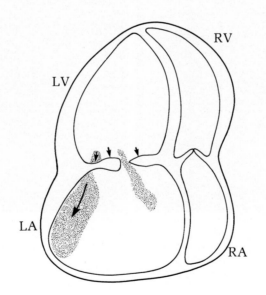

SECTION 7   PROSTHESES

Figure PR-30 **Carpentier ring annuloplasty.** (A and B) Short axis views in a 39-year-old woman who has had MV repair using a Carpentier ring show echoes from the native mitral leaflets anteriorly and brighter echoes of the ring posteriorly (R). The color flow examination in the short axis view (C) shows mosaic signals of turbulence within the orifice which is bounded by the native mitral leaflets and the Carpentier ring. Long axis view (D) shows prominent mosaic signals moving from the LA through the ring and the leaflets into the LV during diastole. R = parts of the Carpentier ring.

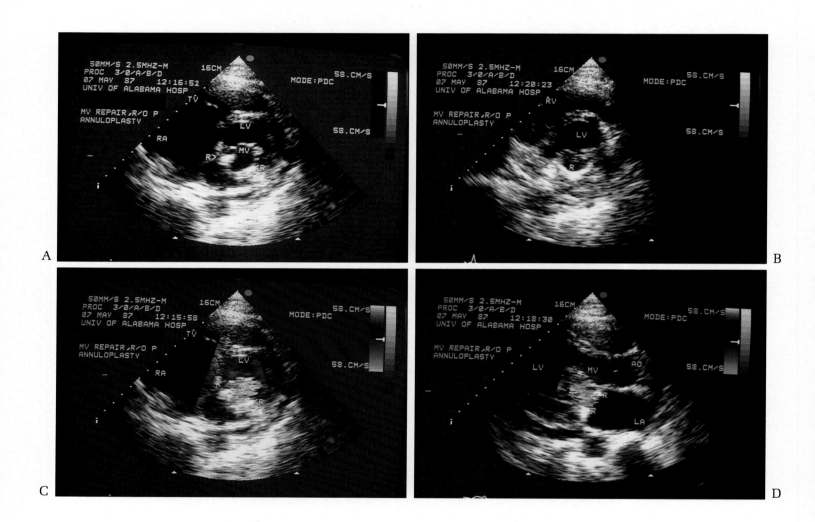

SECTION 7 PROSTHESES

Figure PR-31 **Mitral annuloplasty.** (A) Long axis view in an 18-year-old woman with rheumatic MV disease and mitral annuloplasty shows two jets of flow signals moving into the LV from the LA. The predominantly red jet is directed toward the VS and the predominantly blue is directed toward the LV posterior wall. The blue signals in the AO and in the LVOT represent normal LV outflow. The color M-mode examination (B) through these jets from the apical approach shows, during diastole, mosaic turbulent signals of FA on the atrial aspect of the valve. The mosaic signals during systole in the LA represent MR. The continuous wave cursor (C) placed parallel to the diastolic mosaic signals records a peak velocity of 2.7 m/sec (peak pressure gradient = 29 mm Hg), indicating significant obstruction across the repaired MV. The spectral signals below the baseline during systole represent MR.

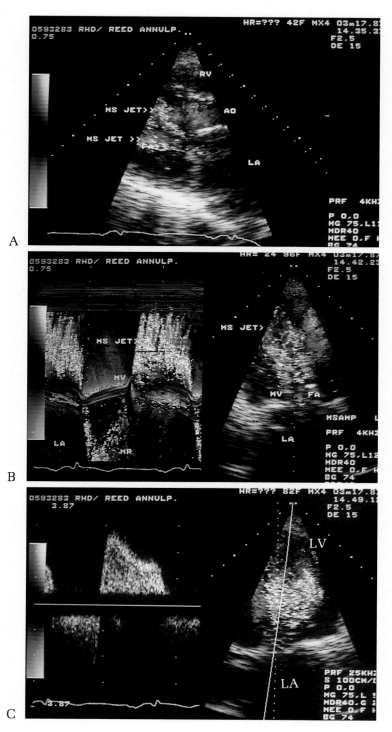

SECTION 7 PROSTHESES

Figure PR-32 **Residual regurgitation following mitral annuloplasty.** Color M-mode examination in a 40-year-old woman with a Carpentier ring annuloplasty reveals the presence of pansystolic MR.

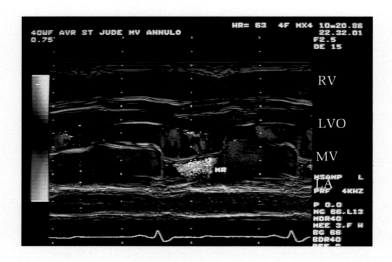

Figure PR-33   **Bjork-Shiley aortic prosthesis.** (A) Schematic illustrates a Bjork-Shiley aortic prosthesis in the open position during systole. (B and C) Long axis views show mosaic signals moving through the prosthesis (AP) into the aortic root during systole. The blue signals in the LVOT indicate normal velocity flow signals, while the mosaic signals in the aortic root imply turbulence.

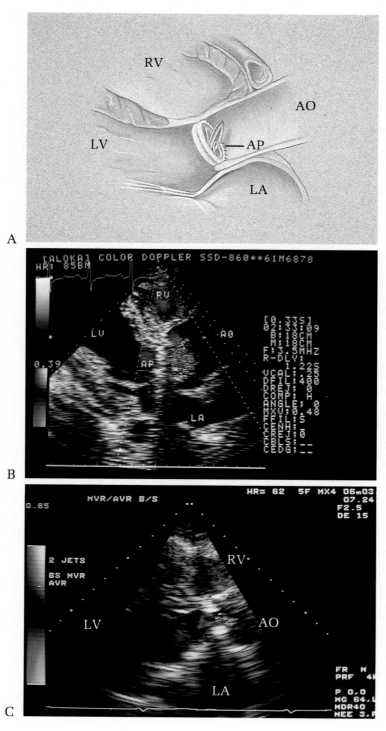

SECTION 7   PROSTHESES

Figure PR-34   **Regurgitation from a Bjork-Shiley aortic prosthesis.** Long axis view in a 38-year-old female who received a Bjork-Shiley aortic prosthesis (AP) in 1983 shows mosaic signals completely filling the LVOT during diastole, indicating severe AR.

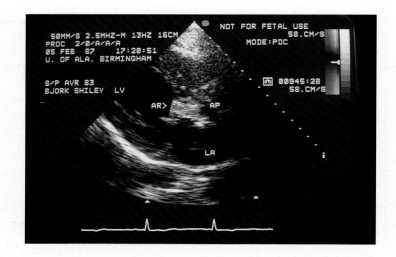

Figure PR-35 **Regurgitation from a Bjork-Shiley aortic prosthesis.** A 33-year-old man had a Bjork-Shiley AV replacement in 1984 because of severe AR resulting from bacterial endocarditis. Apical view displays a broad band of mosaic signals originating from the Bjork-Shiley prosthesis during diastole, indicating severe AR. AP = aortic prosthesis.

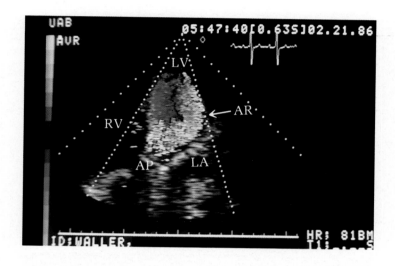

SECTION 7 PROSTHESES

Figure PR-36 **Paravalvular regurgitation from a Bjork-Shiley aortic prosthesis.** (A) Autopsy specimen shows a large gap (arrows) at the suture line of the Bjork-Shiley valve, indicating dehiscence of the prosthesis. Long axis views in a 36-year-old man (B) and a 30-year-old man (C) with Bjork-Shiley AV replacement show eccentric jets of bluish-green and bluish-red signals originating from the side of the anterior stent of the prosthesis, indicating PMR. BS = Bjork-Shiley prosthesis.

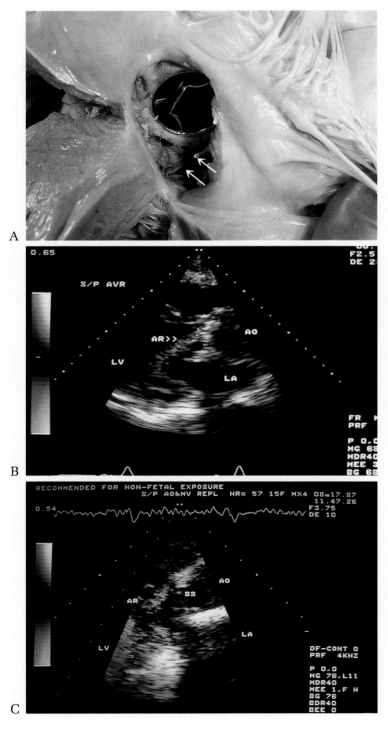

SECTION 7 PROSTHESES

Figure PR-37 **Paravalvular regurgitation from the Bjork-Shiley aortic valve prosthesis.**
(A and B) Diastolic frames of the long axis view in a 45-year-old man who has had bacterial
endocarditis after AV replacement show two jets of AR in the LVOT, originating from the
Bjork-Shiley prosthesis (AP). The green jet which originates from the extreme anterior aspect of
the prosthesis probably represents paravalvular regurgitation while the blue jet which originates from the center of the prosthesis represents valvular regurgitation. The blue and red
signals on the aortic aspect of the prosthesis represent flow acceleration (FA). The apical
4-chamber view (C) shows a circular echolucent area in the LVOT, and the apical view (D) shows
an additional localized echolucent area in the superior portion of the prosthesis. These echolucent areas indicate the possible presence of abscess cavities (AB). Color flow examinations (E and
F) show a jet of yellow signals along the VS and another jet of yellow signals towards the anterior
mitral leaflet. The location of these diastolic signals near the extreme anterior and posterior
aspects of the prosthesis implies the presence of two distinct areas of paravalvular AR in this
patient. AVP = aortic valve prosthesis; BS = Bjork-Shiley prosthesis.

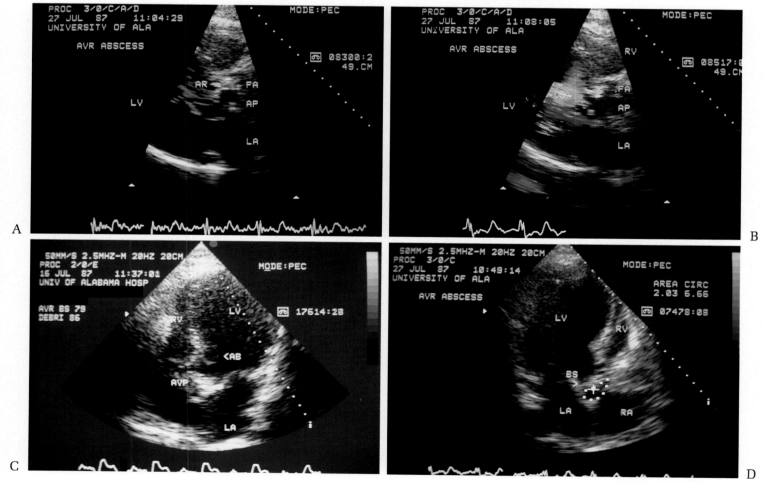

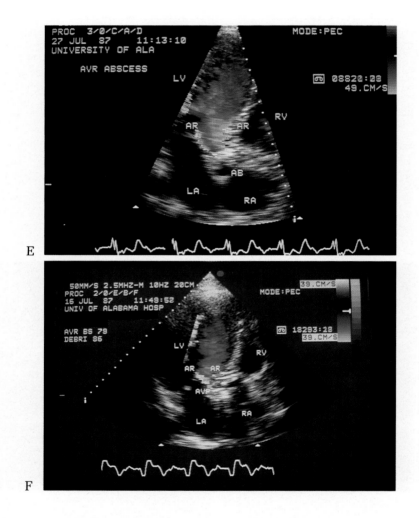

E

F

SECTION 7 PROSTHESES

Figure PR-38 Normal St. Jude aortic prosthesis. (A and B) Long axis views in a 33-year-old man who had a St. Jude's AV replacement in 1987 show red (A) and blue (B) normal velocity flow signals in the LVOT moving through a St. Jude's prosthesis into the aortic root. Both the red and blue signals change into mosaic signals in the aortic root, indicating the presence of turbulence. Long axis view (C) in another adult patient shows mosaic turbulent signals moving from the LVOT through the St. Jude prosthesis into the aortic root. The suprasternal examination in the same patient as C (D) reveals mosaic turbulent signals moving through the AP. The blue signals in the proximal AA represent aliasing and the distal red signals indicate normal velocity flow farther downstream.

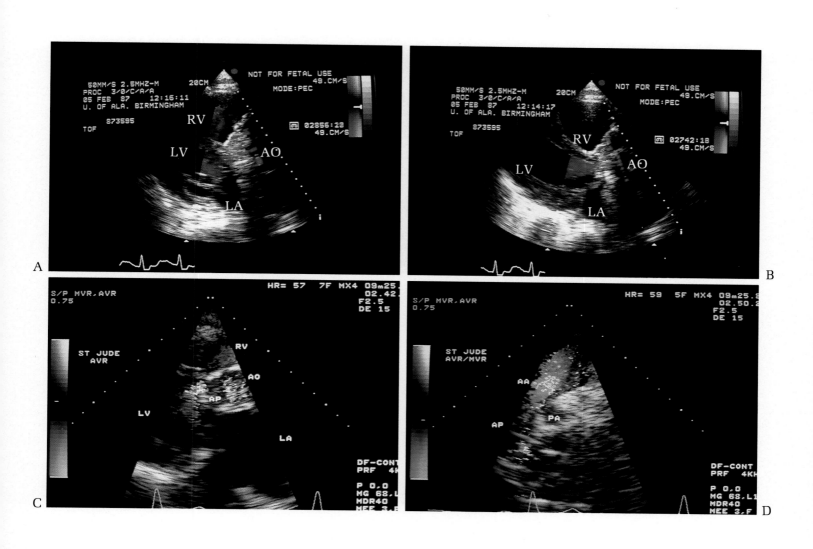

SECTION 7   PROSTHESES

Figure PR-39   **Normal aortic prosthesis viewed from right parasternal position.** The right parasternal view in a patient with a St. Jude aortic prosthesis reveals mosaic signals in the AA, and the continuous wave cursor placed parallel to these signals records a peak velocity of 1.92 m/sec. This translates into a peak pressure gradient of 15 mm Hg using the Bernoulli equation, and thus this patient has no prosthetic obstruction. AVR = aortic valve replacement.

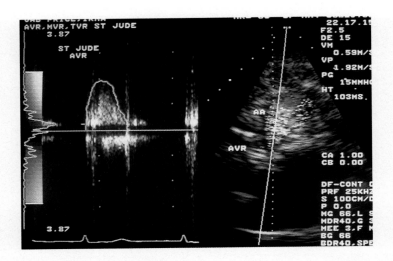

SECTION 7   PROSTHESES

Figure PR-40   **St. Jude aortic prosthesis: Obstruction.** (A) Long axis view in a 57-year-old woman shows mosaic signals representing flow through the AP. The continuous wave cursor is placed through these flow signals to record a peak pressure gradient of only 24 mm Hg, which is considerably less than the 54 mm Hg obtained from the suprasternal transducer position (B). Even though the continuous wave cursor appears to be parallel to the flow signals in the 2D color image (A), it may not be parallel to these signals in all planes because of the 3-dimensional nature of the prosthetic jet. Therefore, the transducer needs to be slightly angled further to be parallel to the "core" of the jet.

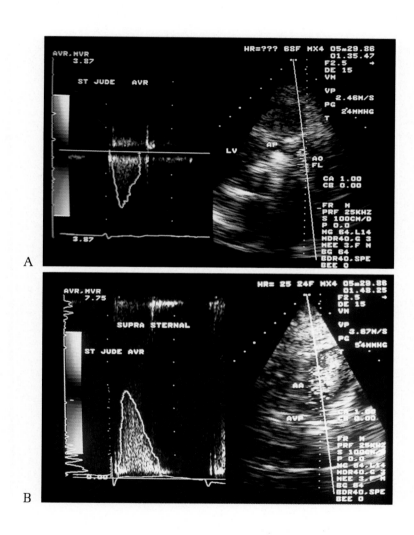

SECTION 7 PROSTHESES

Figure PR-41 Regurgitation from the St. Jude aortic prosthesis. Long axis view in a patient who had an aortic graft with a St. Jude prosthesis (AP) for an aortic aneurysm shows a narrow jet of red signals in the LVOT during diastole, implying AR. The narrow width of the regurgitation flow signals suggests that the aortic leak is small.

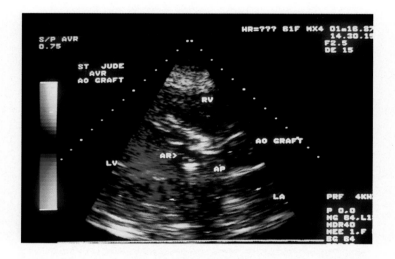

SECTION 7 PROSTHESES

Figure PR-42 **Paravalvular regurgitation from the St. Jude aortic prosthesis.** The long axis view (A) in a 57-year-old man who received a St. Jude AP in 1985 shows a narrow jet of red signals originating from the posterior side of the sewing ring, indicating the presence of mild paravalvular regurgitation. Minimal angulation of the transducer as shown in B reveals additional paravalvular regurgitant signals, blue in color, originating from the anterior side of the sewing ring. These signals in the same patient are seen more prominently on a different color Doppler system (C).

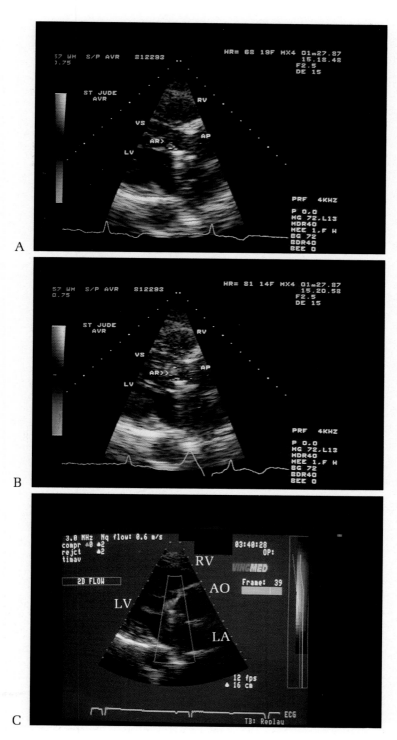

Figure PR-43 **Regurgitation from the St. Jude aortic prosthesis.** (A and B) Long axis views in a 43-year-old man with a St. Jude aortic prosthesis (AVR) shows predominantly green signals moving between the prosthesis and the anterior wall of the aorta, implying paravalvular regurgitation (PAR). (C) Long axis view shows additional bluish-green signals of valvular regurgitation (VAR) originating from the central portion of the prosthesis and moving posteriorly towards the anterior mitral leaflet.

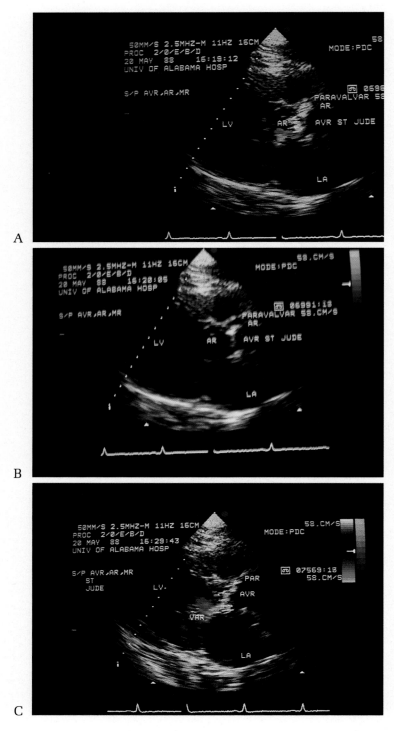

SECTION 7 PROSTHESES

Figure PR-44 **Regurgitation from the St. Jude aortic prosthesis.** (A) Suprasternal examination in a patient with a St. Jude's aortic prosthesis displays mosaic signals in the proximal and blue signals in the distal AA resulting from turbulence and complete aliasing, respectively. At the level of the aortic arch (ARCH), small flecks of blue color resulting from aliasing appear within the expected red signals. Color M-mode examinations (B and C) at the level of the AA show antegrade (forward flow) blue and mosaic signals during systole and retrograde (reverse flow) blue signals of AR during diastole. Color M-mode examination of the DA (D) shows retrograde red signals of AR during diastole. The systolic blue signals indicate forward flow in the DA and the red signals within them represent aliasing. FF = forward flow; BF = backflow.

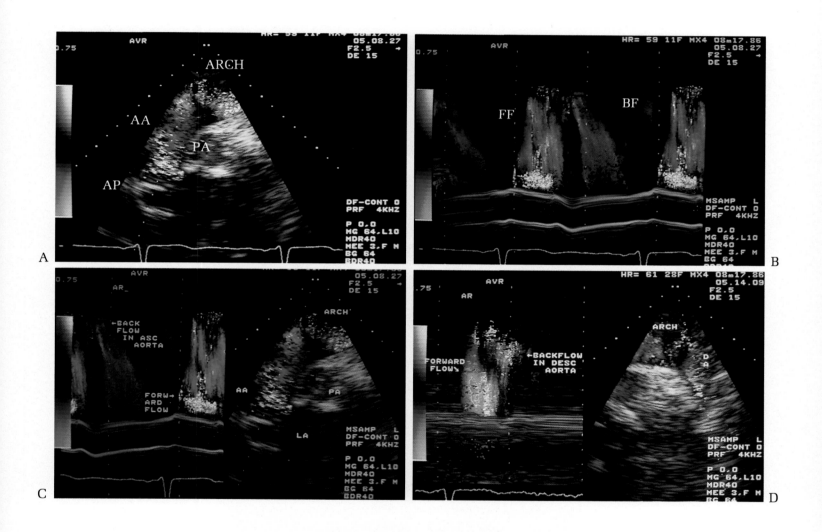

SECTION 7 PROSTHESES

Figure PR-45 **Normal porcine aortic prosthesis.** (A) Long axis view in a 41-year-old man shows two stents of the porcine aortic prosthesis (AP) with thin leaflets in the open position. Color flow examination (B) shows red signals moving through the AP into the aorta while the aortic short axis view (C) shows the three stents of the prosthesis and flow signals within the aorta.

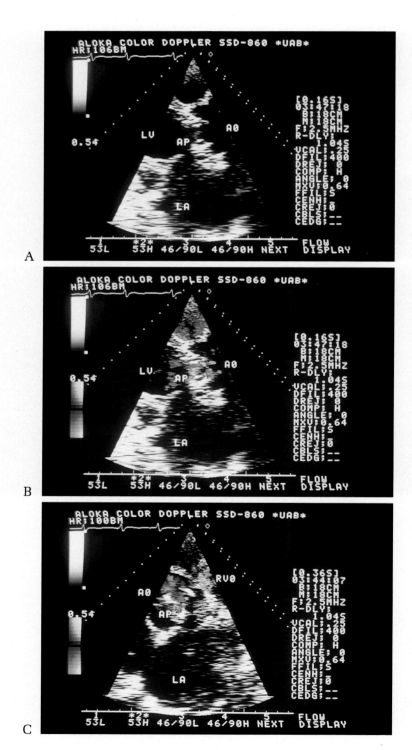

SECTION 7 PROSTHESES

Figure PR-46 **Carpentier-Edwards aortic prosthesis viewed from the right parasternal position.** Examination of the AP in a woman patient from the right parasternal view is shown in A, B, and C. Mosaic systolic signals resulting from turbulent flow through the prosthesis are shown in B. The continuous wave cursor (C) placed parallel to these signals records a peak velocity of 3.07 m/sec, which translates into a peak pressure gradient of 38 mm Hg. The pulse Doppler sample volume is placed in the flow signals in the LVOT in the apical view (D) to measure a peak velocity of 1.39 m/sec. The LVOT diameter measured in the long axis view (E) equals 1.8 cm, and using the continuity equation, an effective prosthetic valve area of 1.15 cm² is calculated, indicating mild to moderate prosthetic obstruction.

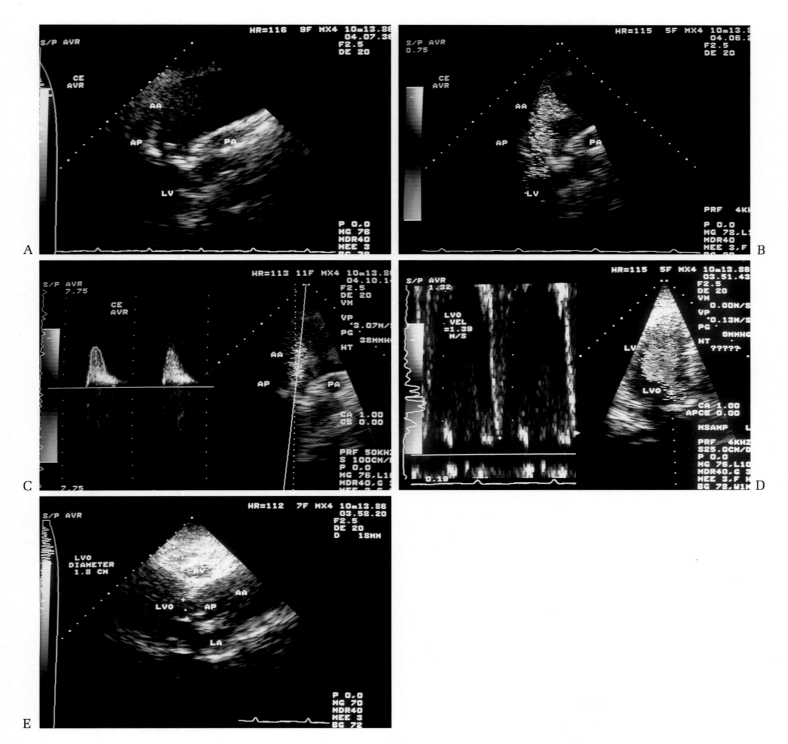

SECTION 7 PROSTHESES

Figure PR-47 **Porcine aortic prosthesis.** The arrows in the long axis views (A and B) and the short axis view (C) in a 28-year-old woman point to the aortic prosthesis stents. The closed porcine leaflets are seen in A between the stents. The color Doppler examination in B displays mosaic colors moving through the prosthesis into the aortic root, representing turbulence, which is schematically shown in the long axis view (D). Examination of the porcine prosthesis from the suprasternal/right parasternal view is shown in E and F, and schematically in G. Color flow examination shows mosaic systolic signals resulting from turbulence in the AA, and the continuous wave cursor placed parallel to these signals records a peak velocity of only 2.10 m/sec (H). The pulse Doppler sample volume is placed in the LVOT in the apical view (I) to measure a peak velocity of 0.77 m/sec. The inside diameter of the LVOT measured in the long axis view (J) equals 1.6 cm, and using the continuity equation, an effective prosthetic valve area of 1.0 cm² is calculated, indicating moderate obstruction of the prosthesis.

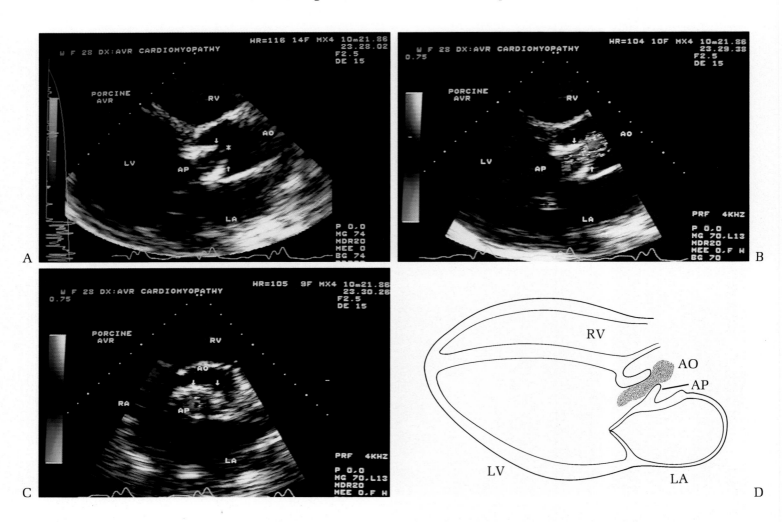

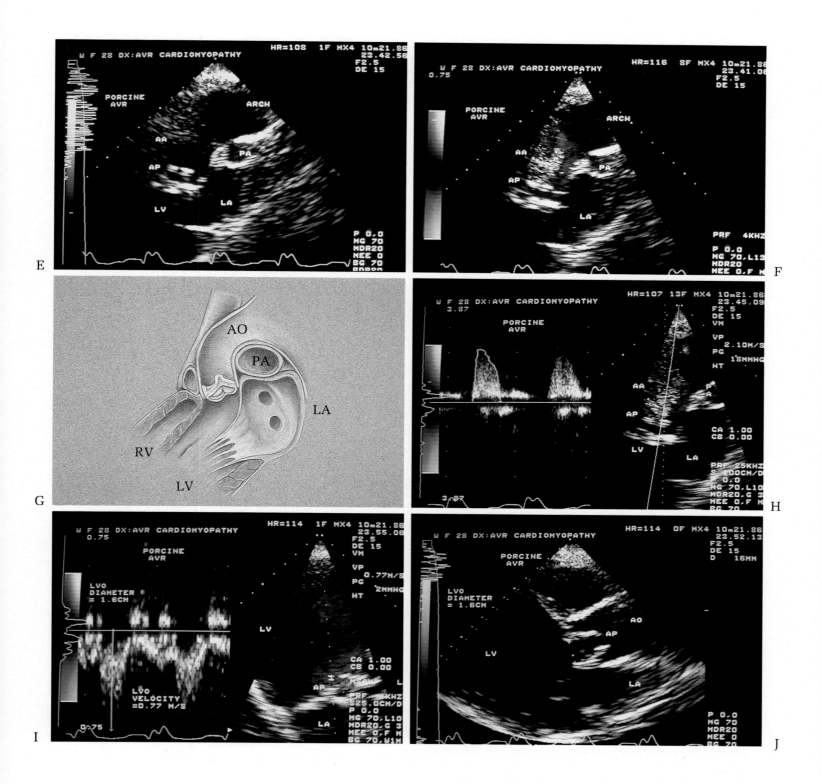

SECTION 7 PROSTHESES

Figure PR-48 **Significant regurgitation from porcine aortic prosthesis.** (A, B, and C) Long axis views in this patient show mosaic signals of valvular regurgitation originating centrally from the porcine AP. These signals merge with the mitral inflow (MI) further downstream. The jet appears to be wider in B and C than in A because slight angling of the transducer allows better alignment of the ultrasound beam with the regurgitant flow. The apical view (D) displays a wide jet of significant AR. In E, the continuous wave cursor is placed parallel to the mosaic signals of AR to obtain a high peak pressure gradient of 72 mm Hg with the velocity waveform showing a slow deceleration, implying normal left ventricular end-diastolic pressure.

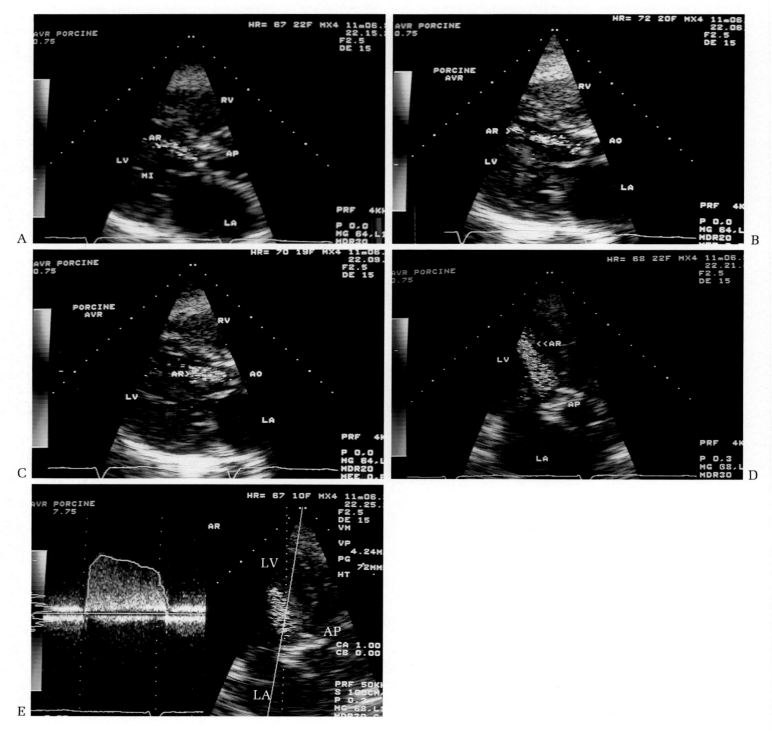

Figure PR-49 **Significant regurgitation from a porcine aortic prosthesis.** Long axis view in a 35-year-old man who had a porcine AV replacement in 1980 shows mosaic signals filling approximately 60% of the LVOT, indicating moderately severe AR. These regurgitant signals are directed along the anterior mitral leaflet.

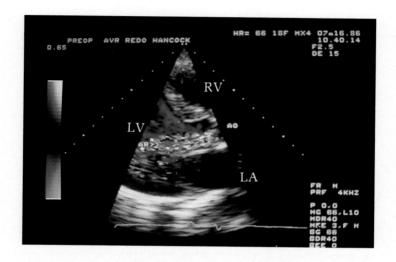

SECTION 7   PROSTHESES

Figure PR-50 **Regurgitation from porcine aortic valve prosthesis.** (A, B, and C) Long axis views in a 50-year-old man with porcine AV and MV replacements shows mosaic signals (FL) through the porcine AP during systole. The mitral MP is also seen in these views. The diastolic frame (C) shows mosaic signals filling almost the entire LVOT immediately below the prosthesis, implying severe AR.

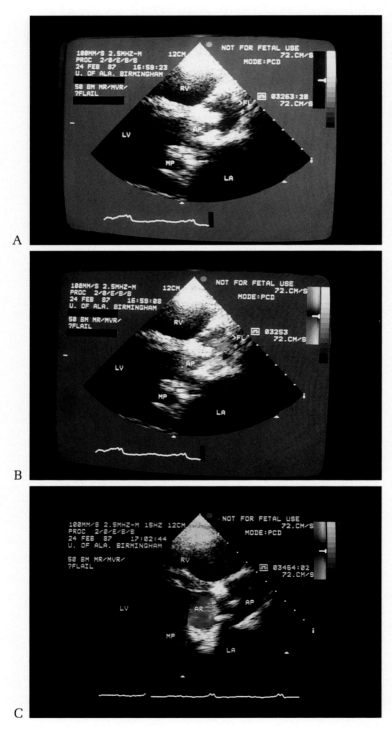

SECTION 7   PROSTHESES

Figure PR-51   **Severe aortic regurgitation from prolapse of porcine aortic leaflet.** A 35-year-old man had a porcine AV replacement in 1979. Long axis views (A and B) in this patient using different color Doppler machines show one leaflet (L) of the AP prolapsing into the LVOT and mosaic signals of severe AR (A) completely filling the LVOT. The degenerated porcine prosthesis was replaced with a St. Jude valve.

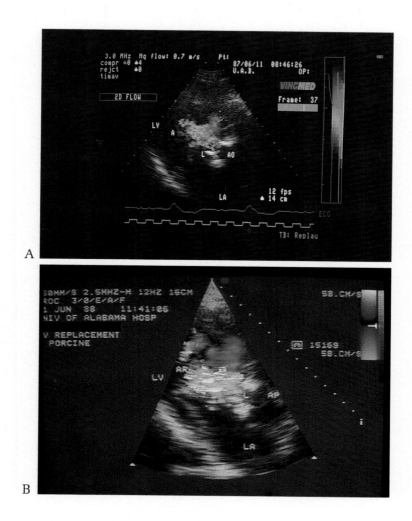

SECTION 7 PROSTHESES

Figure PR-52 **Regurgitation from a porcine aortic prosthesis.** A 65-year-old man had a porcine AV replacement in 1987 because of infective endocarditis and severe AR. The long axis views (A and B) reveal mosaic and red signals filling most of the LVOT, implying persistence of severe AR. The mosaic signals are directed initially towards the VS and then posteriorly towards the mitral leaflets as shown in B. An abscess cavity drained at surgery is shown in A and labeled "C." AP = aortic prosthesis.

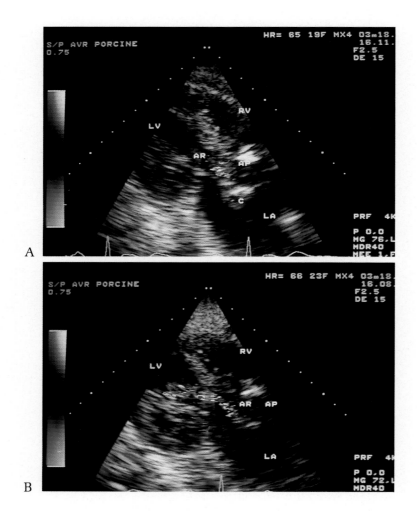

SECTION 7 PROSTHESES

Figure PR-53 **Regurgitation from porcine aortic prosthesis.** (A) Long axis view in a 57-year-old man who had a porcine AV replacement in 1976 shows a mosaic jet originating from the side of the anterior stent during diastole, indicating a paravalvular leak at this site. The paravalvular aortic leak is shown schematically in B. AP = aortic prosthesis.

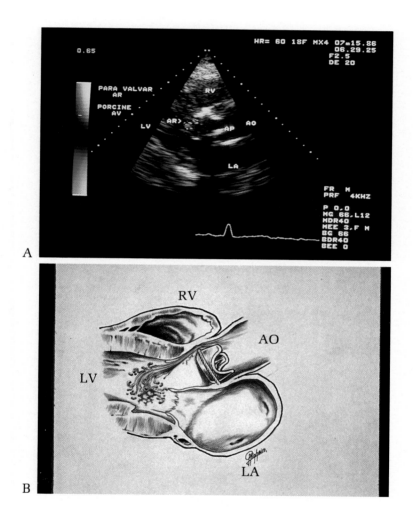

SECTION 7 PROSTHESES

Figure PR-54 **Regurgitation from porcine aortic prosthesis.** (A) Long axis view in a 66-year-old woman who had a porcine AV replacement in 1980 shows two distinct jets of AR. The red jet (J1) originates at the extreme anterior aspect of the prosthesis, and the blue jet (J2) at the extreme posterior aspect. Their origins imply that both of these jets represent paravalvular regurgitation. Slight angling of the transducer (B) shows two jets of bluish-green signals in the LVOT during diastole, implying significant AR.

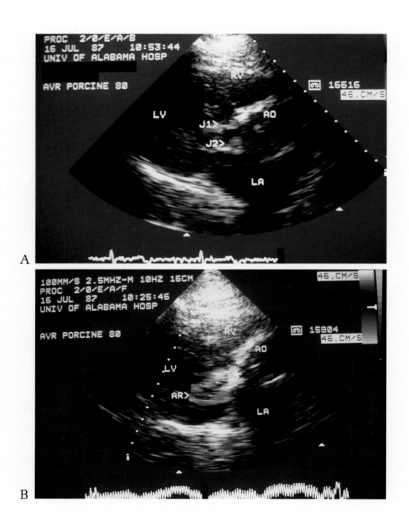

Figure PR-55 **Homograft aortic valve replacement.** (A) Long axis view in a 26-year-old man with a homograft aortic valve (HAV) shows a narrow band of red signals during diastole, indicating mild AR. These signals of AR occur throughout the diastolic period as shown by color M-mode examination (B).

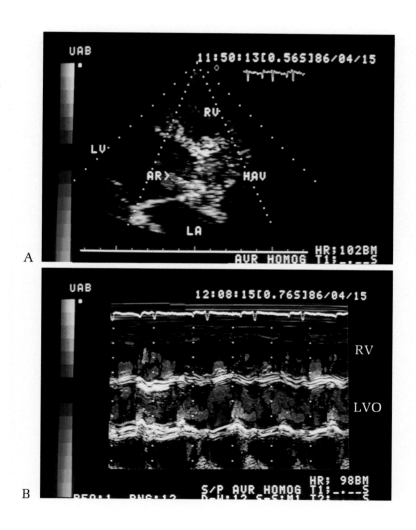

SECTION 7 PROSTHESES

Figure PR-56 **Homograft aortic valve replacement.** A 60-year-old man had an AV homograft replacement (AVR) in 1987 for bacterial endocarditis. The apical long axis view shows a narrow band of mosaic signals originating from the homograft valve during diastole, indicating mild AR. The echolucent area superiorly represents a debrided and drained abscess cavity (AB) in this patient.

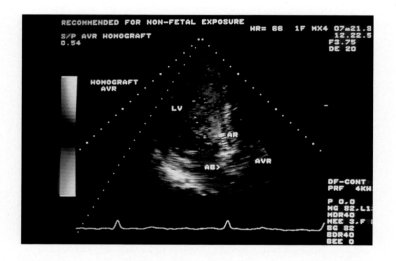

SECTION 7   PROSTHESES

Figure PR-57   Normal St. Jude tricuspid prosthesis. (A) Aortic short axis view in a 55-year-old woman with Ebstein's anomaly and a St. Jude TP shows three discrete flow jets (J1, J2, and J3) in the RV. Two of these jets (J1 and J3) originate from the open St. Jude leaflets, while the third (J2) originates from the central area of the valve, as schematically illustrated in B.

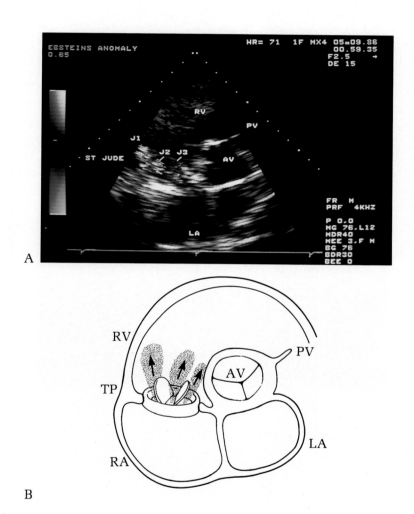

SECTION 7 PROSTHESES

Figure PR-58 **Normal porcine tricuspid prosthesis.** (A) Short axis view in a 46-year-old man shows mosaic signals resulting from turbulence moving across the TP into the RV, while the apical view (B) reveals blue and red signals moving across the TP into the RV. These blue signals in the center of the jet are caused by aliasing. The schematic (C) illustrates flow through a normal porcine prosthesis in the tricuspid position in an apical view.

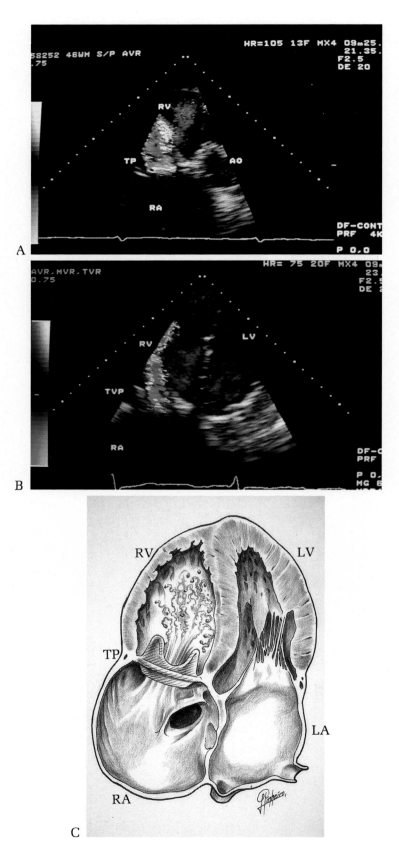

SECTION 7 PROSTHESES

Figure PR-59 **Normal porcine tricuspid prosthesis.** (A and B) Color M-mode examination from the apical view in a 66-year-old woman who had mitral commissurotomy and a porcine TV replacement in 1986 shows red signals during diastole moving through the prosthesis into the RV. The blue color within the red signals in B represents aliasing, and the beat-to-beat variation in the tricuspid inflow color results from atrial fibrillation. TP = tricuspid prosthesis, F = tricuspid inflow.

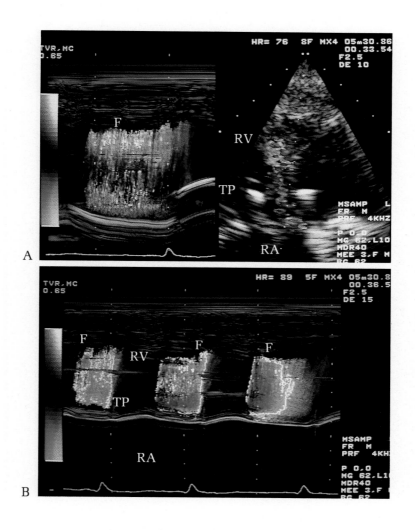

SECTION 7 PROSTHESES

Figure PR-60 **Obstructed porcine tricuspid prosthesis.** (A) Right ventricular inflow view in a 14-year-old child with a tricuspid heterograft shows thickened porcine prosthetic leaflets (THV) and a prominent jet of mosaic signals (SJ) moving through a restricted prosthetic orifice (EO) into the RV. Note that the flow signals are very narrow at the valve orifice level but widen considerably downstream in the RV. In B, the continuous wave cursor (C), passed through the stenotic jet (J), records a peak pressure gradient of 20 mm Hg across the TP, indicating significant obstruction.

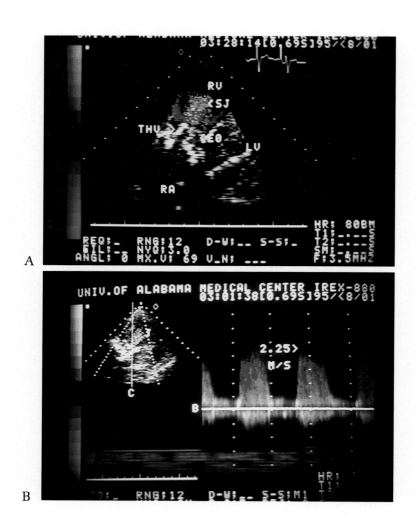

SECTION 7 PROSTHESES

Figure PR-61 **Left ventricular-aortic conduit.** (A and B) Apical views in this patient show a
conduit (CON) placed at the left ventricular apex (AP). Normal low-velocity blue signals moving
through the conduit during systole are shown in A, while the diastolic frame (B) shows normal
left ventricular inflow signals in red and the absence of regurgitation from the conduit. Clinically, this patient has a normally functioning conduit. An autopsy specimen from another
patient (C) shows an LV–AO conduit (arrows).

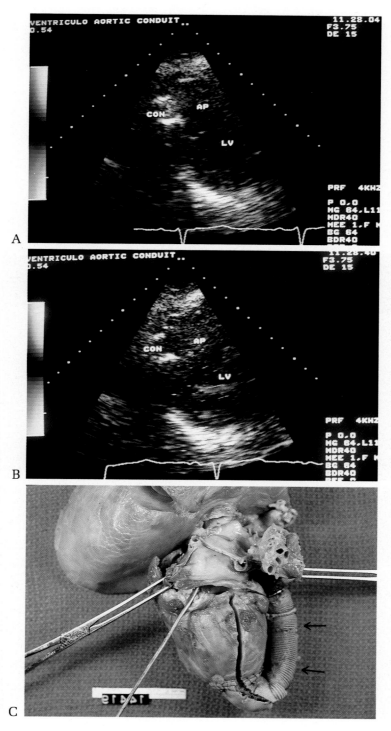

SECTION 7 PROSTHESES

Figure PR-62 **Severe regurgitation from a left ventricular-aortic conduit.** A 30-year-old man had both a Bjork-Shiley AV replacement and a porcine valved conduit from the left ventricular apex to the AO implanted in 1980. The apical views (A–D) in this patient show the conduit clearly situated at the left ventricular apex. The systolic frame (A) displays blue and yellow signals in the region of the conduit resulting from high-velocity turbulent and aliased flow moving into the conduit, while the mosaic signals observed in B (also in systole) in the region of the conduit result from turbulence. The dark red signals in both A and B farther upstream in the LV indicate normal velocity flow directed toward the conduit. The diastolic frames (C and D) display a large area of blue signals originating from the conduit, implying considerable conduit regurgitation, while the late diastolic frame (D) also displays red signals which represent a swirling of the regurgitant signals as they move towards the left ventricular inflow and then back towards the apex. The conduit regurgitation is clearly illustrated in schematic E and the swirling effect is well demonstrated in schematic F. C = conduit, CP = conduit prosthesis.

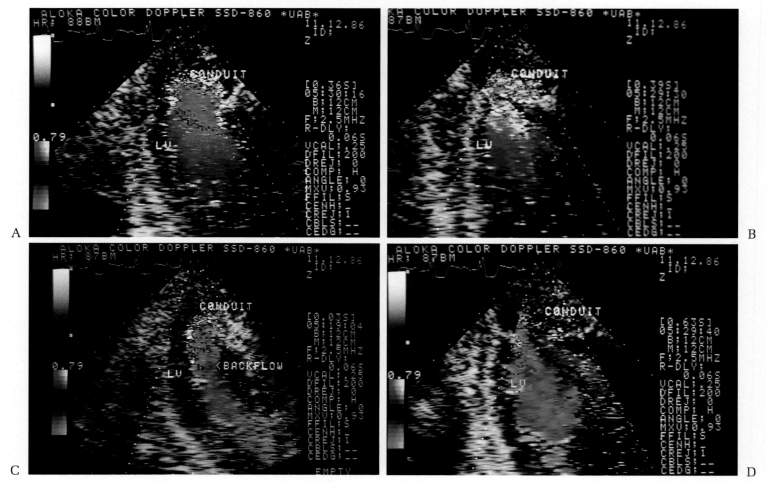

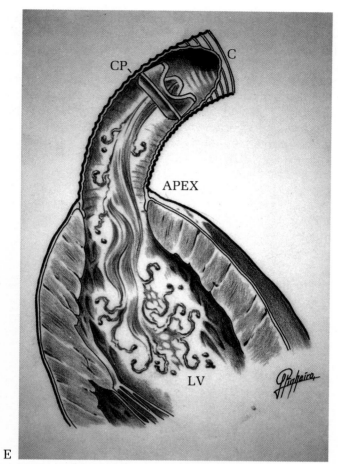

E

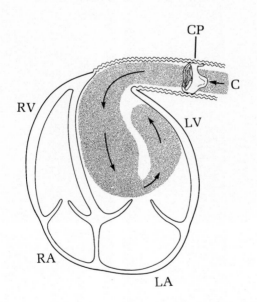

F

Figure PR-63   **Alleviation of conduit regurgitation by St. Jude valve replacement.** The malfunctioning porcine valve of the left ventricular-aortic conduit implanted in the 30-year-old man in Figure PR-62 was replaced by a St. Jude valve. Apical views (A–G) in this patient show the conduit clearly situated at the left ventricular apex. Systolic frames (A and B) show blue and reddish-yellow signals moving into the conduit. These blue signals result from aliasing. The late diastolic frame (C) displays red signals, which represent mitral inflow, and blue signals, which represent flow moving from the left ventricular apex towards the outflow tract. No diastolic flow signals moving from the conduit to the apex are seen in this frame, implying the absence of conduit regurgitation. The expanded apical view (D) clearly displays the rugae of the corrugated conduit (arrows) and the St. Jude valve within it. The color Doppler examination (E) shows blue and yellow signals within the conduit, indicating turbulence. The continuous wave cursor (F) passed through the flow signals in the conduit records a peak velocity of 3.0 m/sec, which translates into a peak pressure gradient of 36 mm Hg, implying the absence of significant conduit obstruction. The diastolic frame (G) of the conduit (C) displays a narrow jet of red signals (L), indicating a minimal leak through the St. Jude prosthesis (P).

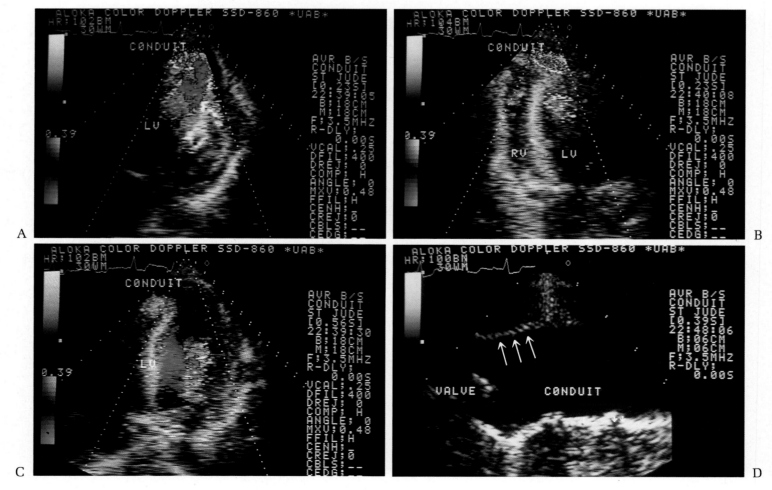

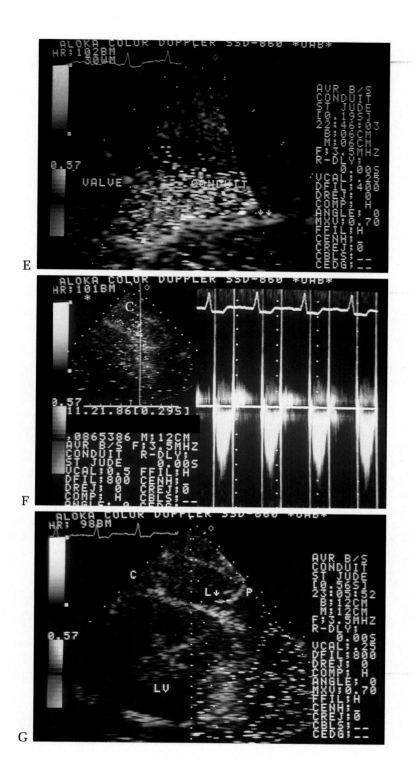

Section 8

CARDIOMYOPATHY AND CONSTRICTIVE PERICARDITIS

HYPERTROPHIC CARDIOMYOPATHY

Color Doppler examination supplements 2D and conventional Doppler assessment in patients with hypertrophic cardiomyopathy. In general, color Doppler displays turbulent mosaic signals in the narrowed LVOT, which indicates the presence of a subaortic obstruction. These mosaic signals may extend into the aortic root and proximal ascending aorta. Color M-mode examination also shows mosaic signals in the LVOT between the systolic anterior movement of the MV and the VS.

In addition, both of these techniques show mosaic signals in the LA originating from the MV during systole, indicating the presence of associated MR. This associated MR, as shown by the color M-mode, develops later during systole after the occurrence of the systolic anterior movement of the MV. In most patients with hypertrophic cardiomyopathy, associated MR does not occur during early systole but after turbulent flow is observed in the LVOT. In some patients with hypertrophic cardiomyopathy, however, MR is shown to be pansystolic and thus to occur before, or occasionally simultaneously with, the appearance of the turbulent flow signals in the LVOT. The severity of the MR in patients with hypertrophic cardiomyopathy can be evaluated by planimetering the maximum area of the mitral regurgitant flow and expressing it as the ratio to the left atrial area measured in the same frame. Most patients with hypertrophic cardiomyopathy show moderate MR, but mild or severe MR may be observed in some patients. Other associated lesions such as TR or AR can also be assessed by color Doppler.

In a patient with hypertrophic cardiomyopathy, absence of mosaic signals in the LVOT implies the absence of turbulence and, thus, the absence of any resting pressure gradient. Amyl nitrate inhalation during a color Doppler study in patients with hypertrophic cardiomyopathy usually results in increased MR, causing the mitral regurgitant area to become conspicuously larger. Amyl nitrate inhalation may also cause increased turbulence in the LVOT because of the increased obstruction and pressure gradient across it.

Using color-guided continuous wave Doppler, the continuous wave cursor is aligned parallel to the direction of the turbulent flow signals in the LVOT to measure reliable peak and mean pressure gradients across the LVOT. Care has to be taken not to misinterpret the high-velocity signals in the LVOT for MR, especially in the apical imaging plane, and vice versa. This can be avoided by inspecting the spectral waveform. The velocity acceleration as displayed by spectral waveform obtained from the LVOT is slower than the deceleration, but the spectral waveform obtained from the MR shows both the acceleration and deceleration slopes to be rapid and practically equal.

Other abnormal flow patterns may also be observed in the LVOT and in the region of the apex. For example, prominent flow signals can be observed in the apical region moving towards the body of the ventricle during systole in many patients with this entity, especially those with a small and narrow left ventricular cavity. During systole, the pumping action of the apical region pushes the blood flow toward the base of the ventricle. In some patients with significant hypertrophy in the apex and milder hypertrophy in the basal and middle portions of the ventricle, an abnormal antegrade high-velocity flow followed by a retrograde high velocity flow is seen during the isovolumic relaxation period. These abnormal flow patterns in the apical region appear to be related to asynchronous or asymmetric contraction and relaxation of the LV, caused by the apex contracting more vigorously and relaxing more rapidly and earlier than the basal region. This asymmetric contraction results in a suctioning effect which draws blood into the left ventricular apex during the early portion of the isovolumic relaxation period. The reason for the retrograde flow in the apex during the latter portion of the isovolumic relaxation period is not known, but it may represent a swirling back of the earlier-occurring rapid antegrade flow. We have also seen these abnormal flow patterns in a patient with left ventricular dysfunction presumably caused by alcoholic congestive cardiomyopathy, who showed basal dyskinesis with vigorous contraction of the apical region.

A color-guided pulsed Doppler examination of the left ventricular apex in these patients shows a normal diastolic spectral waveform with the D or E wave larger than the A wave. The spectral waveform obtained from the mitral inflow area in these patients shows the A wave to be larger than the E wave, indicating decreased left ventricular "compliance."

Another abnormal flow pattern is shown as mosaic turbulent signals in the RV, originating from a right ventricular obstruction produced by a hypertrophied VS and hypertrophied crista supraventricularis.

DILATED CARDIOMYOPATHY

In a patient with congestive or dilated cardiomyopathy, color Doppler can be used to assess the presence and severity of regurgitation from the mitral, aortic, tricuspid, and pulmonary valves and to observe abnormal flow patterns resulting from chamber dilatation and poor ventricular function. In our experience, most patients with dilated cardiomyopathy have abnormal low velocity flows at the mitral and tricuspid inflow and left ventricular outflow levels and near akinetic walls. Low velocity flows are also seen in the apical regions of both ventricles and may account for the presence of clots often seen in this entity.

CONSTRICTIVE PERICARDITIS

Color Doppler examination does not appear to improve the 2D and conventional Doppler assessment of patients with constrictive pericarditis. It may, however, facilitate the pulsed Doppler interrogation of the hepatic veins because it provides a reference for the placement of the pulsed Doppler sample volume by displaying the flows in these veins.

REFERENCES

Hypertrophic Cardiomyopathy

1. Hatle, L.: Noninvasive assessment and differentiation of left ventricular outflow with Doppler ultrasound. Circulation 64:381, 1981.
2. Nishimura, R.A., Tajik, A.J., Reeder, G.S., and Seward, J.B.: Evaluation of hypertrophic cardiomyopathy by Doppler color flow imaging: Initial observations. Mayo Clin. Proc. 61:631, 1986.
3. Sasson, Z., Hatle, L., Appelton, C.P., Jewell, M., Alderman, E.L., and Popp, R.L.: Intraventricular flow during isovolumic relation: Description and characterization by Doppler echocardiography. J. Am. Coll. Cardiol. 10:539, 1987.
4. Maron, B.J., Spirito, P., Green, K.J., Wesley, Y.E., Bonow, R.O., and Arce, J.: Noninvasive assessment of left ventricular diastolic function by pulsed Doppler echocardiography in patients with hypertrophic cardiomyopathy. J. Am. Coll. Cardiol. 10:733, 1987.
5. Stewart, W.J., Schiavone, W.A., Salcedo, E.E., Lever, H.M., Cosgrove, D.M., and Gill, C.C.: Intraoperative Doppler echocardiography in hypertrophic cardiomyopathy: Correlations with the obstructive gradients. J. Am. Coll. Cardiol. 10:327, 1987.

Dilated Cardiomyopathy

1. Gardin, J.M., Seri, L.T., Elkayam, U., Tobis, J., Childs, W., Burn, C.S., and Henry, W.L.: Evaluation of dilated cardiomyopathy by pulsed Doppler echocardiography. Am. Heart J. 10:1057, 1983.
2. Switzer, D.F., and Nanda, N.C.: Color Doppler evaluation of valvular regurgitation. Echocardiography: A Review of Cardiovascular Ultrasound 2:533, 1985.
3. Dittrich, H., Hoit, B., and Sahn, D.: Spatial patterns of mitral flow in patients with congestive cardiomyopathy determined by real time two-dimensional echo Doppler color flow mapping (Abstract). J. Am. Coll. Cardiol. 5(2):426, 1985.
4. Meese, R.B., Adams, D., and Kisslo, J.: Assessment of valvular regurgitation by conventional and color flow Doppler in dilated cardiomyopathy. Echocardiography: A Review of Cardiovascular Ultrasound 3:505, 1986.

Constrictive Pericarditis

1. Agatston, A.S., Rao, A., Price, R.J., and Kinney, E.L.: Diagnosis of constrictive pericarditis by pulsed Doppler echocardiography. Am. J. Cardiol. 54:929, 1984.
2. Pandian, N., Kirdar, J., Isner, J., Gardin, J., McInerney, K., Caldeira, M., Fulton, D., and Hatle, L.: Doppler echocardiography in constrictive pericarditis and correlation with computed tomography and pathology (Abstract). J. Am. Coll. Cardiol. 7:205A, 1986.

SECTION 8   CARDIOMYOPATHIES AND CONSTRICTIVE PERICARDITIS

This section provides an illustrated overview of the value of color Doppler in the evaluation of hypertrophic cardiomyopathy. A patient with constrictive pericarditis is also presented.

Figure CM-1   **Hypertrophic cardiomyopathy.** (A) Autopsy specimen shows asymmetrical hypertrophy of interventricular septum, narrow LVOT, and the MV apparatus in contact with the VS. B is a closeup view of the same specimen. Another autopsy specimen (C) shows marked hypertrophy of the VS, LV posterior wall (LVPW), and RV free wall (RVFW).

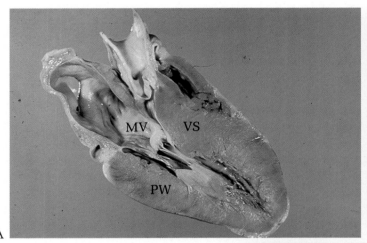

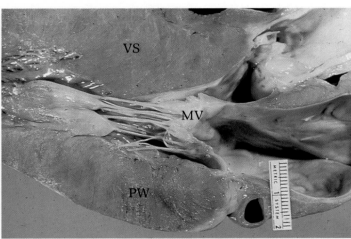

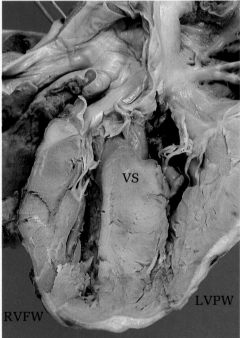

SECTION 8 CARDIOMYOPATHIES AND CONSTRICTIVE PERICARDITIS

Figure CM-2 **Hypertrophic cardiomyopathy.** (A) Long axis view in a 33-year-old woman shows asymmetric ventricular septal hypertrophy. Color Doppler examination (B) shows a mosaic pattern of signals in the narrowed LVOT indicating turbulence due to subaortic obstruction. In C, mosaic-colored systolic signals occupying more than 40% of the LA represent severe MR. Schematics (D,E) show asymmetric ventricular septal hypertrophy, narrow LVOT, prominent systolic anterior movement of the MV, and turbulent flow in the LVOT, AO, and MR. F and G represent color M-mode studies which show the mosaic-colored MR signals in LA appearing later in systole as compared to turbulence in the LVOT (also represented by mosaic signals). In H and I, the blue area, together with the red area surrounding it, represents aliased flow acceleration, and the adjacent mosaic-colored signals represent turbulence in the LVOT. Mosaic-colored signals occurring later in systole in the LA are due to MR. These findings are typical of hypertrophic cardiomyopathy. S = systolic anterior movement of the MV. J is an M-mode examination showing prominent systolic anterior motion of the MV. K and L are M-mode studies that demonstrate typical midsystolic closure and coarse systolic fluttering of the AV and red, blue, and green flow signals in the aortic root, implying flow disturbance. CW Doppler interrogation of the LVOT (M,N) demonstrates a peak velocity of 3.67 m/sec equivalent to a peak pressure gradient of 54 mm Hg. Thus, this patient has significant LVO obstruction at rest.

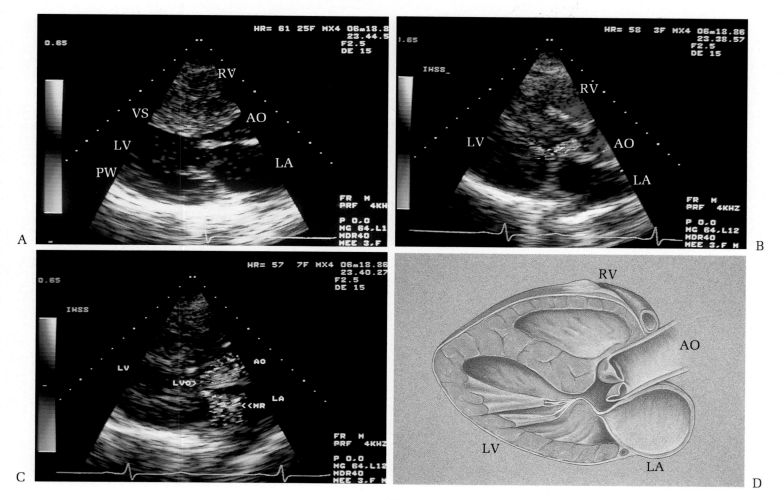

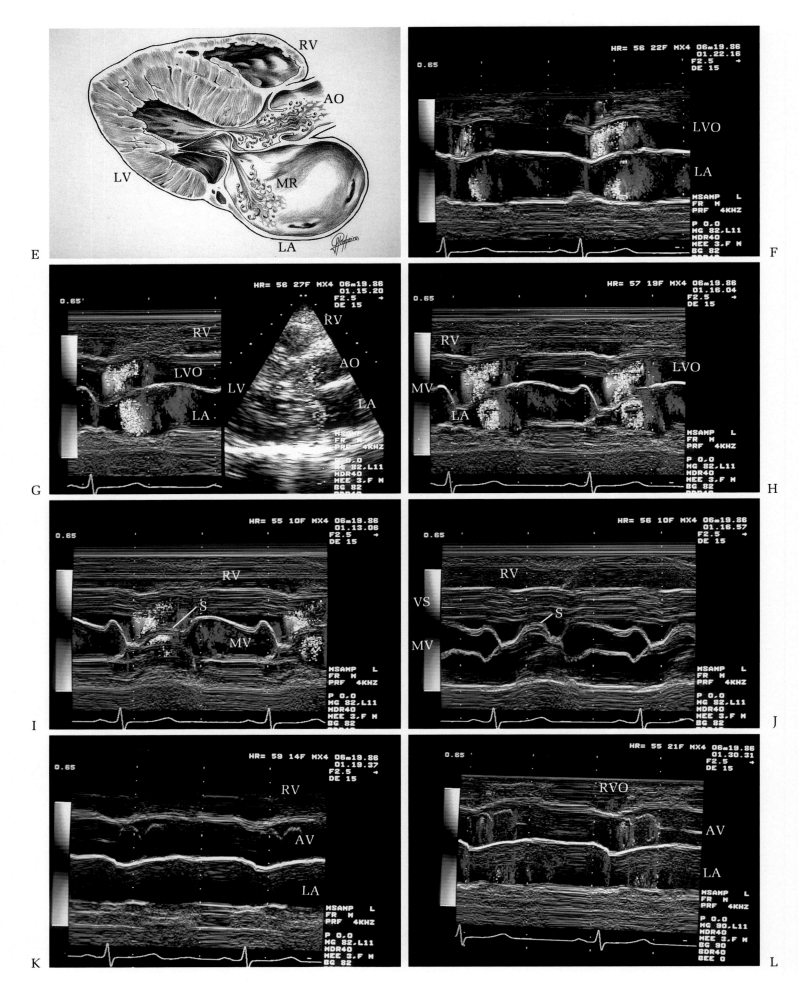

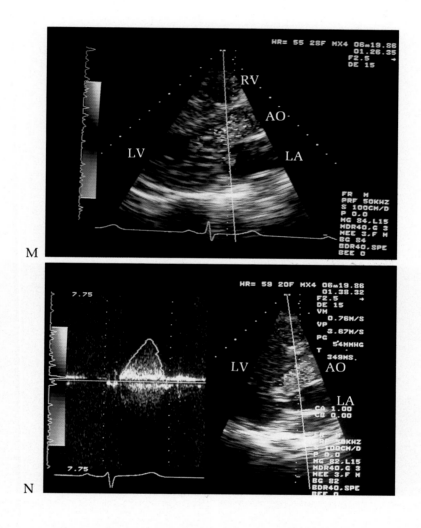

SECTION 8 CARDIOMYOPATHIES AND CONSTRICTIVE PERICARDITIS

Figure CM-3 **Hypertrophic cardiomyopathy.** Long axis views in a 45-year-old woman show systolic mosaic-colored signals in the LVOT due to obstruction (A) and later appearance of mosaic-colored signals in the LA due to MR (B). M-mode and color M-mode studies show abnormal systolic anterior motion of the MV (C), mosaic-colored signals in the LVOT due to obstruction, and bluish-green signals in LA due to MR (D,E,F). Although in D and E, MR appears to occur late in systole, F shows it to be pansystolic. The continuous wave (CW) Doppler cursor line is placed parallel to the direction of disturbed flow in the LVOT (G,H) to obtain a peak velocity of 4 m/sec, which translates into a peak pressure gradient of 64 mm Hg using the Bernoulli equation. In this patient, the spectral waveform shows a slower-velocity acceleration as compared to the deceleration slope characteristic of hypertrophic cardiomyopathy. In valvar stenosis and regurgitation (such as AS and MR), both the acceleration and deceleration slopes are practically equal and rapid.

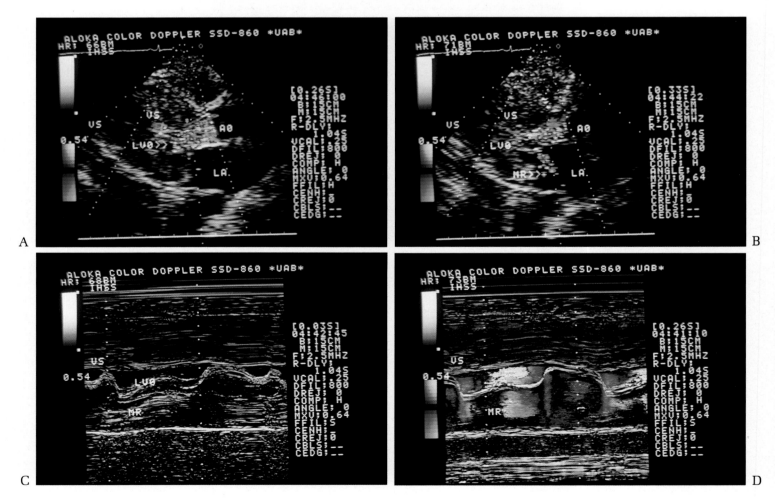

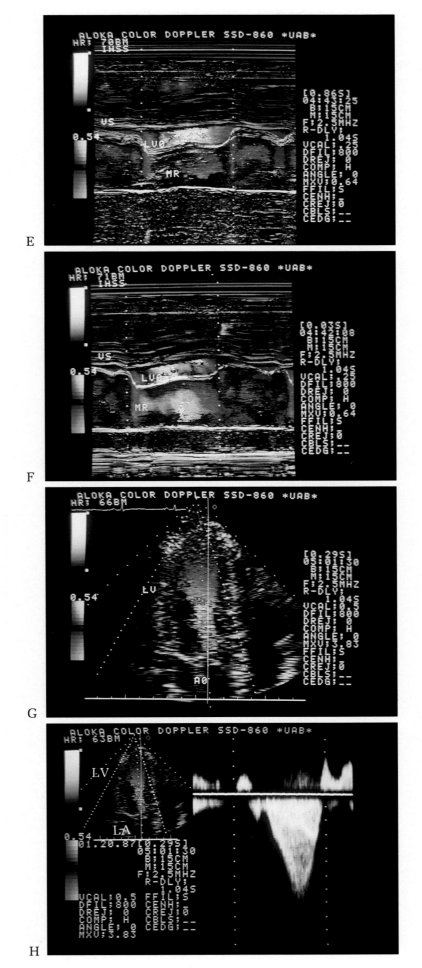

E

F

G

H

SECTION 8   CARDIOMYOPATHIES AND CONSTRICTIVE PERICARDITIS

Figure CM-4   **Hypertrophic cardiomyopathy.** Long axis views in a 46-year-old man show mosaic-colored signals in the LVOT and aortic root, representing turbulence (T) due to obstruction (A) and late systolic appearance of MR (B).

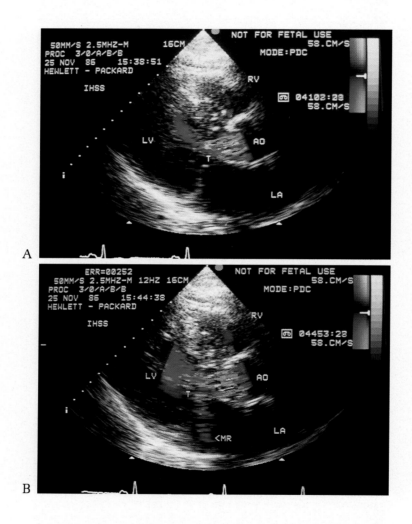

SECTION 8 CARDIOMYOPATHIES AND CONSTRICTIVE PERICARDITIS

Figure CM-5 **Hypertrophic cardiomyopathy without significant obstruction.** 2D and color Doppler studies in an elderly patient demonstrate concentric left ventricular hypertrophy (LVH) (A) and significant MR (B). Mosaic-colored signals signifying turbulence are not conspicuous in the LVOT, and no pressure gradient was detected by CW Doppler examination.

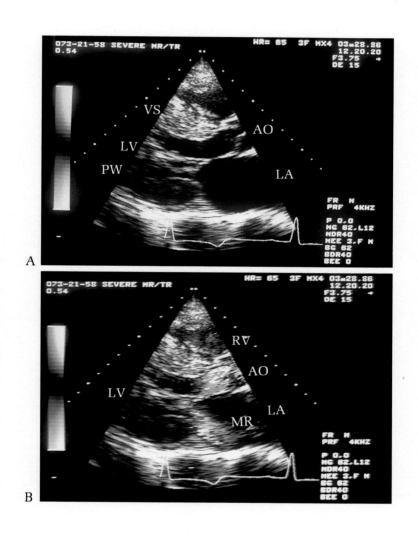

SECTION 8 CARDIOMYOPATHIES AND CONSTRICTIVE PERICARDITIS

Figure CM-6 **Hypertrophic cardiomyopathy.** Long axis views in a woman patient show asymmetric hypertrophy of the LV posterior wall (A, VS is only mildly hypertrophied) and mosaic-colored signals in the LVOT, indicating significant obstruction. Note also the LV cavity obliteration during systole (B).

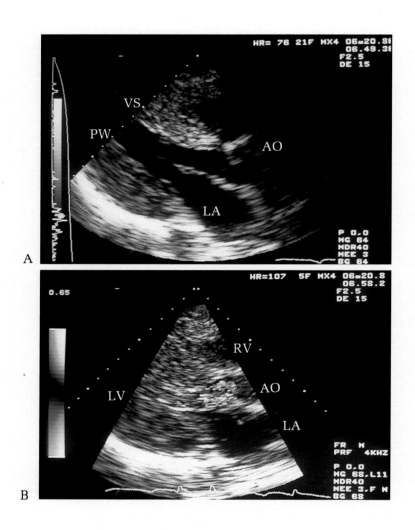

SECTION 8 CARDIOMYOPATHIES AND CONSTRICTIVE PERICARDITIS

Figure CM-7 **Hypertrophic cardiomyopathy.** (A) Long axis view in a 57-year-old man shows a small area of bluish-green signals in LA during systole, indicating mild MR. C = control state. After amyl nitrite inhalation, the bluish area becomes larger because of increased MR (B). The blue flow signals present in the LVOT in the basal state (A) are replaced by red signals because of aliasing from increased velocity and obstruction after amyl nitrite inhalation. The patient was also examined by color-guided continuous wave Doppler and the peak pressure gradient across the LVOT increased from 16 mm Hg at rest to 64 mm Hg with amyl nitrite inhalation. (Reproduced with permission from Switzer and Nanda, Ultrasound in Medicine and Biology, *11*:403 – 416, 1985.)

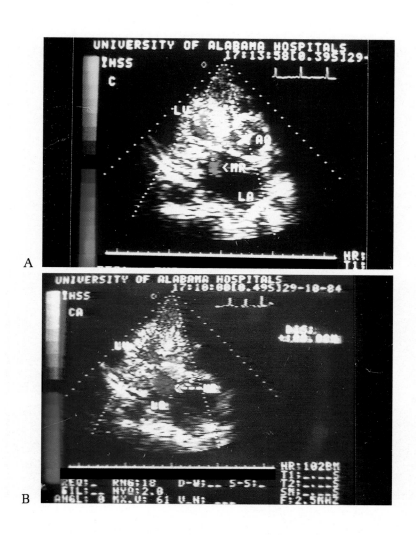

SECTION 8   CARDIOMYOPATHIES AND CONSTRICTIVE PERICARDITIS

Figure CM-8   **Hypertrophic cardiomyopathy: Abnormal flow patterns.** (A) Apical 4-chamber view in a 71-year-old man shows marked apical hypertrophy. (B) Color-guided continuous wave Doppler interrogation demonstrates peak and mean pressure gradients of 29 and 14 mm Hg, respectively. Note the typical conventional Doppler spectral waveform during systole with the acceleration slope slower than deceleration. Also, the A wave is larger than the E (or D) wave near the MV, indicating decreased LV compliance. Conventional Doppler interrogation (C) of prominent flow signals seen in the apex (AP) shows abnormal antegrade (above the baseline) and retrograde (below the baseline) high-velocity flows (arrowheads) during the isovolumic relaxation period. Systolic and diastolic waveforms are normal, with the D (or E) wave larger than the A wave in the apical region. Aortic short axis views (D,E) show a hypertrophied crista supraventricularis (CR) with aliased (blue) flow signals in this region due to mild RV obstruction (no significant RV pressure gradient was found by continuous wave Doppler). F,G,H, and I are taken from a 64-year-old woman with isolated apical hypertrophy and coronary artery disease. The apical view (F) shows mosaic-colored flow signals (F) moving into the LV body from the apex, and pulse Doppler (G) and color M-mode examinations (H and I) reveal high velocities and turbulence in both systole and diastole.

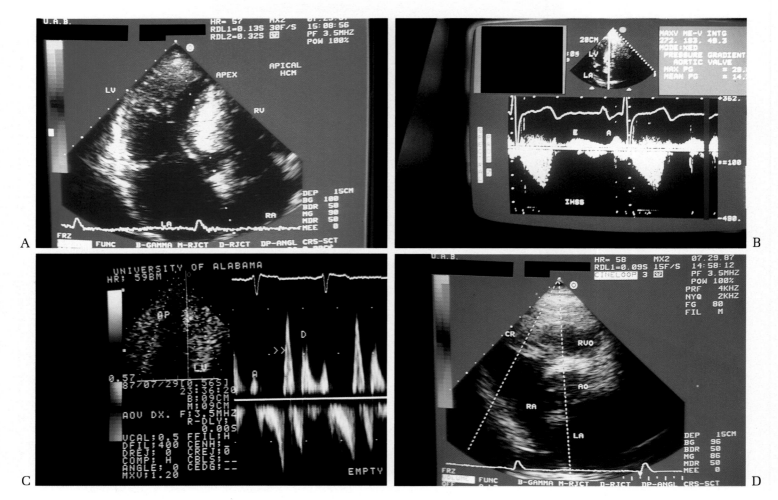

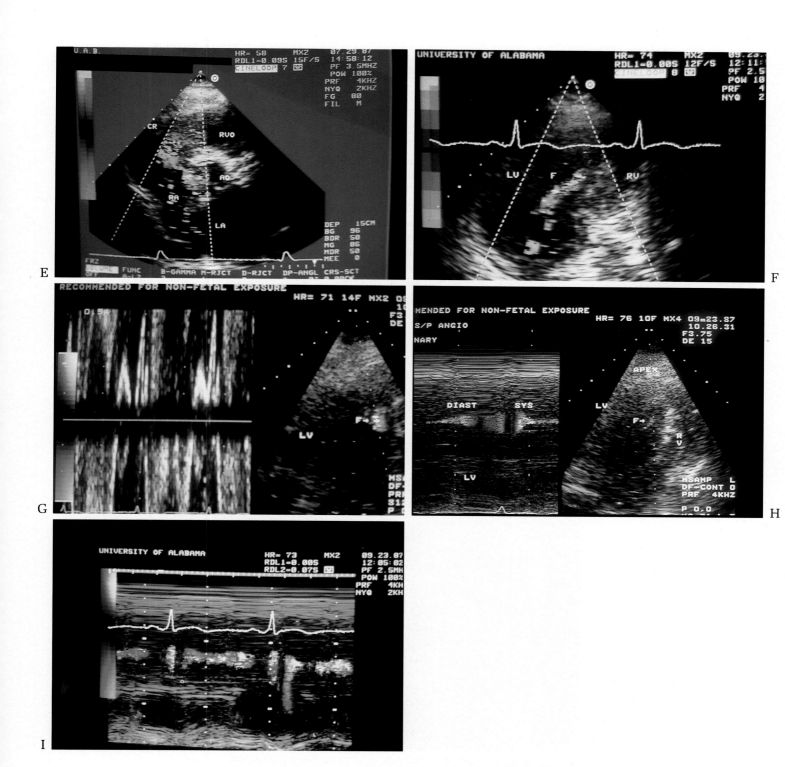

SECTION 8   CARDIOMYOPATHIES AND CONSTRICTIVE PERICARDITIS

Figure CM-9   **Congestive cardiomyopathy: Abnormal flow during isovolumic relaxation period.** 2-D echocardiogram in a patient with LV dysfunction, presumably on the basis of alcoholic congestive cardiomyopathy, shows basal dyskinesis with vigorous contraction of the apex. This patient also demonstrates, on both color and pulse Doppler examinations, relatively high-velocity flow signals moving into the apex during the isovolumic relaxation period (A). AP = apex, AB = abnormal flow. The timing of these signals is identified by their occurrence before MV opening on the color M-mode (B and C) and just before mitral inflow signals on the pulse Doppler tracing (A). The A wave on the mitral inflow is larger than the E (or D) wave, suggesting decreased LV compliance (A). Abnormal flow patterns in the apical region during the isovolumic relaxation period in this patient and in the patient with hypertrophic cardiomyopathy shown in Figure CM-8 appear to be related to asymmetric contraction and relaxation of the LV, with the apex contracting more vigorously and also relaxing more rapidly and earlier than the basal region. The resulting "suction effect" draws blood into the LV apex. The reason for the retrograde movement of blood flow from the apex into the LV body in the later phase of the isovolumic relaxation period seen in the patient with hypertrophic cardiomyopathy is not clear. D and E are autopsy specimens showing marked dilatation of both ventricles in congestive cardiomyopathy.

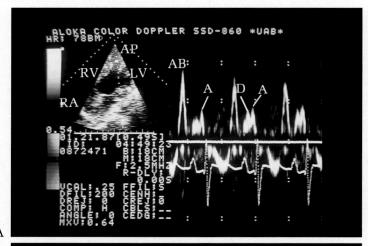

A

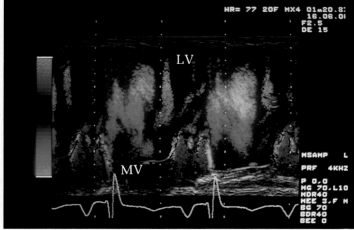

B

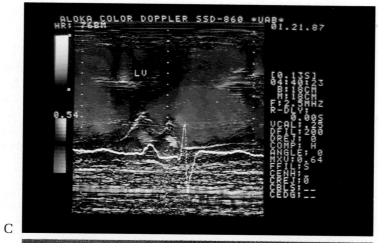

C

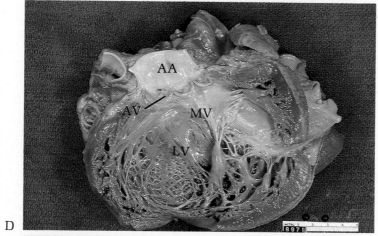

D

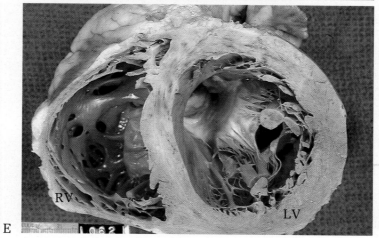

E

SECTION 8 CARDIOMYOPATHIES AND CONSTRICTIVE PERICARDITIS

Figure CM-10 **Constrictive pericarditis.** (A,B) Para-apical 4-chamber and subcostal views in a 29-year-old man demonstrate heavy calcification in the LV free wall and RV diaphragmatic wall pericardium (P). HV = hepatic vein. Pulse Doppler interrogation of LV at various levels (C,D,E) shows a large E wave with rapid acceleration and deceleration slopes and a small A wave consistent with constrictive pericarditis. Pulse and color Doppler interrogation (F,G,H,I) of HV shows prominent abnormal retrograde flow during late systole and late diastole (arrows) and D (diastolic) wave (W) larger than S (systolic) wave. A = A wave. Two to 3 weeks after partial surgical stripping of the pericardium, there was no significant change in the hepatic or IVC waveforms (J,K) or LV inflow waveforms (L,M). Para-apical examination (N,O) shows the presence of a loculated pericardial effusion (PE) behind the LV posterior wall. E = LV endocardium. Although the patient has shown considerable clinical improvement, the Doppler parameters of LV diastolic function have remained unchanged in the initial postoperative period.

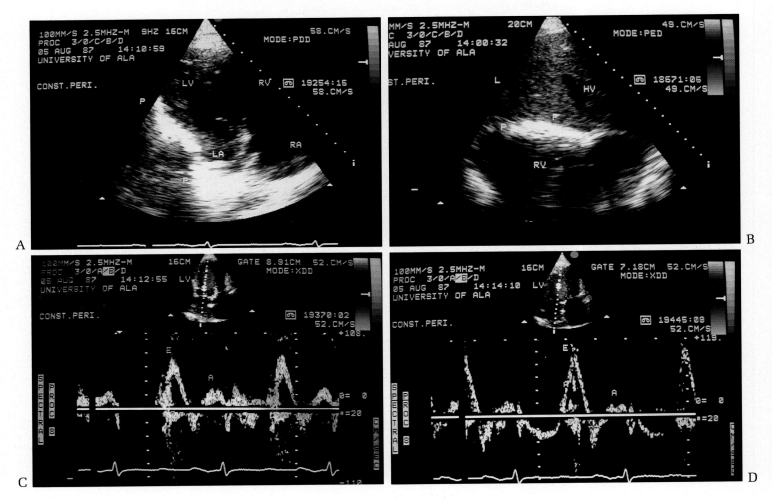

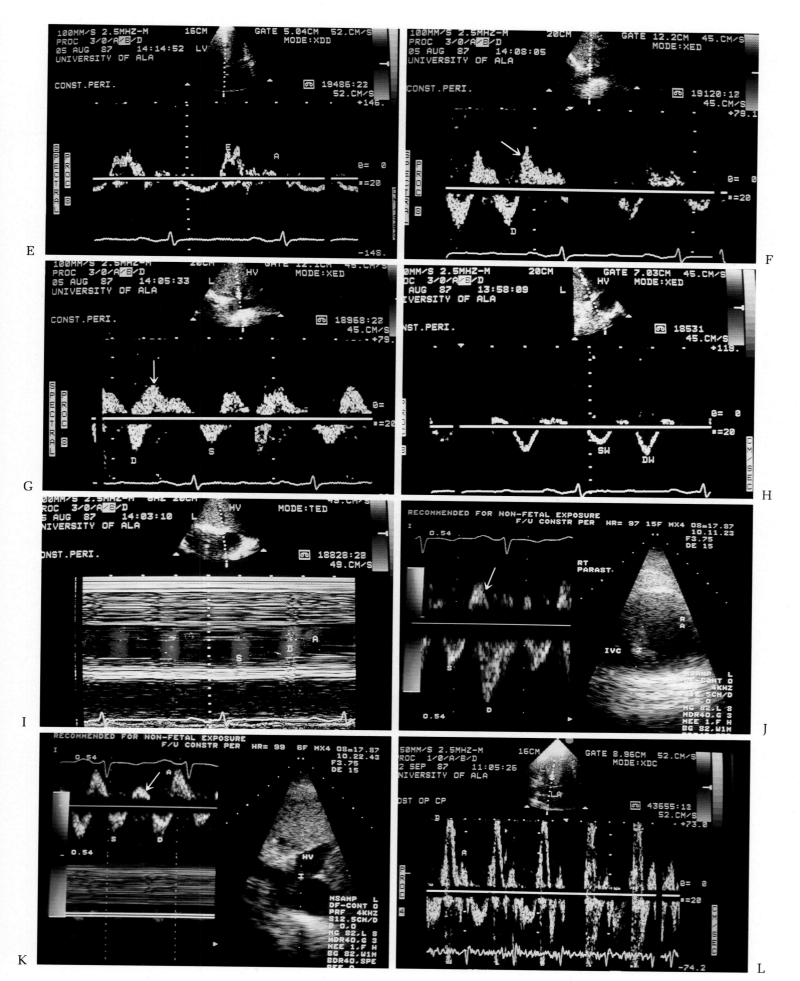

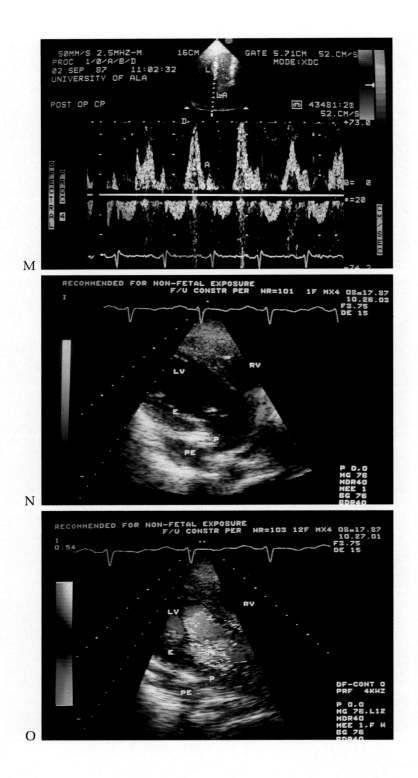

Section 9

ISCHEMIC HEART DISEASE

In our experience, color Doppler has become increasingly useful in the assessment of patients with ischemic heart disease. It evaluates the presence and severity of both mitral and tricuspid regurgitation resulting from ischemic left and right ventricular and papillary muscle dysfunction. Color Doppler examination can also be used to examine patients who have undergone coronary artery bypass surgery or left ventricular aneurysmectomy, to assess the presence and severity of residual MR.

Combined with exercise, color Doppler can also be used to evaluate patients with proven or suspected coronary artery disease. In one study conducted in our laboratory, we were able to induce MR in a significant proportion of patients with coronary artery disease during supine bicycle exercise. Although ghosting artifacts were observed, we were able to distinguish these artifacts from the mitral regurgitant signals in most of these patients. In general, we found that the development of MR indicated the presence of ischemic heart disease, especially in patients with 3-vessel disease, and that patients with 2- or 1-vessel disease and those without obvious coronary artery disease did not develop MR during exercise. In addition, in some patients, MR was observed to develop before the onset of wall motion abnormalities and in other patients, MR was seen even though wall motion abnormalities were not detected. This first observation, the development of MR during acute myocardial ischemia, is a well-documented phenomenon. In fact, the MR was the first detectable sign of myocardial ischemia in some patients before they had any complaint of chest pain. The latter observation may have occurred because these patients had only papillary muscle dysfunction. In most patients, the MR usually occurred within 3 minutes of the onset of supine bicycle exercise. Finally, the color Doppler assessment of the severity of MR estimated by the ratio of the maximum area of the regurgitant signals to the left atrial area did not correlate with the severity of the coronary artery disease. The findings of this study need to be confirmed using a much larger study group. Color M-mode is useful in timing the MR occurring in patients with papillary muscle dysfunction. This MR is usually pansystolic, but in some patients, it may be confined to late systole.

A color Doppler examination also complements a 2D examination of the LV in the evaluation of left ventricular aneurysms. Flow signals can be seen moving from the left ventricular chamber into the aneurysm during late systole. This finding helps to differentiate the aneurysm from other "echo-free" spaces around the LV. In patients with left ventricular pseudoaneurysm, high-velocity flow signals can be seen moving from the LV through a narrow opening into the pseudoaneurysm during systole. Because the small opening between the ventricle and the pseudoaneurysm may not be easily detectable and echo dropouts may be present, continuity between the chambers may not always be shown with 2D echocardiography. It is therefore useful to examine these patients using color Doppler to view the flow signals moving into the aneurysmal sac. A color-guided continuous wave Doppler examination can be performed to obtain the pressure gradient from the velocity of the flow moving through the opening into the aneurysm. This may have potential prognostic implications for the rupture of the pseudoaneurysm.

A color Doppler examination of the left ventricular apex in patients with apical aneurysm or dyskinesis shows flow signals moving into the aneurysmal apex during systole and away from it during diastole. Flow signals in the aneurysm may also appear to persist for an inappropriately long time, indicating the presence of relative flow stasis in the aneurysm. In our experience, the incidence of LV apical thrombus formation is higher in patients with very low-velocity flows than those with higher-velocity flows in the apical region.

In patients with inferior wall aneurysms, abnormal low-velocity flows are seen during systole within the aneurysm. High-velocity flow signals moving into the LV apex during the isovolumic relaxation period are seen in patients with proximal inferior wall aneurysms with a well-contracting left ventricular apex. This finding is similar to that seen in patients with hypertrophic cardiomyopathy, and results from asynchronous contraction and relaxation of the basal and apical portions of the left ventricle, producing a suction effect.

Color Doppler can also be used to indicate the presence of a clot in the aneurysm and to differentiate this clot from a false tendon or left ventricular trabeculations. In one patient we studied, a thick linear echo observed in the LV apex was initially suspected to be the edge of a large clot, but color Doppler displayed prominent flow signals freely moving into the apical region, implying the absence of any thrombus. Additional 2D views showed that the thick linear echo was a false tendon in the LV and not the suspected edge of a clot. Because low-velocity flow signals are present in the left ventricular aneurysm, we have found that occasionally a power mode examination that allows a better visualization of these flows is helpful in assessing the flow patterns in these patients. If the color Doppler system is set at a high color threshold or a low gain, the low-velocity signals are cut off, and thus no flow is observed in the aneurysm.

The presence and severity of TR in patients with ischemic right ventricular dysfunction or right ventricular infarction can also be assessed using the subcostal, right ventricular inflow, aortic short axis, and apical 4-chamber and 2-chamber color Doppler imaging planes. In general, mosaic or reversed flow signals seen moving into the RA during systole and originating from the TV indicate the presence of TR. The severity of this regurgitation is categorized according to the ratio of the maximum regurgitant jet area to the right atrial area measured in the same frame. We have also found TR developing in patients with ischemic heart disease, especially those with 3-vessel coronary artery disease, during supine bicycle exercise. This finding is probably related to the development of exercise-induced ischemic right ventricular dysfunction or right ventricular papillary muscle dysfunction.

Color Doppler examination is very useful in the diagnosis of acute ventricular septal rupture and in differentiating it from mitral chordal or papillary muscle head rupture or avulsion. The examiner is immediately alerted to the presence of ventricular septal rupture when mosaic turbulent signals are observed in the RV. The actual site of the rupture in the ventricular septum can be observed by angling the transducer. If the defect is present in the posterobasal septum, color Doppler may not be able to identify it using any parasternal or apical imaging plane, except the apical inferobasal plane. Color Doppler is also used to examine these patients after the ventricular septal rupture is repaired to determine if any residual leak is still present. Many patients with acute ventricular septal rupture have coexisting mild MR.

REFERENCES

1. Smith, J.S., Cahalan, M.K., Benefiel, D.J., Byrd, B.F., Lurz, F.W., Shapiro, W.A., Roizen, M.F., Bouchard, A., and Schiller, N.B.: Intraoperative detection of myocardial ischemia in high risk patients: Electrocardiography versus two-dimensional transesophageal echocardiography. Circulation 72:1015, 1985.
2. Konstady, S., Goldman, M.E., Thys, D., Mindich, P., and Kaplan, J.A.: Intraoperative diagnosis of myocardial ischemia. Mt Sinai J. Med. 52:521, 1985.
3. Erbel, R., Mohr-Kahaly, S., Drexler, M., Wittlich, N., Kersting, H., Iverson, S., Oelert, H., and Meyer, J.: Color Doppler echocardiography in emergency diagnosis of ventricular septal rupture after acute myocardial infarction. Z. Kardiol. 75:468, 1986.
4. Zachariah, Z.P., Hsiung, M.C., Nanda, N.C., Kan, M.N., and Gatewood, R.P., Jr.: Color Doppler assessment of mitral regurgitation induced by supine exercise in ischemic heart disease. Am. J. Cardiol. 59:1266, 1987.
5. Zachariah, Z.P., Hsiung, M.C., Nanda, N.C., and Camarano, G.P.: Diagnosis of rupture of the ventricular septum during acute infarction by Doppler color flow mapping. Am. J. Cardiol. 59:162, 1987.
6. Kapur, K.K., Nanda, N.C., Fan, P.H., Bolgar, A.F., Czer L., and Maurer, G.: Color Doppler evaluation of acute ventricular septal rupture (Abstract). Circulation 76 (Supp. IV):IV-527, 1987.
7. Omoto, R., Wong, M., Matsumura, M., Yagamata, S., and Ishiguro, T.: Noninvasive analysis of left ventricular blood-flow dynamics in left ventricular aneurysm by color flow mapping (Abstract). J. Am. Coll. Cardiol. 9:66A, 1987.

SECTION 9 ISCHEMIC HEART DISEASE

Various abnormal flow patterns in the LV in patients with ischemic heart disease are shown and their correlation with 2D echocardiographic findings described.

Figure IS-1 **Papillary muscle dysfunction.** Apical 4-chamber view in an elderly patient shows inferior displacement of the coaptation point of the mitral leaflets beyond the annulus level, suggesting papillary muscle (PM) dysfunction. The blue signals in the LA cavity, originating from the MV and occupying approximately 35% of the LA area, indicate the presence of moderate MR.

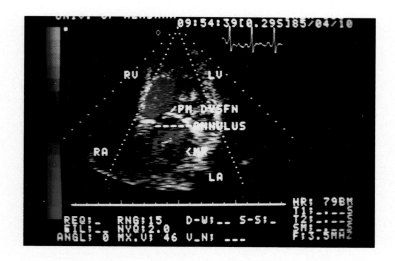

Figure IS-2 **Mitral regurgitation induced by exercise in ischemic heart disease.** In an elderly patient, reversed flow signals in the LA due to MR are absent in a pre-exercise apical 4-chamber view (A). During supine bicycle exercise (B), prominent blue signals (arrow) appear in the LA during systole, indicating development of MR. This occurred approximately 3 minutes into the exercise in this patient with 3-vessel coronary artery disease. (Reproduced with permission from Zachariah et al., Am. J. Cardiol. 59:126, 1987.

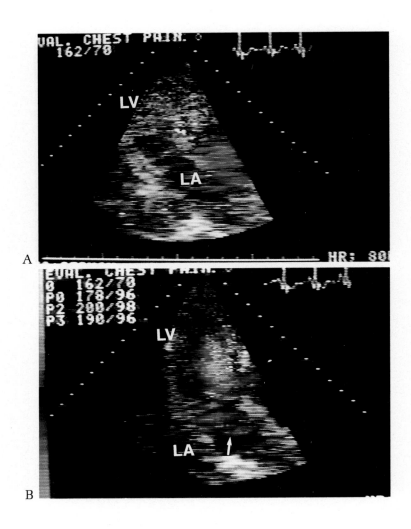

SECTION 9   ISCHEMIC HEART DISEASE

Figure IS-3   **Mitral regurgitation in ischemic heart disease.** Apical 2-chamber view (systole) shows bluish-green signals originating from the MV and occupying most of the LA, indicating significant MR. The coaptation point of the mitral leaflets is displaced inferiorly beyond the level of the annulus, suggesting papillary muscle dysfunction. The proximal inferior wall (IW) shows mild dyskinesis (DYS) in this 67-year-old man with inferior myocardial infarction. FW = LV free wall.

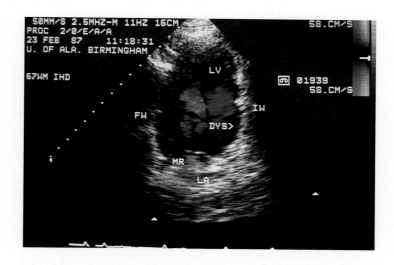

Figure IS-4   **Abnormal flow patterns in ischemic heart disease.** (A,B,C) During systole, abnormal flow signals (SF) are seen moving from the body of the LV into the aneurysmal apex, which contains a large thrombus (TH). This finding is also confirmed by pulse Doppler and color M-mode examinations. Blue signals represent normal flow directed into the LVOT during systole.

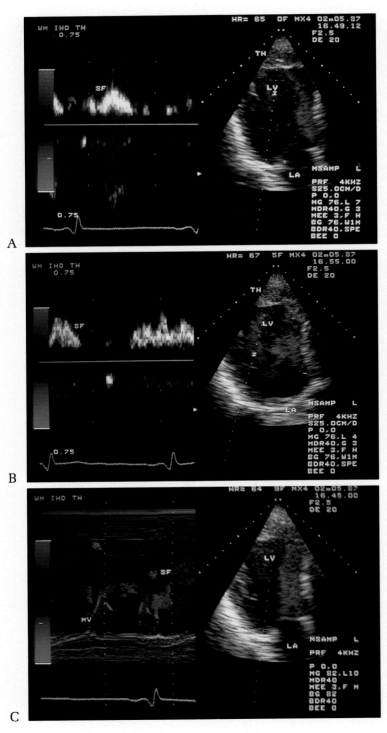

SECTION 9   ISCHEMIC HEART DISEASE

Figure IS-5   **Abnormal flow patterns in ischemic heart disease.** Apical view in a 44-year-old man with LV apical aneurysm shows prominent red signals during systole, indicating abnormal flow moving from the body of the LV into the apex. The red signals during diastole on the color M-mode represent normal mitral inflow.

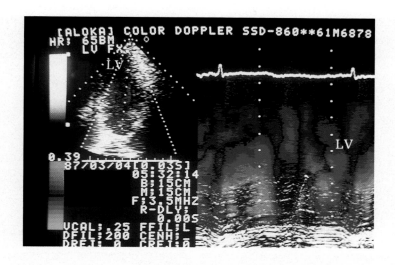

SECTION 9 ISCHEMIC HEART DISEASE

Figure IS-6 **Abnormal flow patterns in ischemic heart disease.** (A,B) Long axis views in a 32-year-old woman with myocardial infarction show an LV aneurysm (AN) with VS thinning and mosaic-colored MR signals in the dilated LA. Examination of the LV apex shows prominent dyskinesis (DYS) with swirling of blood flow within it (C,D). Color M-mode study (E) demonstrates flow signals moving towards the aneurysmal apex (red) during systole and away from it (blue) during diastole. PW = posterior wall.

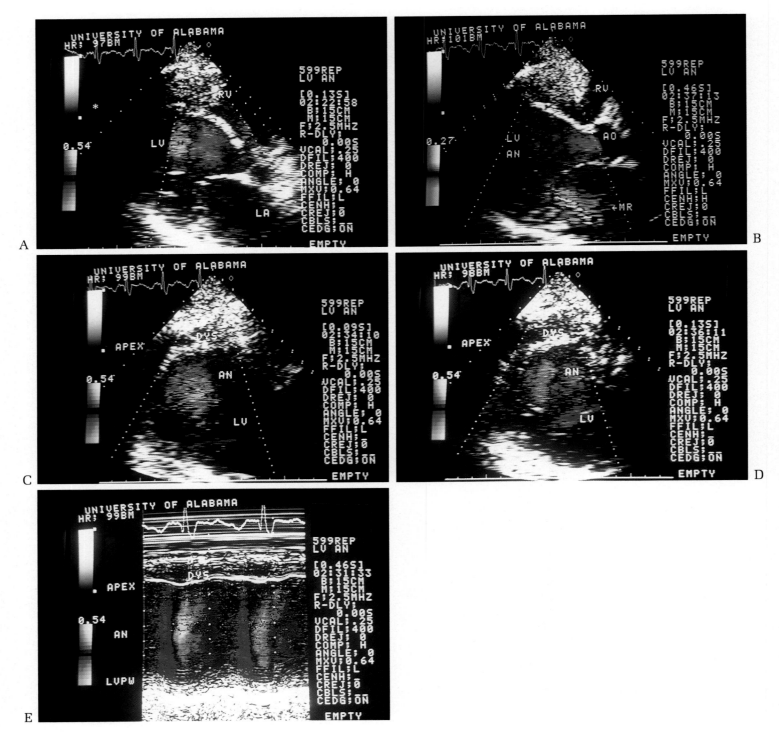

SECTION 9   ISCHEMIC HEART DISEASE

Figure IS-7   **Abnormal flow patterns in ischemic heart disease.** (A) Apical view in an elderly man with myocardial infarction shows abnormal systolic flow signals (F) originating at the junction of proximal normally moving VS and distal dyskinetic VS and directed towards the LV apex. Color M-mode and pulse Doppler examination (B,C,D) confirm this finding. E and F represent other frames showing prominent systolic movement of blood flow (red) into the aneurysmal apex.

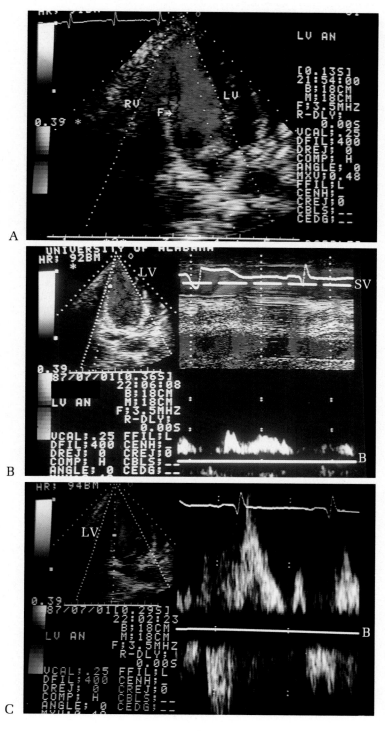

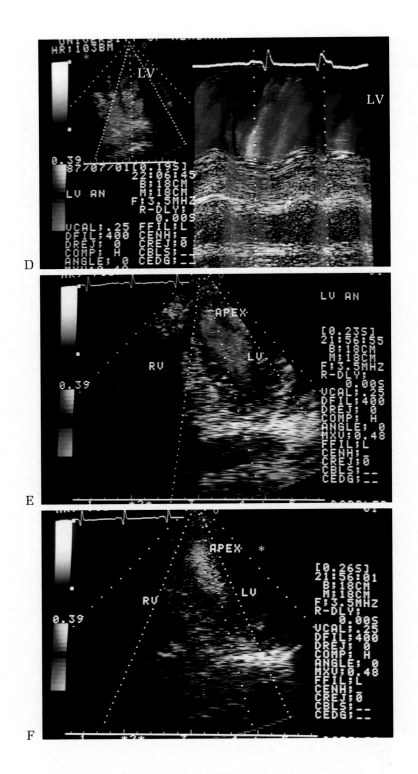

Figure IS-8 **Abnormal flow patterns in ischemic heart disease.** (A) Standard color Doppler and (B,C) power mode examination using different equipment demonstrate swirling of blood flow in the LV aneurysm in the apical 4-chamber view in this 52-year-old man. Flow signals appeared to persist for an inappropriately long time, indicating flow stasis in the aneurysm (A). TH = thrombus.

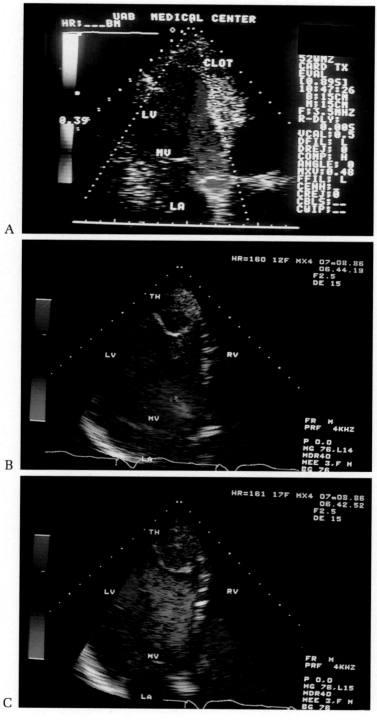

SECTION 9   ISCHEMIC HEART DISEASE

Figure IS-9   **Abnormal flow patterns in ischemic heart disease.** (A,B,C) Swirling of blood flow is noted in the LV in this 35-year-old man with extensive myocardial infarction and large LV clots (arrows).

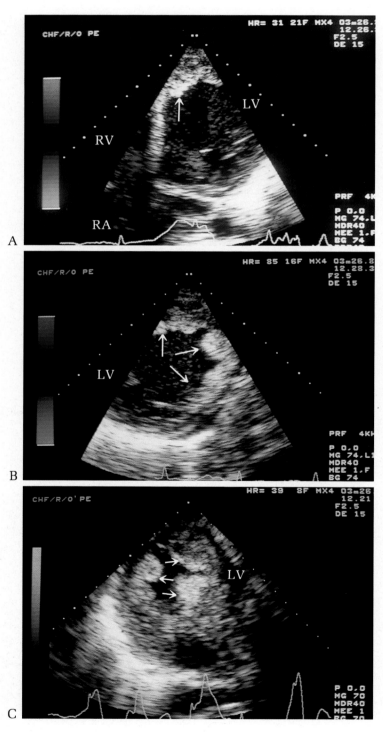

SECTION 9   ISCHEMIC HEART DISEASE

Figure IS-10   **Abnormal flow patterns in ischemic heart disease.** (A) Apical 4-chamber view in a 79-year-old man shows blood flow signals moving into the LV apex beyond a thick linear echo (FT), which was suspected to be the edge of a large clot located in the apical region. Color Doppler demonstration of prominent flow signals freely moving into this area suggests absence of thrombus and other 2D views show the linear echo to be a false tendon (FT) in the LV. B and C show prominent blood flow signals moving into the LV apex during systole. D and E demonstrate mosaic-colored MR signals in the LA. F, G, and H show spontaneous contrast echoes in the large LV aneurysm related to stasis of blood flow (red).

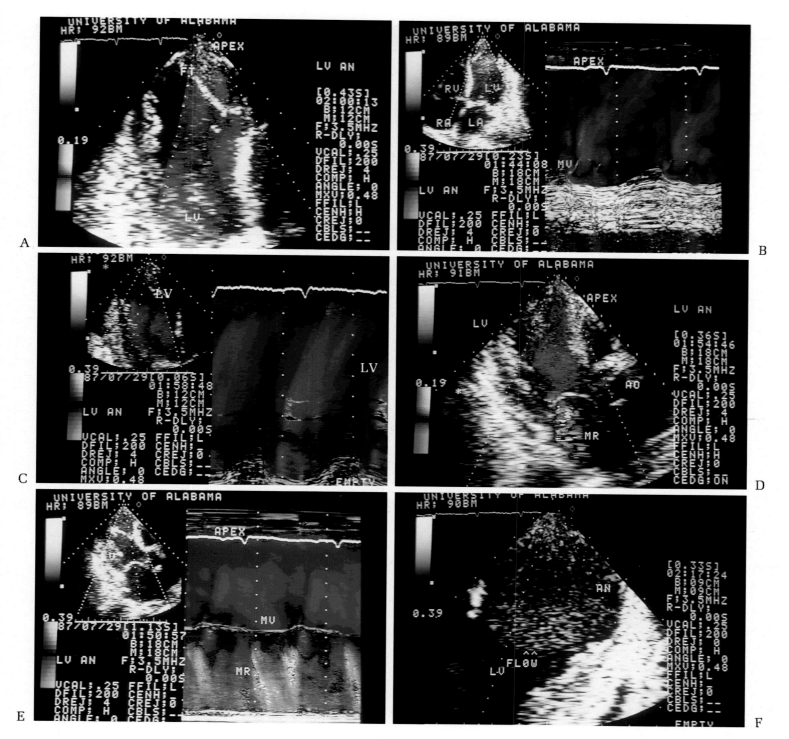

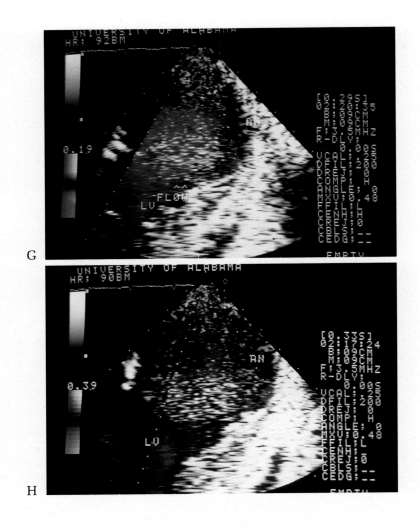

G

H

SECTION 9   ISCHEMIC HEART DISEASE

Figure IS-11   **LV posterior wall aneurysm.** Power mode examination in a 71-year-old man shows flow signals moving from the LV into the large true aneurysm (AN). In this frame, the posterior papillary muscle (PM) obscures the large opening of the aneurysm, which was more clearly visualized in other views. The vertical arrow points to a large clot in the aneurysmal sac.

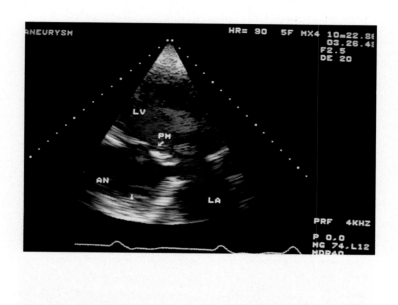

Figure IS-12   **LV inferior wall aneurysm.** (A) Apical 2-chamber view in a 73-year-old woman shows a large inferior wall aneurysm (AN) and a few mosaic-colored signals in the LA, indicating minimal MR. The paucity of color Doppler signals in the aneurysm is related to low blood flow velocities. (B) Apical 2-chamber view in an 81-year-old woman shows prominent flow signals during systole which move from the body of the LV into the aneurysm (blue), and then swirl back into the LV (reddish-brown).

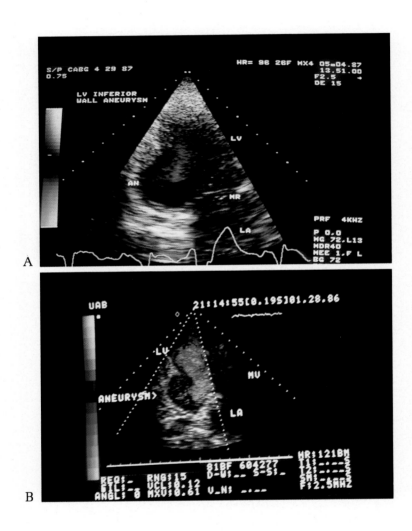

Figure IS-13 **LV pseudo-aneurysm.** (A) Modified long axis view in an elderly man shows mosaic and blue signals entering the large pseudo-aneurysm through a narrow neck (arrow). (B) Color-guided continuous wave Doppler interrogation of the aneurysm neck demonstrates high-velocity signals in systole (FF = blood flow entering aneurysm) and diastole (BF = blood flow moving from aneurysm into LV). AN = aneurysm.

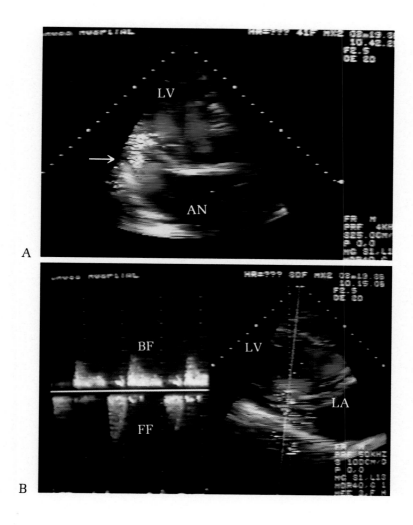

Figure IS-14 **LV aneurysm status post-resection.** Early systolic frame in a 49-year-old man shows a dilated LV with no evidence of MR (A), but during late systole, mild MR is clearly noted, demonstrated by the presence of bluish-green signals in the LA originating from the MV (B).

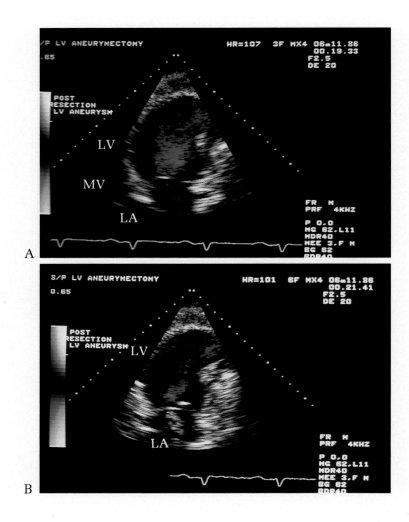

Figure IS-15 **Persistent mitral regurgitation following coronary artery bypass surgery.** Apical 4-chamber view taken after surgery in a 65-year-old woman shows prominent mosaic-colored and blue signals originating from the MV and filling approximately 25% of the LA, indicating the presence of moderate MR, unchanged from the preoperative examination.

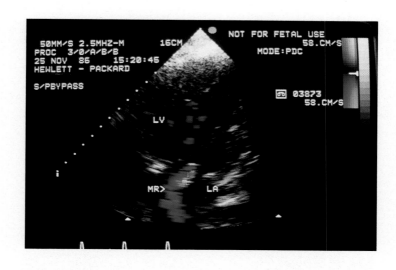

Figure IS-16   **Myocardial infarction.** (A and B) Autopsy specimens. Serial cross sections of the LV (A) show extensive fibrosis in the LV walls and septum due to old myocardial infarction. A large clot (C) is also present. B shows a large clot (C) contained within an LV apical aneurysm.

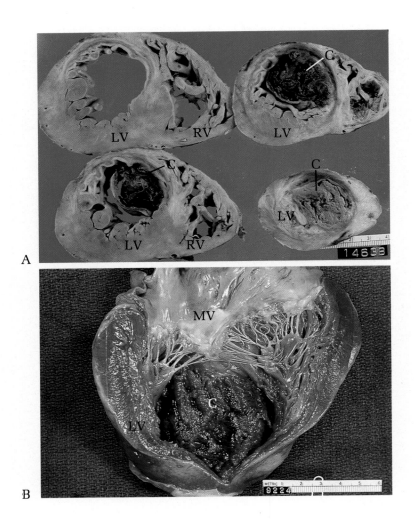

Figure IS-17   **Exercise-induced RV dysfunction in triple vessel coronary artery disease.**
(A) Subcostal examination in an elderly man shows a few bluish-green signals in the RA due to
mild TR in a pre-exercise study. (B) Three minutes into a supine bicycle exercise, the regurgitant
area is much larger, indicating increased severity of TR in this patient, consistent with RV
papillary muscle dysfunction induced by exercise.

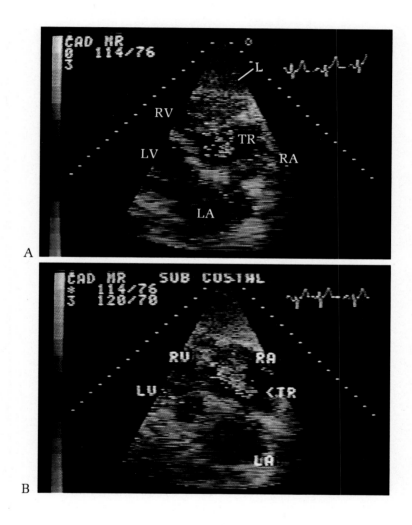

SECTION 9 ISCHEMIC HEART DISEASE

Figure IS-18 **RV infarction.** Autopsy specimen shows recent infarction of the LV and RV diaphragmatic walls (horizontal arrows). The whitish area (oblique arrow) in the RV free wall indicates fibrosis due to old infarction.

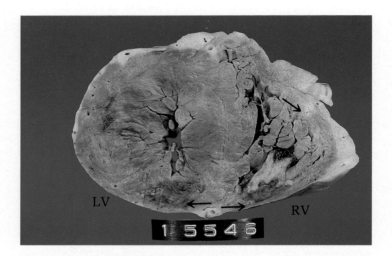

Figure IS-19 **RV infarction.** Subcostal view in a 52-year-old man shows a small area of mosaic-colored signals in the RA, indicating mild TR. RV diaphragmatic wall in this plane shows akinesis.

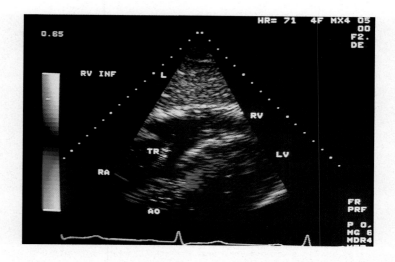

SECTION 9   ISCHEMIC HEART DISEASE

Figure IS-20   **RV infarction.** (A,B,C) Short axis views at various LV levels and (D) subcostal examination in a 71-year-old woman with inferior myocardial infarction show RV free wall aneurysm (AN) and mosaic-colored signals filling more than 40% of RA during systole, indicating severe TR. DYS = dyskinesis.

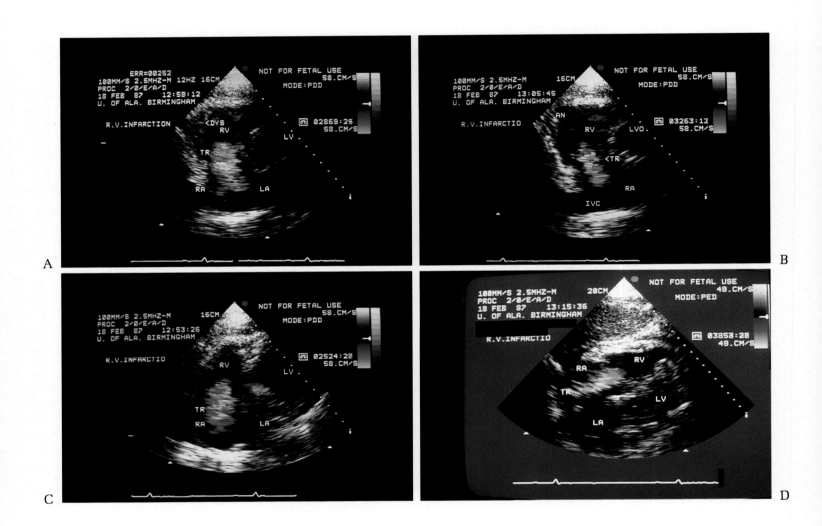

Figure IS-21   **Ventricular septal rupture.** Autopsy specimen shows a large ventricular septal rupture after acute myocardial infarction.

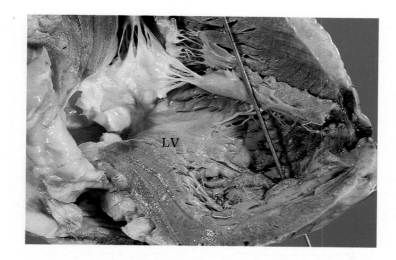

SECTION 9 ISCHEMIC HEART DISEASE

Figure IS-22 **Ventricular septal rupture.** (A) Apical infero-basal plane in a 76-year-old woman with acute diaphragmatic myocardial infarction shows mosaic-colored signals (arrows) moving from the LV into the RV through the VSD. This defect, present in the postero-basal septum, was not visualized by 2D echo or color Doppler in any other parasternal or apical views. (B) Subcostal 2D examination also did not visualize the defect, but mosaic-colored flow signals are clearly seen moving from the LV into the RV. D = defect. (C) Postoperatively, a narrow band of mosaic-colored signals is seen moving through the surgically inserted patch into the RV, consistent with a small residual leak. The much larger area of flow disturbance noted farther downstream in the RV body does not suggest a large residual leak, but is related to postoperative improvement in LV pressure, resulting in a high-pressure gradient across the small defect in the patch. The patient is doing well clinically.

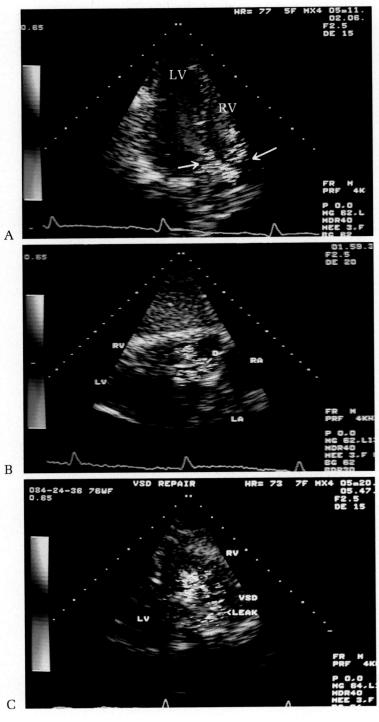

Figure IS-23 **Ventricular septal rupture.** (A,B,C) Parasternal 4-chamber view in a 76-year-old woman with diaphragmatic wall myocardial infarction shows mosaic-colored signals moving through a VSD, well visualized on 2D examination. The red signals on the left side of the defect represent flow acceleration.

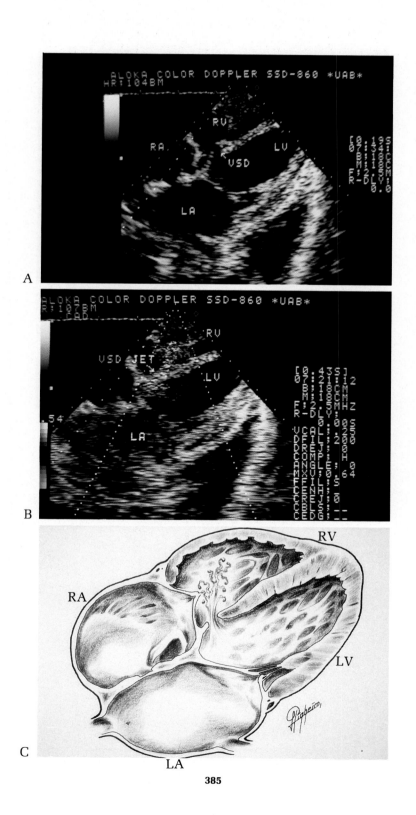

Figure IS-24   **Apical ventricular septal rupture.** (A,B) Modified apical views in a 66-year-old man show a wide band of mosaic-colored signals moving from the LV into the RV through a large defect in the echogenic surgical patch, indicating significant leakage. C is a schematic showing apical ventricular septal rupture.

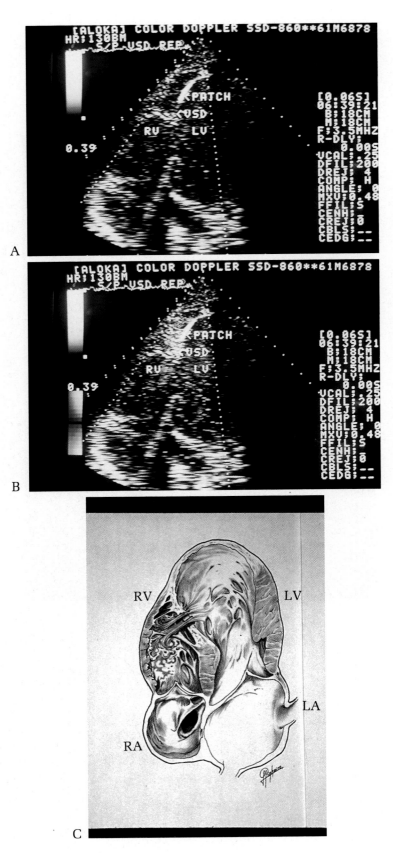

Section 10

CONGENITAL HEART DISEASE

ATRIAL SEPTAL DEFECT

Color Doppler has proven a useful supplement to 2D and conventional Doppler examination in the assessment of atrial septal defects (ASD). Pulse Doppler can generate unreliable flow information when the sample volume is not properly placed in the flow through the defect. Color Doppler avoids this by showing the hemodynamics of the flow in and around the defect. To conduct Doppler examination, the pulse Doppler sample can then be positioned in the visualized flow signals, allowing accurate flow information to be easily obtained.

An ASD is diagnosed by color Doppler detecting flow signals moving from the LA to the RA through an area of discontinuity in the AS. This is often seen in the apical 4-chamber view and the aortic short axis view. "Echo dropouts," however, occur in this midportion or fossa ovalis region of the AS in these views. The hemodynamics of the flow in this region must therefore be studied by Doppler to assess the presence of an ASD. A large number of color flow signals in the right heart may suggest the presence of this defect and thus indicate the need for a more comprehensive conventional and color Doppler examination in multiple imaging planes to confirm the presence or absence of an ASD.

The types of ASD are specified by the location of the ASD in the AS (Fig. 10-1). A secundum ASD is located in the middle of the AS, and the sinus venosus ASD is located at the origin of the superior or inferior vena cava. Ostium primum ASD shows the defect located at the base of the AS. The right parasternal transducer position, with the patient turned in the right lateral decubitus position, has proved invaluable in the assessment of this defect because the flow direction is aligned parallel to the ultrasonic beam. Also, in this position, a secundum ASD can be easily differentiated from a sinus venosus defect because, in the secundum defect, intact AS can be observed between the defect and the origin of the superior vena cava (SVC).

2D color flow imaging cannot be used in timing the duration of flow through the defect with respect to the cardiac cycle because the associated slow frame rates cause time delays in the processing of the flow information. Color M-mode imaging, however, can be used by placing the M-line cursor through the ASD flow signals in the 2D image to categorize and record the exact timing of shunt duration. Most patients with uncomplicated ASD show flow through the ASD during both systole and diastole, and in some patients, this flow is observed continuously through the entire cardiac cycle. These flows have velocities that are usually higher during diastole than systole.

Sometimes a patient showing a septal dropout on 2D color flow imaging can be misdiagnosed as having an ASD because the slow frame rates associated with this technique can cause overlapping of flow patterns in the atria in the region of the septal dropout. This creates the appearance of flow continuity between the two atrial chambers. Because this, in our experience, occurs only during systole, this pattern often serves to differentiate this color image from that obtained in the presence of a true ASD, in which this pattern is also seen during diastole. In addition, in such cases, the right parasternal view fails to reveal the presence of a defect.

An ASD may also be suspected when a flow jet in the RA in the vicinity of the AS is clearly noted even though the defect itself is not viewed with 2D imaging. A confident diagnosis cannot be made, however, unless the transducer is angled carefully to show flow signals moving through this defect. Prominent flow signals moving from the SVC and the inferior vena cava (IVC) in the vicinity of the AS may sometimes cause confusion, and the examiner must be careful not to misinterpret these flow signals as resulting from an ASD.

In an elderly patient of ours, a fairly high velocity flow jet was clearly noted in the RA in the vicinity of the aortic root and the AS, but no defect could be imaged by 2D echocardiography using apical or left parasternal transducer positions. In this patient, the right para-

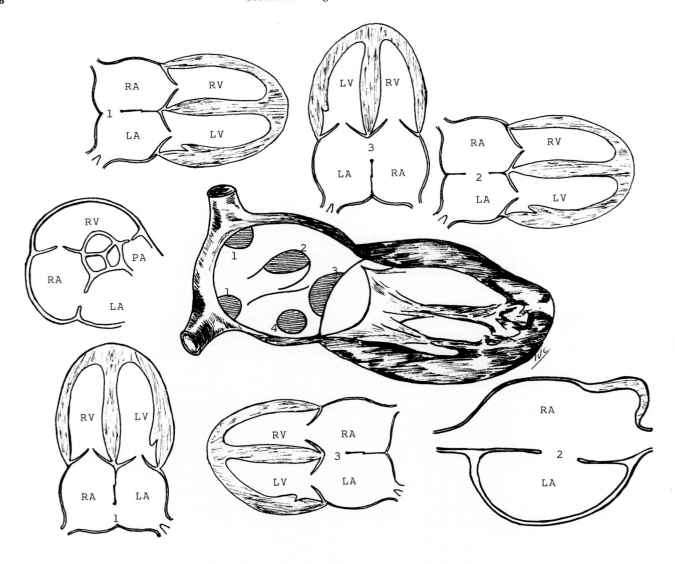

1 – ''Sinus Venosus'' defects
2 – Secundum atrial septal defect
3 – Ostium Primum* atrial septal defect
4 – Communication at the site of the coronary sinus**

*This so-called ostium primum atrial septal defect is in
  fact a type of atrioventricular defect.

**This interatrial communication is characterized by drainage
  of the left superior vena cava to the roof of the left atrium.

Figure 10-1   Diagram illustrates the position of the different types of interatrial communications with the main echocardiographic views to identify them.

sternal window was small and not helpful because the AS, especially near the SVC entrance, could not be visualized in these imaging planes. Because of the presence of prominent flow signals in the RA during both systole and diastole and because the fossa ovalis and the basal portion of the AS were shown to be intact in the standard imaging planes, we suspected that the patient probably had a sinus venosus ASD. This was confirmed subsequently by catheterization and angiocardiography.

Ostium primum ASD is best diagnosed by 2D echocardiography as a defect in the basal portion of the AS using the apical or low left parasternal transducer positions, but color Doppler best defines the characteristics of the shunt flow in this type of ASD. The flow signals through the shunt often present a typical "butterfly" appearance resulting from blood moving from both atria into the respective ventricles and shunting occurring from the LA into the RA. Color Doppler is also useful in assessing the presence and severity of associated TR and MR, which have important prognostic and surgical implications. MR signals can often be seen moving into the LA through the cleft in the anterior mitral leaflet.

The width of the flow signals moving through the ASD also correlates with the width seen on the angiocardiogram and with the size of the defect noted during surgery or autopsy. In patients with ASD and significant pulmonary hypertension, left-to-right shunting is not prominently seen even though the defect can be clearly visualized on 2D examination. This often indicates the presence of pulmonary hypertension, which can be confirmed by placing the continuous wave cursor through the tricuspid regurgitant jet and recording high velocity signals. When the pulmonary artery pressure is normal, continuous wave examination of the tricuspid regurgitant jet reveals low-velocity signals.

VENTRICULAR SEPTAL DEFECT

Large VSDs can be easily diagnosed by 2D echocardiography. The small defects, however, may be difficult to distinguish from the "echo dropouts" which probably result from the parallel orientation of the ultrasonic beam to the tissue. These "dropouts" are commonly observed in routine 2D imaging, but conventional Doppler can be used to help differentiate these "echo dropouts" from true VSD. Because the VS is a large, curved structure and these defects can occur anywhere in this structure, some small VSDs may not be easily recognized in the available standard and nonstandard 2D imaging planes. Multiple VSDs, especially when they are located close together, are also not easily characterized by either 2D or conventional Doppler examination.

We have used color Doppler to supplement the 2D and conventional Doppler examinations in the assessment of VSD. The VS can be scanned in multiple planes with color Doppler to identify turbulence in the RV near the VS. Observation of turbulence in the RV can indicate the presence of this defect. When turbulent blood flow is identified, the transducer is moved and angled to define its site of origin, thus giving a more confident diagnosis of the presence and exact location of the VSD.

Small VSDs may show turbulent flow in only one or two planes, and thus the color setting must remain on when scanning the VS in the different planes to avoid missing these VSDs. The multiple defects, especially when they are located close together, can also be observed using color Doppler. The discrete and separate jets originating from each defect are easier to distinguish with the color flow. As many as three or four separate proximate defects in the same patient have been detected by this technique.

A discrete area of systolic or diastolic flow acceleration on the left side of the septum also indicates the presence of a VSD. This area corresponds to the site of defect on the left side. Some irregular and serpiginous VSDs have their sites of communication between the two ventricles so that they are not directly opposite. In these clinical situations, the left ventricular site of the defect can be easily identified by the location of the flow acceleration. The width of the flow signals moving through the VS is a good indicator of the size of the defect in patients in whom the VSD is not clearly visualized on 2D echocardiographic study. It is particularly useful to look for these signals in diastole because they are laminar because of the relatively low pressure gradient between LV and RV and often clearly outline the anatomic course of the defect and its communication with both ventricles. This is not the case when they are in systole.

Depending on the locations of the defect, VSDs are categorized as perimembranous, muscular, and doubly committed defects (Fig. 10-2). Perimembranous and muscular defects are further divided into subtypes depending on their extensions. A brief description of each defect and its subtypes has been included in Table 10-1.

First, the short axis view at the level of the AV and high LVOT is studied. Perimembranous defects are seen adjacent to the origin of the septal leaflet of the TV. All three extensions can be diagnosed in this view. With an inlet extension of the perimembranous defect, initial systolic flow signals are noted only along the septal leaflet of the TV. Because the flow signals move inferiorly along the VS, they are not observed to extend laterally along the anterior TV leaflet. Some perimembranous VSDs may, however, be large and extend not only toward the inlet but also toward the outlet and trabecular portions of the VS. With an outlet extension, the flow jet is seen moving anteriorly and to the left towards the RVOT and the PV. The trabecular extension is less common, but can be identified by the jet moving laterally towards the free wall of RV. The so-called AV canal type of VSD simply represents a perimembranous defect with a large inlet and posterior extension to the crux cordis (junction of the postero-inferior part of the AS with AV groove).

Muscular defects also can be detected in the parasternal short axis view by the turbulent flow originating more anteriorly in the muscular septum than the turbulent flow of the perimembranous defects. When this flow is directed toward the PV or the right ventricular free wall, this defect is diagnosed as muscular outlet or muscular trabecular, respectively. Unlike perimembranous defects, muscular defects are separated from the septal TV leaflet attachment and the PV by an intact septum. Muscular outlet VSDs, especially if they are small, may be mistaken for severe pulmonic stenosis or right ventricular obstruction because a continuous wave Doppler interrogation reveals high velocities and hence high pressure gradients in the region of the RVOT in the absence of associated pulmonary hypertension. Therefore, a meticulous 2D and color Doppler examination for a VSD should be performed in all patients suspected of having pulmonic stenosis or RVOT obstruction because of Doppler detection of high velocities in the region of the pulmonary artery or outflow tract.

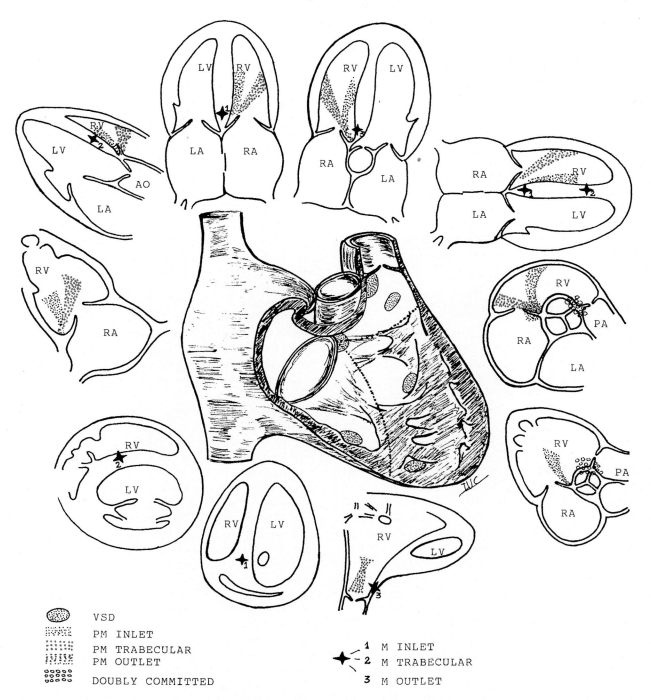

Figure 10-2   Diagram illustrates the position of the different types of ventricular septal defects and the main echocardiographic views to identify them.

Doubly committed VSDs are also observed in the short axis view and are located adjacent to the PV leaflets. They are diagnosed by the absence of intact septum between the VSD and the PV attachment. Color Doppler examination, in these cases, demonstrates prominent flow signals moving through the defect into the PA.

After the short axis view, other views are studied to further assess the presence and type of VSD. In a modified long axis view or an RV inflow plane, an inlet extension of a perimembranous VSD may be diagnosed by noting the VSD jet moving in the RV along the septal leaflet of the TV. The modified parasternal long axis view in which the septal leaflet of the TV can also be visualized is useful in recognizing an inlet extension, by noting the initial systolic flow jet moving along the septal leaflet of the TV and along the VS. Each frame must be carefully examined to track this VSD jet during early systole. A small perimembranous defect with an inlet extension is not evident in the standard parasternal long axis view. Large perimembranous defects, especially

Table 10-1 Ventricular Septal Defects

Type	2D Echo	Color Doppler
Perimembranous VSD A portion of the defect involves the membranous septum (a small fibrous portion of the cardiac septum located directly beneath the AV at the junction of right and noncoronary cusps and related to septal TV leaflet attachment). May have inlet, trabecular, or outlet extension. Inlet as well as posterior extension to crux cordis may be present (AV canal type of defect).	Best seen in short axis (aortic/LVO), modified long axis, or RV inflow views. May be seen in other views, especially if large or multiple extensions are present. No intact septum between VSD and septal TV leaflet attachment. Fibrous tag or aneurysm may be present at defect site. AV canal type of VSD may be visualized in the apical 4-chamber view.	RV turbulence adjacent to septal TV leaflet. Flow signals moving through the septum and presence of systolic/diastolic flow acceleration help localize small defects. Shunting into RA through septal TV leaflet may occur in some cases. Inlet extension: Flow signals seen along septal TV leaflet or VS. Trabecular extension: Flow signals directed laterally toward RV free wall. Outlet extension: Flow signals directed anteriorly and to the left toward the PA.
Muscular VSD. The defect is in the muscular portion of the VS. Membranous septum is not involved. Muscular septum is divided into 3 parts—inlet, trabecular, and outlet. The portion of the VS to which the septal TV leaflet chordae are attached is the inlet septum. The portion of the VS having prominent trabeculations including the body of trabecula septo-marginalis is the trabecular septum. The muscular septum separating the subaortic and subpulmonic area is the outlet (infundibular) septum. Muscular defects may be inlet, trabecular, or outlet in type.	All standard and nonstandard planes may need to be utilized. Rotating the transducer from the apical position will scan the anterior and posterior portions of the VS in a supero-inferior orientation. Muscular inlet: Seen in the proximal VS in apical 4-chamber view or in LV short axis view (near TV but separated from septal TV attachment by intact septum.) Muscular trabecular: May be seen in any view. Defects may be present in anterior or posterior VS and in the proximal, middle or distal (apical) VS. Muscular outlet: Often seen best in the short axis view (aortic/LVO). Intact septum present between the VSD and septal TV leaflet attachment and intact septum also separates the VSD from PV attachment.	Origin of RV flow disturbance, site of flow signals moving from LV to RV, and site of flow acceleration help localize the VSD. Muscular inlet: Flow signals along the proximal VS. Muscular trabecular: No characteristic flow direction. Muscular outlet: Flow signals directed anteriorly and to the left toward the PA.
Doubly committed (subarterial) VSD. The aortic and pulmonary valves form a boundary of the defect. The outlet (infundibular) septum is hypoplastic or absent.	Best seen in the aortic short axis view or subcostal views such as RV inflow-apical-outflow plane. No intact septum present between VSD and PV attachment.	Flow signals are seen moving through VSD into PA.

with multiple extensions, may be visualized in many views, e.g., apical 4-chamber, long axis, and subcostal views. But these perimembranous defects, when small, may be seen only in the high LVOT short axis view.

As mentioned previously, relatively small muscular defects may be difficult to recognize by 2D examination because the VS is a very large structure and the 2D examining plane cuts only a thin slice through it. Therefore, multiple transducer angulations are needed with the color flow turned on to identify these defects. A useful routine is to examine the VS first in standard planes such as the parasternal long axis, apical 4-chamber, and short axis views at multiple levels and then use nonstandard planes in which the transducer is angled in multiple directions from the apical and para-apical positions to view extensively both the anterior and posterior muscular portions of the septum. Angling the transducer anteriorly from the apical position to view the aorta tends to scan the anterior portion of VS. The posterior angulation of the transducer which obtains the apical inferobasal plane visualizes the most posterior aspect of the VS. In this plane, the beam exits through the basal walls of both ventricles, causing the atria to not be visualized. Also, when the transducer is gradually rotated counterclockwise from the apical 4-chamber position to obtain the apical 2-chamber and apical long axis views, a large portion of the VS is scanned anteroposteriorly and superoinferiorly. The apical portion, especially the apical posterior portion, of the VS must be viewed because some defects which are congenital as well as acquired due to septal rupture in acute myocardial infarction may occur in this region. In addition, subcostal views including 4-chamber, short axis, and long axis views, and the right ventricular inflow-apical-outflow plane, are useful in visualizing muscular defects. The subcostal RV inflow-apical-outflow plane can also show the doubly committed defects.

In approximately one third of the patients with perimembranous VSD with inlet extensions, the VSD jet can flow through a fenestration or deficiency in the septal leaflet of the TV into the RA. This may be misdiagnosed as TR. This can be easily differentiated from the usual TR, however, because this regurgitant jet is usually centrally located and originates at the tip of the TV leaflets, while the flow through the perimembranous VSD into the RA originates from the medial aspect of the septal leaflet of the TV. This flow pattern, when present, is a good indicator of the presence of a perimembranous VSD with an inlet extension.

Fibrous tags or a membranous septal aneurysm occasionally seen partially covering a perimembranous defect may deflect the flow jet and cause confusion in classifying the defect by both angiocardiography and color flow mapping. This has presented us with problems in 1 of 5 patients in whom we have visualized the fibrous tag.

Characterization of VSD has surgical importance because parts of the conduction system are located very close to the perimembranous area and the inlet portion of the VS, and depending on the type and extension of the VSD, it may be damaged during operation. Knowledge of the locations of the openings on left and right sides of the VS and the full extent of the VSD is also helpful in planning the surgical approach. Perimembranous and muscular VSDs are known to close spontaneously, and these defects may be examined in a serial manner by echocardiography to assess any reductions in their size. Residual VSDs after surgical patch repair, which has a highly echogenic appearance, can also be detected by color flow imaging.

Dr. Ritter's group has shown that measurement of RV pressures in patients with VSD is more accurate when the continuous wave cursor is guided by color Doppler to parallel the VSD flow signals. High-velocity systolic VSD jets indicate normal RV pressure, while low-velocity VSD jets indicate significant pulmonary hypertension.

Color M-mode examination conducted by placing the M-line cursor through the VSD flow signals reveals the direction of the flow across the VSD during both systole and diastole. This examination is more accurate for timing the onset and duration of the shunt flows than color 2D examination because of the faster frame rates available for color M-mode examination. This shunt flow direction depends on the relative pressures in the two ventricles. A small uncomplicated VSD shows predominantly left-to-right shunting throughout the cardiac cycle. Moderate-sized VSDs, which have a systolic pressure difference of approximately 15 mm Hg or more between the two ventricles, also show predominantly left-to-right shunting during most of the cardiac cycle, but right-to-left shunting may occur briefly during the isovolumic relaxation period. Large VSDs associated

with mild to moderate elevation of pulmonary vascular resistance show bidirectional shunting, which is left to right during early to mid systole and diastole and right to left during late systole and the isovolumic relaxation period. Large VSDs associated with severely elevated pulmonary vascular resistance show left-to-right shunting only during diastole and very early systole. During the rest of systole and the isovolumic relaxation period, right-to-left shunting occurs. The RV systolic pressure in these patients is usually greater than 80% of the LV systolic pressure. In general, the duration and velocity of the right-to-left shunting increases with increasing RV systolic pressure.

A combination of 2D and color flow imaging is very useful in accurately characterizing the types and subtypes of VSD by identifying exactly their sites of origin and extensions. In general, echocardiographic findings correlate well with angiography, which tends to misdiagnose doubly committed defects.

PATENT DUCTUS ARTERIOSUS

The presence of patent ductus arteriosus (PDA) is indicated by the color Doppler display of mosaic turbulent signals in a prominent or dilated PA during diastole and systole. The aortic short axis, high left parasternal, and suprasternal views are the best 2D echocardiographic views in which to observe this flow pattern. The communication between the descending aorta and the PA can also be observed in these views.

In addition, a mosaic jet of antegrade or forward flow moving from the distal PA toward the PV, indicating the presence of a PDA, can be observed by careful angulation of the transducer. This jet is most often directed toward the lateral wall of the PA, but sometimes can be seen oriented medially or centrally in the PA. This jet tends to swirl back as it moves up the PA during late diastole and systole. Because of its decreased velocity and turbulence, this backward or retrograde flow is displayed by nonturbulent blue signals. This swirling pattern is often observed during both systole and diastole.

Careful transducer angulation also may show the bifurcation of the PA and the continuity of flow signals between the descending aorta and the PA. This provides another way of detecting the presence of a PDA. A bounded echo-free space representing the PDA may be also outlined by these continuous flow signals moving from the descending aorta into the PA.

A PDA causes a localized area of accelerated flow in the descending aorta near or at the origin of the ductus. This helps in locating the site of the aortic end of the ductus. After this end is located, the transducer can then be angled to detect and outline the entire ductus. The size of the PDA can be estimated by measuring the width of this flow moving from the descending aorta into the PA. It can also sometimes be estimated by measuring the width of the area of flow acceleration near the aortic end of the ductus because the flow acceleration often takes the shape of the ductus. A long, tortuous ductus arteriosus may not be profiled in its entire length, but the width of the flow through it may still be delineated.

PDA is often associated with a dilated PA. If the PDA is very small, PA dilatation may not be obvious. Both the mitral-pulmonic and the aortic short axis imaging planes are useful in delineating the ductal flow because the former visualizes the anterior and posterior walls and the latter visualizes the medial and lateral walls of the main PA. Associated PV regurgitation may also be present and observed in these planes.

A color M-mode examination accurately times the shunt flow with respect to the cardiac cycle by placing an M-line cursor in a PDA jet. In patients whose PA pressure is normal or less than 2/3 of the systemic pressure, continuous mosaic antegrade signals are noted in the PA. In patients with a PA pressure greater than ⅔ of the systemic pressure, however, only systolic antegrade flow may be noted. Color Doppler examination therefore may help in detecting the presence and development of pulmonary hypertension.

OBSTRUCTIVE LESIONS

Although imaging echocardiography can identify the presence of obstructive congenital cardiac lesions, it does not always allow these lesions to be accurately quantified. Continuous wave Doppler, however, is excellent for assessing the severity of obstructive lesions by its measurement of the velocity increase immediately distal to the stenosis. This velocity increase can be translated into a pressure gradient across the stenosis using the Bernoulli equation. Experimental work has shown a one-to-one correlation between simultaneous Doppler and cardiac catheterization measurements of pressure gradients in human subjects. This work has been further extended to calculate the area of the obstructed orifice using the continuity equation, which involves the additional measurement of the cross-sectional area and the estimation of the velocity time integral in the chamber proximal to the stenosis. Accurate Doppler assessment of stenosis results when the Doppler ultrasonic beam is aligned parallel to the direction of the flow. If the beam is not appropriately aligned, the peak velocities can be significantly underestimated, leading to inaccurate assessment of the severity of the lesion.

The actual flow cannot be visualized during a continuous wave Doppler examination using either the freestanding probe, which does not show the 2D images, or the imaging probe, which generates 2D anatomical images. Because flows are not visualized during a continuous wave Doppler examination, the transducer is angled in various directions by trial and error to obtain maximum velocity. When this velocity is obtained, the Doppler ultrasonic beam is assumed to be optimally aligned parallel to the flow direction. When the stenotic jet has an eccentric orientation, however, parallel alignment of the Doppler beam to the jet in a given 2D

imaging plane may not be possible. Color Doppler overcomes this limitation of continuous wave Doppler by displaying the flow direction. This facilitates the placement of the Doppler cursor parallel to the flow direction. Because the cursor originates from the top of the wedge-shaped sector image, parallel orientation through a markedly eccentric jet may not be possible from one given imaging plane. A Doppler examination using multiple imaging planes may be required in such instances. Because the stenotic jet has a 3-dimensional configuration, an attempt must be made to position the Doppler beam parallel to the "core" of the jet that has the highest velocity. Thus, even after the required orientation is achieved in a 2D imaging plane, the transducer must still be angled in small increments to accurately interrogate the "core" of the jet. Correct alignment of the cursor provides reliable estimate of the peak velocity and thus the peak pressure gradient and the severity of the stenotic lesion. In our experience, the addition of color Doppler to a continuous wave Doppler examination considerably improves the ability to assess the severity of various congenital stenotic lesions.

Another estimation of the severity of a stenotic lesion using color Doppler can be made by directly measuring the proximal width of the flow signals at the origin. These flow signals represent the stenotic jet as it emerges from the valve, and hence their width is expected to approximate closely the width of the stenotic orifice. In practice, excellent correlations have been obtained between the color jet widths and stenotic orifice areas, but to obtain such results, the jet width must be measured at the origin and not distally where the flow signals widen considerably. These signals widen distally because the jet, as it emerges from the valve, creates turbulence in the poststenotic chamber or vessel.

Multiple views must be taken of the stenotic jet to measure its true dimensions. A stenotic orifice is generally assumed to be circular in shape, allowing the width measured in any plane to be used to assess the severity of the lesion. This assumption, however, may not be true for all clinical situations, and in cases of irregularly shaped stenotic orifice or buttonhole stenosis in which the two dimensions of the orifice are markedly different, erroneous assessment of the severity of a stenotic lesion can occur if the jet is measured in only one plane.

The color-guided Doppler cursor alignment gives a more reliable spectral waveform of congenital mitral stenosis. The pressure-half-time computed from this spectral waveform can be used to calculate the effective mitral orifice area.

In conclusion, one advantage of color Doppler assessment of obstructive lesions is that the continuous wave Doppler cursor can be easily placed parallel to the stenotic jet visualized by color Doppler. This allows a more reliable estimation of the pressure gradients. Another advantage is that the proximal stenotic jet width can be measured because of the visible flow signals. This provides a completely independent assessment of the severity of the stenosis. In general, a narrow jet width indicates severe stenosis and a wider jet width indicates less severe stenosis. These advantages give two completely independent methods to evaluate the obstructive lesions present. Therefore, color Doppler is an excellent supplement to the continuous wave Doppler and 2D assessment of stenotic lesions in patients with congenital heart disease.

COMPLICATED LESIONS

The anatomical components of complicated congenital anomalies can be well delineated by imaging echocardiography. Color Doppler identifies the presence and timing of shunts across septal defects and helps in the evaluation of the various stenotic and regurgitant lesions present in the anomaly. Specific complicated lesions have been listed below with a brief description of color Doppler findings for each.

1. Complete atrio-ventricular canal defect (atrio-ventricular septal defect). This anomaly is characterized by the absence of atrio-ventricular septum (septum between the septal TV attachment and anterior MV leaflet attachment), deficiency of the adjacent atrial and inlet VS and common atrio-ventricular annulus (either with common or partitioned atrio-ventricular orifices). This anatomical defect is well seen using 2D echocardiography. Therefore, color Doppler does not help in diagnosing this lesion, but shows the various abnormal flow patterns seen in the entity. Shunting from the LA into the RA and from the LV into the RV are clearly delineated by color Doppler. These flow patterns produce a "butterfly" appearance. Associated right and left atrioventricular valve regurgitations are also clearly revealed by color Doppler. In some patients, left ventricular to right atrial shunt flow through the defect may be shown.

The severity of the atrio-ventricular valve regurgitation is also reliably assessed by color Doppler. Mild regurgitant signals fill less than 20% of the respective atrial area, and severe atrio-ventricular valve regurgitation occupies more than 40% of the atria. Other associated lesions such as muscular VSD defect, secundum ASD, or PDA are also well delineated by color Doppler.

PA pressure can be estimated by aligning the continuous wave Doppler beam parallel to the right sided atrioventricular valve regurgitant jet. The obtained peak velocities can be translated into peak pressure gradients across the valve by using the modified Bernoulli equation. Assuming a right atrial pressure of 10 mm Hg, the right ventricular and PA-systolic pressures can then be obtained. Therefore, pulmonary hypertension, a complication of this defect, can be diagnosed and its severity assessed reliably.

2. Tetralogy of Fallot. Color Doppler is useful in showing the shunt flow across the VSD and any associated AR. When color Doppler is used with 2D echocardiography, the type and extension of VSD is delineated. Color M-mode conducted by passing an M-line cursor through the shunt reliably assesses the timing and direction of the shunt flow. In general, right-to-left shunting occurs during middle and late systole, and left-to-right shunting occurs during diastole and very early systole.

In some patients, associated AR occurs in both the LV and RV. Color Doppler is useful in diagnosing the presence of this associated AR and in comparing the severity of AR in the two ventricles. AR is indicated by the presence of mosaic high-velocity flow signals during diastole just underneath the AV. They are easily distinguished from the lower-velocity shunt flow signals across the VSD. The low velocities in the shunt flow result from the flow moving through the large defect and, hence, a very small or almost no gradient exists between the two ventricles.

Infundibular and pulmonary valve stenosis may be evaluated by the color-guided continuous wave Doppler technique using the modified Bernoulli equation. The proximal width of the stenotic jet at the level of the obstruction correlates well with the assessed severity of the stenosis. Other lesions such as associated ASD are also easily identified by color Doppler.

3. Double outlet RV. Color Doppler examination of this defect shows flow patterns similar to those observed in tetralogy of Fallot. Color Doppler is used to evaluate atrioventricular valve and semilunar valve regurgitation and to observe shunt flow through the VSD.

4. Single ventricle. Both the tricuspid and mitral inflow signals are observed moving into the single ventricle by color Doppler, which also reliably evaluates the presence and severity of associated atrio-ventricular valve regurgitation.

5. Transposition of the great vessels. Associated defects such as VSD and ASD, tricuspid and mitral regurgitation, subpulmonic and pulmonary valve stenosis, and semilunar valve regurgitation can be delineated by color Doppler echocardiography. Flow in the intra-atrial baffle, which is often surgically placed to achieve physiological correction in this anomaly, and the presence of baffle leak and obstruction can also be detected.

6. Tricuspid atresia. In this anomaly, flow signals are clearly seen moving through the atrial and ventricular septal defects by color Doppler. Flow signals move into the LV through the open MV during diastole, but no flows are seen moving through the thickened and atretic TV. This finding helps to provide a more confident diagnosis of tricuspid atresia and differentiates it from severe tricuspid stenosis. The presence and severity of associated MR can also be evaluated. MR is often observed because of the enlarged LV and the dilatation of the mitral annulus.

7. Pulmonary valve atresia. Associated ventricular and atrial septal defects are shown by color Doppler in this entity. Systemic-to-pulmonary-artery shunts are also characterized by observing turbulent flow in the pulmonary artery, aorta, or cephalic branches arising from the aorta from suprasternal or right parasternal imaging planes. The Blalock-Taussig shunt may also be well visualized. In clinically suspected cases, PV atresia

can be ruled out when flow signals are observed moving through the PV.

8. Ebstein's anomaly of the tricuspid valve. This anomaly is characterized by an apparent displacement of the septal and/or other leaflets of the TV towards the right ventricular apex, resulting from plastering of the proximal portion of the involved leaflet(s) to the VS or right ventricular wall. The degree of this displacement determines the relative sizes of the atrialized RV and the functional right ventricular chamber. In general, the septal tricuspid leaflet origin appears to be inferiorly displaced, while the anterior leaflet has a normal origin from the annulus. The anterior leaflet, however, is considerably elongated and has a "snake-like" motion. The septal leaflet of the TV may demonstrate restricted mobility when it is anchored to the VS by chordal attachments. These valvular abnormalities frequently cause considerable TR, although an occasional patient may also show evidence of mild TV stenosis. A patent foramen ovale or an ASD may be present in this anomaly, and because of increased right atrial pressure may result in right-to-left shunting at the atrial level.

With color Doppler, TR can be readily identified and its severity reliably assessed by noting the proportion of the RA occupied by the reversed flow signals.

Because the right ventricular systolic pressure is often low and the right atrial pressure high, the tricuspid regurgitant jet may have a low velocity. This low-velocity regurgitation is easily detected on color flow mapping as low velocity reversed flow signals (deep blue). With conventional Doppler, however, these low velocity signals may not be recognized as due to TR because of the absence of aliasing, and the severity of regurgitation may thus be markedly underestimated.

Color-guided continuous wave Doppler interrogation of the tricuspid inflow and regurgitant jets aids in obtaining the pressure gradients across the TV in diastole and systole, respectively. The diastolic gradient permits accurate evaluation of any tricuspid stenosis present, while the systolic gradient allows estimation of the right ventricular and pulmonary artery systolic pressures.

Color Doppler also aids in characterizing the direction and timing of flows across an associated ASD or patent foramen ovale.

REFERENCES

Atrial Septal Defect

1. Kyo, S., Omoto R., Takamoto, S., and Takanawa, E.: Quantitative estimation of intracardiac shunt flow in atrial septal defects by real-time two-dimensional color flow Doppler. Circulation 70:39, 1984.
2. Omoto, R., Yokote, Y., Takamoto, S., Kyo S., Tamura, F., Asano, H., Namekawa, K., Kasai, C., Kondo, Y., and Koyano, A.: Diagnostic significance of real-time two-dimensional Doppler echocardiography (2-D Doppler) in congenital heart diseases, acquired valvular diseases, and dissecting aortic aneurysms. J. Cardiol. 14:103, 1984.
3. Suzuki, Y., Kambara, H., Kadota, K., Tamaki, S., Yamazota, A., Nohara, R., Osakada, G., and Kawai, C.: Detection of intracardiac shunt flow in atrial septal defect using

a real-time two-dimensional color-coded Doppler flow imaging system and comparison with contrast two-dimensional echocardiography. Am. J. Cardiol. 56:347, 1985.
4. Takamoto, S., Kyo, S., Adachi, H., Matsumura, M., Yokote, Y., and Omoto, R.: Intraoperative color flow mapping by real-time two-dimensional Doppler echocardiography for evaluation of valvular and congenital heart disease and vascular disease. J. Thorac. Cardiovasc. Surg. 90:802, 1985.
5. Swensson, R.E., Sahn, D.J., and Vales-Cruz, I.M.: Color flow Doppler mapping in congenital heart disease. Echocardiography: A review of cardiovascular ultrasound 2:545, 1985.
6. Ritter, S.B.: Color Flow Mapping. A Visual Text of Congenital and Acquired Heart Disease. Johnson and Johnson Ultrasound Inc, Ramsey, NJ, and Lea & Febiger, Philadelphia, PA, 1986.
7. Ritter, S.B.: Two-dimensional Doppler color mapping in congenital heart disease. Clin. Cardiol. 9:12:591, 1986.
8. Reeder, G.S., Seward, J.B., Hagler, D.J., and Tajik, A.J.: Color flow imaging in congenital heart disease. Echocardiography: A review of cardiovascular ultrasound 3:533, 1986.
9. Colvin, E., Nanda, N.C., and Bargeron, I.M.: Color Doppler flow mapping in atrioventricular septal defects (Abstract). Circulation 72 (Supp III):III-436, 1985.
10. Shah, R.M., and Roitman, D.I.: Doppler color flow mapping in congenital heart disease (Abstract). Circulation 72 (Supp III):III-28, 1985.
11. Fan, P.H., Philpot, E., and Nanda, N.C.: Color Doppler echocardiography in congenital heart disease. Diagnostic Imaging 9:288, 1987.
12. Helmcke, F., Aggarwal, K.K., Nanda, N.C., Moos, S., Daruwala, D.F., and Gupta, A.: Color Doppler assessment of shunt flow across large atrial septal defects (Abstract). J. Am. Coll. Cardiol. 11:240A, 1988.

Ventricular Septal Defect

1. Stevenson, J.G., Kawabori, I., Dooley, T.K., and Guntheroth, W.G.: Diagnosis of ventricular septal defect by pulsed Doppler echocardiography: Sensitivity, specificity, and limitation. Circulation 58:322, 1978.
2. D'Arcy, B.J., and Nanda, N.C.: Two-dimensional echo features of right ventricular infarction. Circulation 65:167, 1982.
3. Stevenson, J.G., Kawabori, I., and Brandestini, N.: Color coded Doppler visualization of flow within ventricular septal defects: Implications for peak pulmonary artery pressure (Abstract). Am. J. Cardiol. 49:944, 1982.
4. Santamaria, H., Soto, B., Ceballos, R., Bargeron, L.M., Jr., Coghlan, H.C., and Kirklin, J.W.: Angiographic differentiation of types of ventricular septal defects. A.J.R. 141:273, 1983.
5. Ortiz, E., Robinson, P.J., Deanfield, J.E., Franklin, R., Macartney, F.J., and Wyse, R.K.H.: Localisation of ventricular septal defects by simultaneous display of superimposed colour Doppler and cross section echocardiographic images. Br. Heart J. 54:43, 1985.
6. Marx, J.R., Allen, H., and Goldberg, S.J.: Doppler echocardiographic estimation of systolic pulmonary artery pressure in pediatric patients with interventricular communications. J. Am. Coll. Cardiol. 6:1132, 1985.
7. Takamoto, S., Kyo, S., Adachi, H., Matsumura, M., Hokote, Y., and Omoto, R.: Intraoperative color flow mapping by real-time two-dimensional Doppler echocardiography for evaluation of valvular and congenital heart disease and vascular disease. J. Thorac. Cardiovasc. Surg. 90:802, 1985.

8. Ludomirsky, A., Huhta, J.C., Vick, G.W., Murphy, D.J., Jr., Danford, D.A., and Morrow, W.R.: Color Doppler detection of multiple ventricular septal defects. Circulation 74:1317, 1986.
9. Chung, K.H., Sherman, F.S., Sahn, D.J., Hagen-Ansert, S., Swensson, R.E., and Valdes-Cruz, I.M.: Real-time Doppler color flow mapping for assessment of patch and baffle leaks after surgery for congenital heart defects (Abstract). J. Am. Coll. Cardiol. 7:14A, 1986.
10. Hillel, Z., Thys, D., Ritter, S.B., Goldman, M., Griepp, R., and Kaplan, J.: Two-dimensional Doppler flow echocardiography for the intraoperative monitoring of cardiac shunt flows in patients with congenital heart disease. J. Cardiothorac. Anesth. 1:42, 1987.
11. Moos, S., Helmcke, F., Shah, R., Pinamonti, B., and Nanda, N.C.: Color Doppler in ventricular septal defect with pulmonary hypertension (Abstract). Clin. Res. 35:307A, 1987.
12. Helmcke, F., Pinamonti, B., Colvin, E.C., Moos, S., Adey, C.K., Soto, B., and Nanda, N.C.: Color Doppler evaluation of type of ventricular septal defect (Abstract). Clin. Res. 35:286A, 1987.

Patent Ductus Arteriosus

1. Kyo, S., Takamoto, S., Ueda, K., Emoto, H., Tamura, F., Asano, H., Yokote, Y., Omoto, R., and Takanawa, E.: Clinical significance of newly developed real-time two-dimensional Doppler echocardiography (2-D Doppler) in congenital heart diseases: With special reference to the assessment of the intracardiac shunts. Proceedings of the 43rd Meeting of the Japan Society of Ultrasonics in Medicine, 465, 1983.
2. Kyo, S., Omoto, R., Takamoto, S., Ueda, K., Emoto, H., Asano, H., and Yokote, Y.: Real-time two-dimensional Doppler echocardiography in congenital heart disease. J. Cardiogr. 14:785, 1984.
3. Kyo, S., Shime, H., Omoto, R., and Takamoto, S.: Evaluation of intracardiac shunt flow in premature infants by color flow mapping real-time two-dimensional Doppler echocardiography. Circulation 70:456, 1984.
4. Ritter, S.B., Golinko, R.J., and Copper, R.S.: Systemic to pulmonary artery anastomoses: Pulsed Doppler evaluation of aortic flow properties (Abstract). J. Ultrasound Med. Biol. 3:42, 1984.
5. Reeder, G.S., Currie, P.J., Hagler, D.J., Tajik, A.J., and Seward, J.B.: Use of Doppler techniques (continuous-wave, pulse-wave, and color flow imaging) in the noninvasive hemodynamic assessment of congenital heart disease. Mayo Clin. Proc. 61:725, 1986.
6. Hillel, Z., Thys, D., Ritter, S.B., Goldman, M., Griepp, R., and Kaplan, J.: Two-dimensional color flow Doppler echocardiography: Intraoperative monitoring of cardiac shunt flow in patients with congenital heart disease. J. Cardiothorac. Anesth. 1:42, 1987.
7. Sahn, D.J., and Allen, H.D.: Real-time cross-sectional echocardiographic imaging of the patent ductus arteriosus in infants and children. Circulation 58:343, 1987.
8. Fan, P.H., Philpot, E., and Nanda, N.C.: Color Doppler echocardiography in congenital heart disease. Diagnostic Imaging 9:288, 1987.

Obstructive Lesions

1. Omoto, R.: Color Atlas of Real-Time Two-Dimensional Doppler Echocardiography. Tokyo, Shindan-To-Chiryo Co., Ltd. 1984, and Philadelphia, Lea & Febiger, 1984.
2. Ritter, S.B.: Color Flow Mapping. A Visual Text of Congenital and Acquired Heart Disease. Ramsey, NJ, Johnson and Johnson Ultrasound Inc., and Philadelphia, Lea & Febiger, 1986.
3. Fan, P.H., Philpot, E., and Nanda, N.C.: Color Doppler echocardiography in congenital heart disease. Diagn. Imag. 9:288, 1987.
4. Murphy, D.J., Jr., and Judd, V.E.: Postoperative congenital heart disease. In Ludomirsky, A., and Huhta, J.C. (eds): Color Doppler of Congenital Heart Disease in the Child and Adult. Mount Kisco, NY, Futura Publishing, 1987.

Complicated Lesions

1. Nanda, N.C.: Case Studies in Color Doppler Echocardiography. New York, Igaku-Shoin Medical Publishers, Inc., 1985.
2. Satomi, G., Takao, A., Momma, K., Mori, K., Ando, M., Touyama, K., Konishi, T., Tomimatsu, H., Nakazawa, M., and Nakamura, K.: Detection of the drainage site in anomalous pulmonary venous connection by two-dimensional Doppler color flow mapping echocardiography. Heart Vessels 2:41, 1986.
3. Ritter, S.B., Arnon, R., Steinfeld, L., Kawai, D., and Golinko, R.J.: Anomalous venous drainage: Identification by Doppler color flow mapping (Abstract). Circulation 74:37, 1986.
4. Fan, P.H., Philpot, E., and Nanda, N.C.: Color Doppler echocardiography in congenital heart disease. Diagn. Imag. 9:288, 1987.

SECTION 10 CONGENITAL HEART DISEASE
A. ATRIAL SEPTAL DEFECTS

Figure CA-1 **Atrial septal defect.** (A) Autopsy specimen from an elderly patient shows a large ASD (arrow) of the secundum variety. (B) Autopsy specimen shows a fenestrated ASD (arrow). This patient also shows rupture of the sinus of Valsalva into the RA and vegetations (V) in its vicinity. Small thrombi are also present in the right atrial appendage (RAA). (C) Schematic shows flow through an ASD.

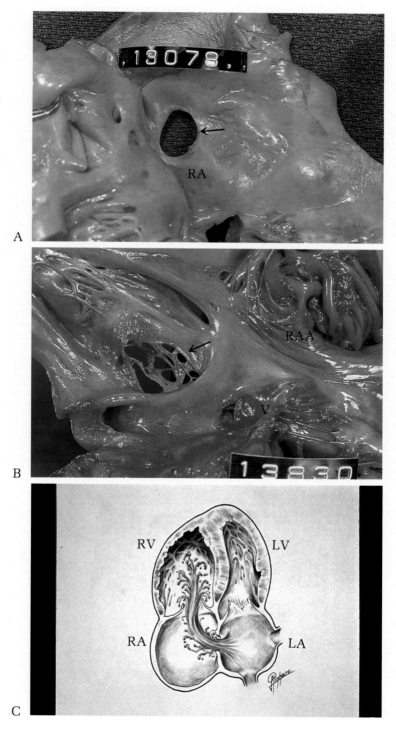

Figure CA-2 **Secundum atrial septal defect.** (A) Apical 4-chamber view in a 40-year-old woman shows a large defect (D) in the AS. B and C are color flow studies showing flow signals moving from the LA into the RA through the defect.

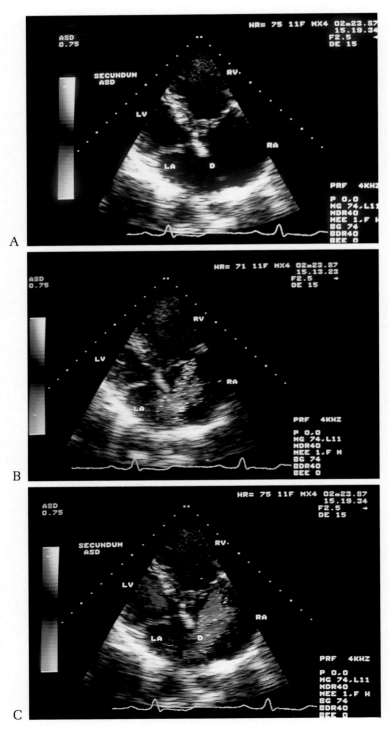

SECTION 10   CONGENITAL HEART DISEASE

Figure CA-3   **Secundum atrial septal defect.** (A) Color flow study in an adult shows flow moving from the LA into the RA and RV through the ASD, imaged from a para-apical transducer position. The mosaic pattern of colors noted in the RA and RV is due to high-velocity flow and turbulence. (B,C) Aortic short axis views in another adult patient show the large defect (D) and flow moving through it into the right heart. (D) Modified apical 4-chamber view in another patient (38-year-old woman) shows prominent flow signals (red with bluish-green due to aliasing) moving into the RA through a secundum defect that reopened after septal repair 10 years ago. The defect was reclosed (E,F). Apical 4-chamber views in a 23-year-old woman show prominent flow signals moving from the LA into the RA and RV through a large secundum defect during diastole.

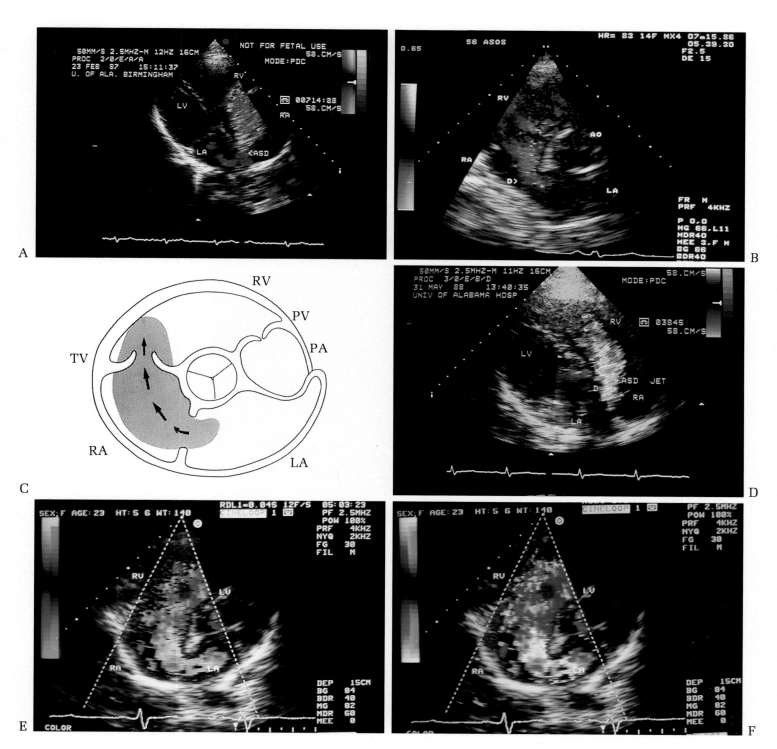

Figure CA-4 **Secundum atrial septal defect.** (A) Examination of the HV. Color Doppler M-mode shows egress of flow into the hepatic vein (H) during late systole (red) in an 18-year-old man. This finding results from the proximity of the opening of the IVC to the secundum defect so that blood flow entering the RA through the defect easily finds its way into the IVC and HV. Early and mid-systolic flow moving towards the RA (blue with yellow in it due to aliasing) and flow (red) moving into the HV during atrial systole (A) represent normal flow patterns. Late systolic flow into the HV in ASD (AB) is easily differentiated from moderate or severe tricuspid incompetence, which results in predominantly early to mid-systolic retrograde flow into HVs. (B) Pulse and color Doppler interrogation of the HV in another patient with secundum ASD shows prominent late systolic flow (AB) into the HV. B = Doppler baseline; D = D wave; S = S wave.

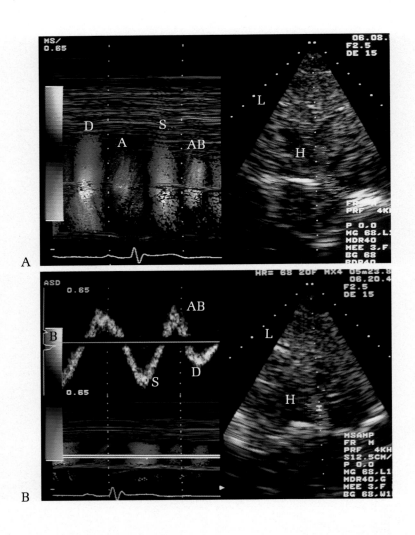

Figure CA-5   **Secundum atrial septal defect mimic.** (A) Apical 4-chamber view in a 27-year-old woman shows a large dropout in the region of the AS. There was no clinical or electrocardiographic evidence for an ASD and the 2D echocardiogram did not show RV enlargement or evidence of right-sided volume overload. (B) Color flow study from the same patient shows flow toward the transducer in both atria in systole. The flow in the LA probably represents pulmonary venous return, and in the RA, IVC drainage. Note that the two flow streams are very close to each other in the region of the septal dropout. (C) The transducer was slightly angled to produce an appearance of systolic flow moving from the LA into the RA through the septal dropout. This finding was noted in one isolated plane only and was absent during diastole, excluding the presence of an ASD.

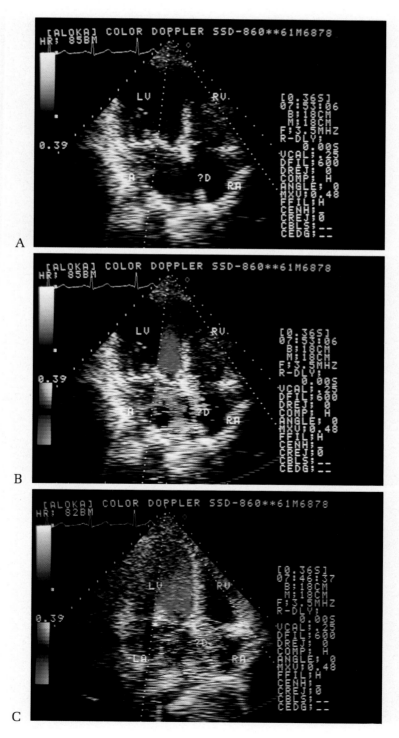

Figure CA-6 **Secundum atrial septal defect.** (A) Schematic shows secundum ASD imaged from the right parasternal transducer position. (B) Real-time 2D examination shows a large ASD in a 7-year-old girl. (C) Color flow study shows streaming of blood flow (red) from two posteriorly placed left superior and inferior PVs into the RA through the defect. (D) The blue flow signals near the AS represent flow from the two anteriorly placed right superior and inferior PVs. Schematic (D) shows atrial flow directions in this patient. Color M-mode (E) shows flow signals (F) moving through the defect into RA in both systole and diastole. CS = coronary sinus.

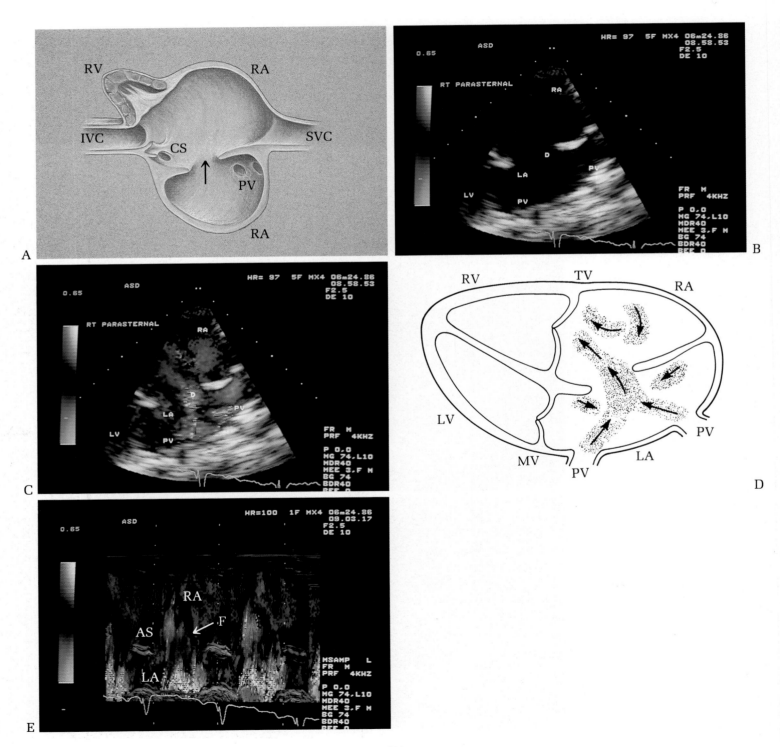

SECTION 10   CONGENITAL HEART DISEASE

Figure CA-7   **Secundum atrial septal defect.** (A) Right parasternal approach in a 15-year-old girl demonstrates prominent flow signals (red with some blue due to aliasing) moving from the LA into the RA through the large ASD, D. Intact septum between the defect and SVC opening excludes the presence of a sinus venosus type of ASD. The secundum ASD is also clearly diagnosed in a 57-year-old woman from the right parasternal approach (B,C). Intact AS on either side of the defect excludes the presence of both sinus venosus and ostium primum defects. CS = coronary sinus.

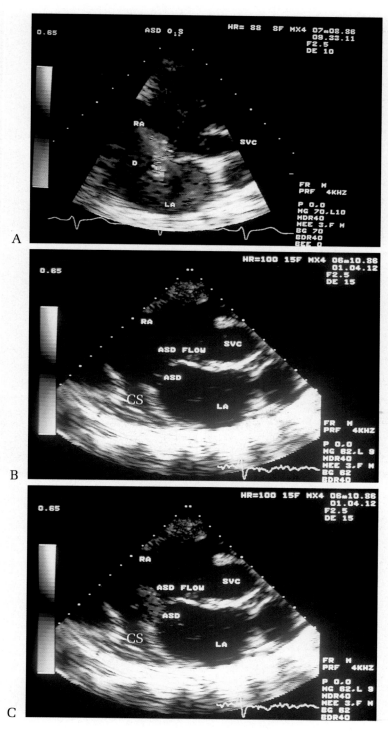

Figure CA-8 **Secundum atrial septal defect.** Para-apical 4-chamber (A,B) and right parasternal (C,D) views in a 5-year-old girl show two areas of discontinuity in the AS, but color Doppler examination demonstrates flow signals (red with some blue due to aliasing) passing from the LA into the RA through only one, thus identifying it as a true defect (D).

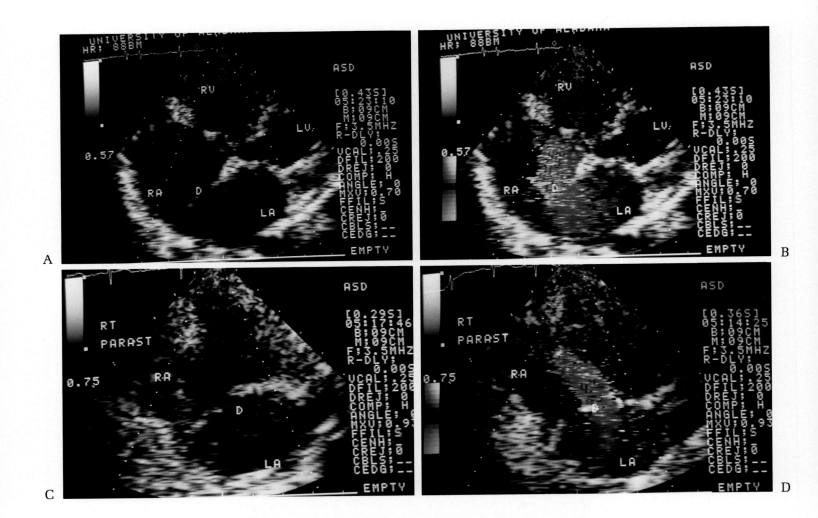

Figure CA-9   Patent foramen ovale/small secundum atrial septal defect. (A) Right parasternal examination in a 20-year-old man who underwent pulmonary valvotomy in childhood shows a very small defect (D) in the middle of the AS. EV = Eustachian valve. In B, a narrow flow jet is noted moving from the LA through the defect into the RA, corresponding with the small defect seen on the 2D examination. Minimal transducer angulation (C) shows localized areas of thickening bordering the small defect, and a small flame-shaped jet. An M-line cursor, used to time the duration of flow through the defect, shows left-to-right shunting (F) in both systole and diastole (D,E). Greenish-colored signals during diastole result from turbulence. F is an autopsy specimen from another patient, showing a patent foramen ovale (arrows).

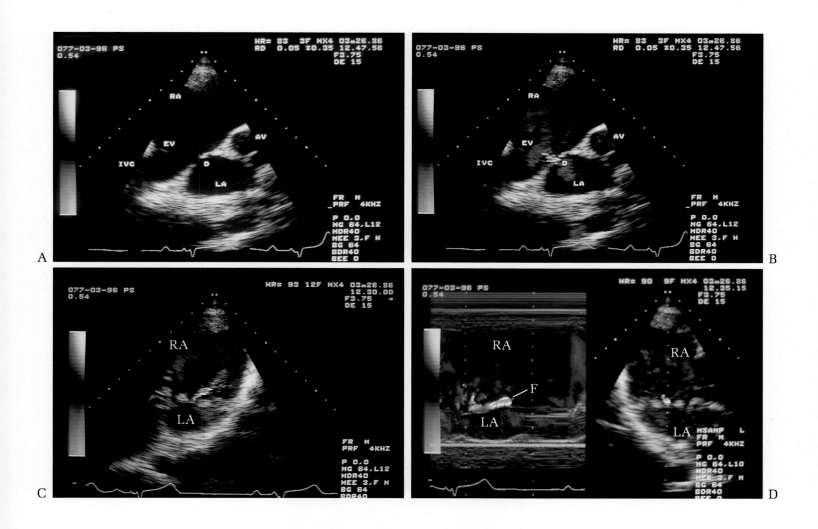

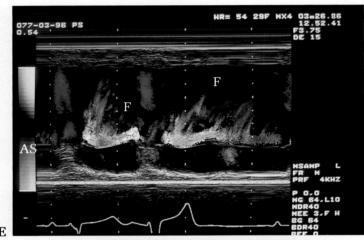

E

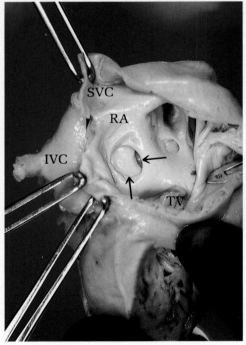

F

Figure CA-10 **Secundum atrial septal defect associated with tricuspid regurgitation.** (A) Short axis view at the level of the high LVOT in a young woman shows a wide band of flow signals moving from the LA into the RA, indicating a large defect. Small areas of blue-colored signals within the large yellowish red shunt flow represent aliasing. Greenish signals originating from the TV and moving superiorly into the RA next to the shunt signals represent TR in this end-systolic frame. Apical 4-chamber view (B,C) in a 71-year-old woman shows shunting from the LA into the RA through a large defect and mosaic-colored systolic signals in the RA due to TR.

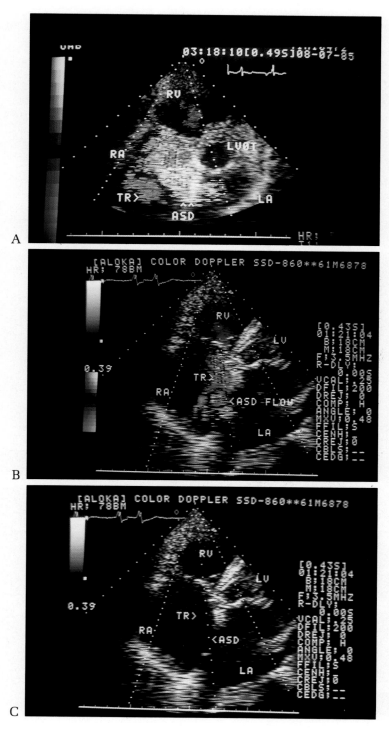

Figure CA-11   **Secundum atrial septal defect associated with pulmonary hypertension.** (A,B) Left-to-right shunting is noted through the large defect (D) imaged in a low parasternal 4-chamber view in a 37-year-old woman. (C) Color M-mode examination demonstrates shunting (red signals) in late systole and green signals due to TR in early systole in RA. Blue signals moving from the RA into the LA represent right-to-left shunting in this patient (D). Mosaic signals in RA originating from the TV during systole represent TR (E). Some of the associated red signals in RA may be related to the swirling of the TR jet and can be confused with left-to-right shunting (E). Measurement of PA pressure is shown in F. The continuous wave Doppler cursor line is placed parallel to the TR jet direction in the same patient and a peak velocity of 4.72 m/sec is obtained; this translates into a peak pressure gradient of 89 mm Hg using the Bernoulli equation. The right ventricular pressure is thus estimated as 99 mm Hg, which is in the systemic range in this patient.

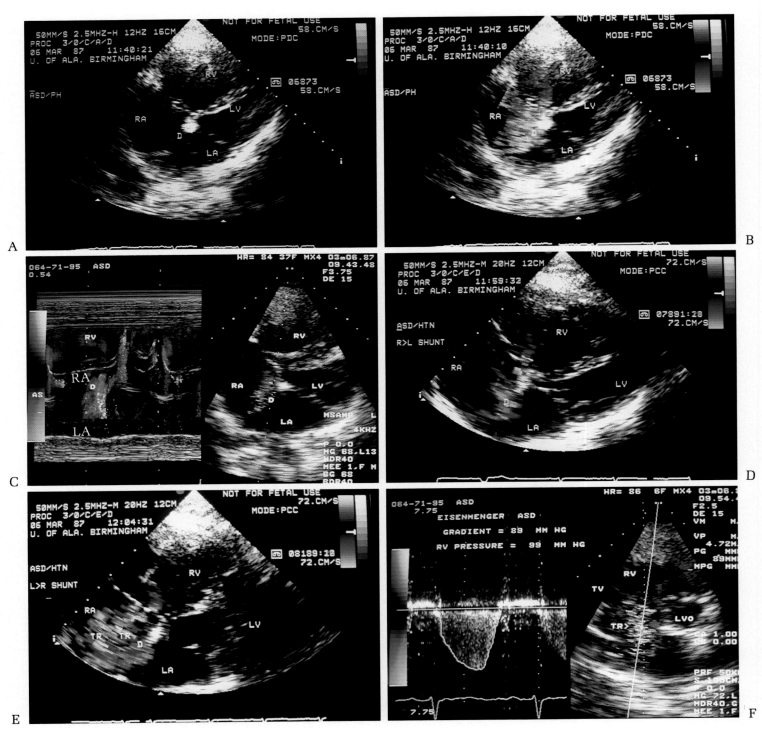

Figure CA-12   **Secundum atrial septal defect associated with atrial septal aneurysm.** (A,B) Subcostal 4-chamber examination in an 8-month-old infant shows a well-defined atrial septal aneurysm (arrow) and left-to-right shunting through the defect.

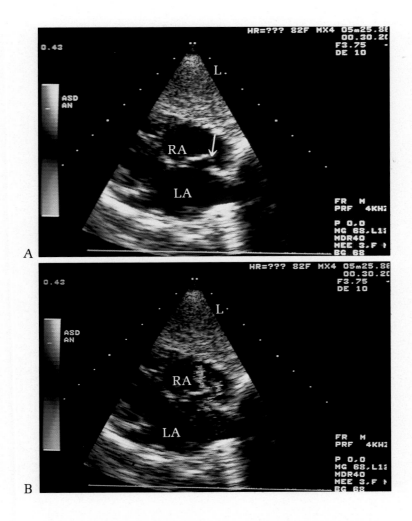

Figure CA-13   **Secundum atrial septal defect associated with ventricular septal defect.** (A,B, and C) Para-apical and parasternal 4-chamber views in a 1-month old infant show left-to-right shunting through an ASD and a muscular VSD (arrows).

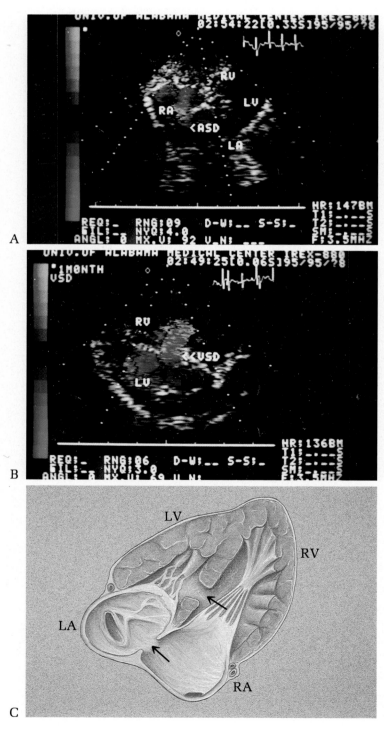

SECTION 10 CONGENITAL HEART DISEASE

Figure CA-14 **Secundum atrial septal defect associated with partial anomalous pulmonary venous drainage into the left azygos vein.** (A) Para-apical view shows some residual left-to-right shunting in a 48-year-old woman who had previously undergone repair of a large secundum ASD. (B) Right supraclavicular examination shows flow disturbance, characterized by both bluish-green and red color signals in the SVC. Pulse Doppler interrogation also reveals abnormal retrograde signals in the SVC in systole, consistent with partial anomalous pulmonary venous drainage into this area. C is an autopsy specimen from another patient showing all pulmonary veins (PV) draining into the azygos vein (AZ). ABN FL = Abnormal flow signals.

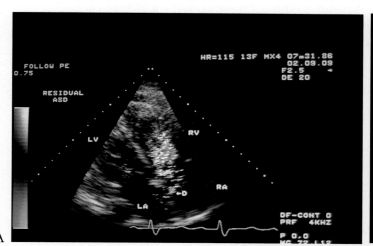

A

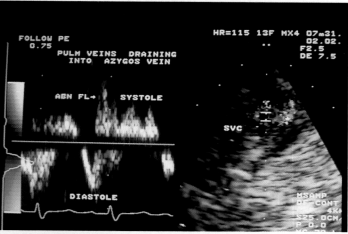

B

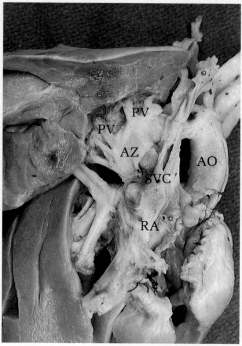

C

Figure CA-15 **Ostium primum atrial septal defect.** (A,B,C,D,E) Apical 4-chamber views in a 25-year-old man show blood flow signals (red) moving from the LA into the RA through a defect (D, horizontal arrow) at the base of the AS and flow signals moving from both atria into the respective ventricles producing a typical "butterfly" appearance. In B, flow signals are also seen moving into the RA through a smaller associated secundum ASD (oblique arrow). Color M-mode also shows left-to-right shunting through the defect. Measurement of the PA pressure is shown in F and G. The continuous wave Doppler cursor line is placed in the small TR jet and a peak velocity of 2.72 m/sec is obtained. This translates into a peak pressure gradient of 30 mm Hg using the Bernoulli equation and a calculated systolic PA pressure of 40 mm Hg. Thus there is no significant elevation of PA pressure in this patient. Color M-mode echocardiogram of the MV (H) shows blue signals in the LA during systole, indicating MR. Note the prolonged mitral septal apposition in diastole and a narrow LVOT, both typical of this entity. Another color M-mode echocardiogram (I) was obtained by placing an M-line cursor through the area of the cleft in the anterior MV leaflet seen on the 2D image. A dropout in the M-mode recording of the MV, consistent with imaging of the cleft (C) in diastole, enlarged RV, and abnormal anterior ventricular septal motion during systole are visualized. Color M-mode recording also shows blue signals in late diastole in the LA, indicating diastolic MR resulting from first degree atrio-ventricular block present in this patient (J). K is an autopsy specimen from another patient showing a large ostium primum ASD (arrow). Note its location at the base of the AS.

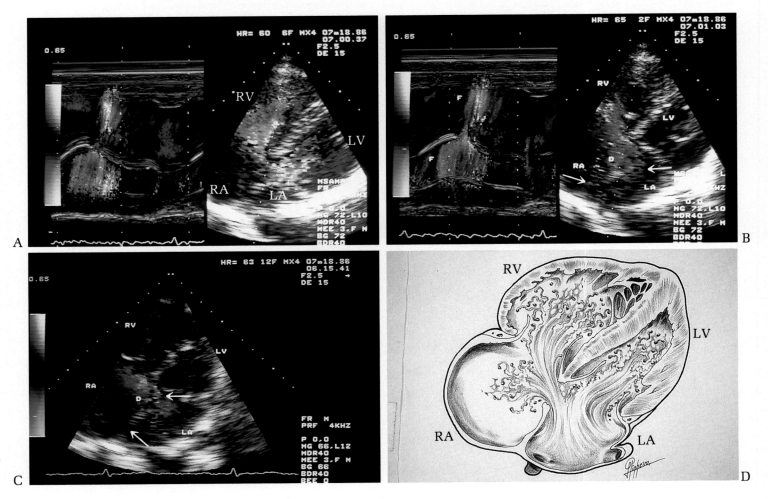

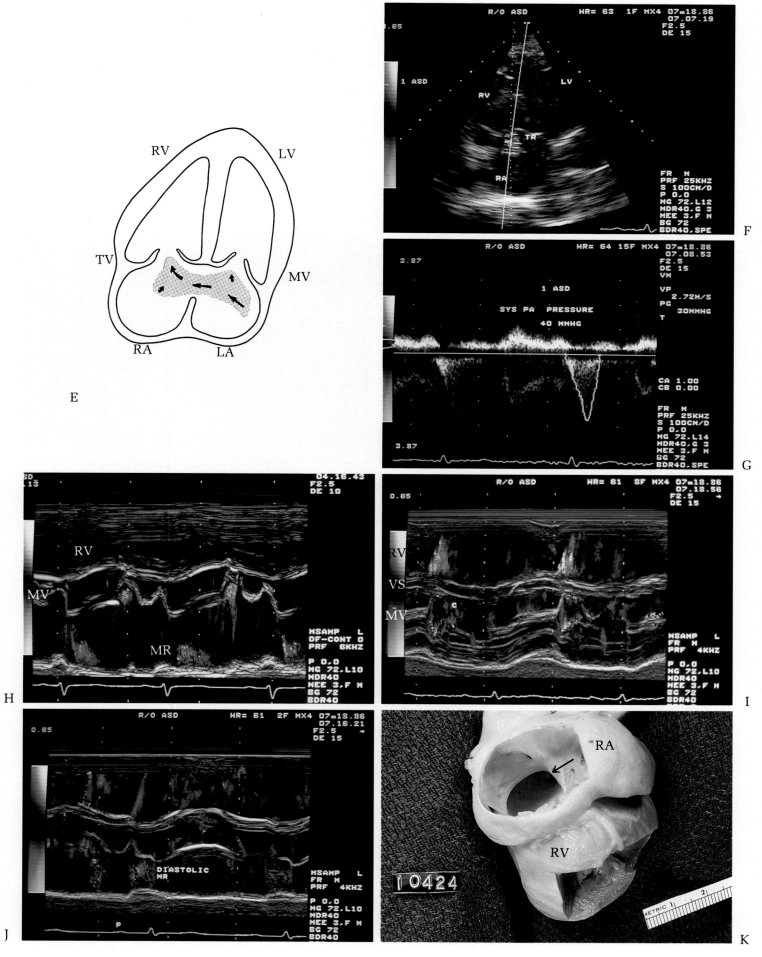

SECTION 10   CONGENITAL HEART DISEASE

Figure CA-16   Ostium primum atrial septal defect. (A,B) Left ventricular short axis views at the level of the MV in a 29-year-old woman show a prominent cleft (C) in the anterior leaflet and an intact posterior cusp. (C,D,E,F) Left ventricular short axis views at the level of the MV in another young woman who had an ostium primum ASD repaired in childhood, showing a large cleft (C) in the anterior mitral leaflet and prominent blue and greenish-blue signals of MR moving through the cleft into the LA during systole. The parasternal long axis view (G) demonstrates mosaic-colored signals occupying most of the LA in systole, indicating severe MR. H is an autopsy specimen from another patient showing a large cleft (arrow) in the anterior mitral leaflet.

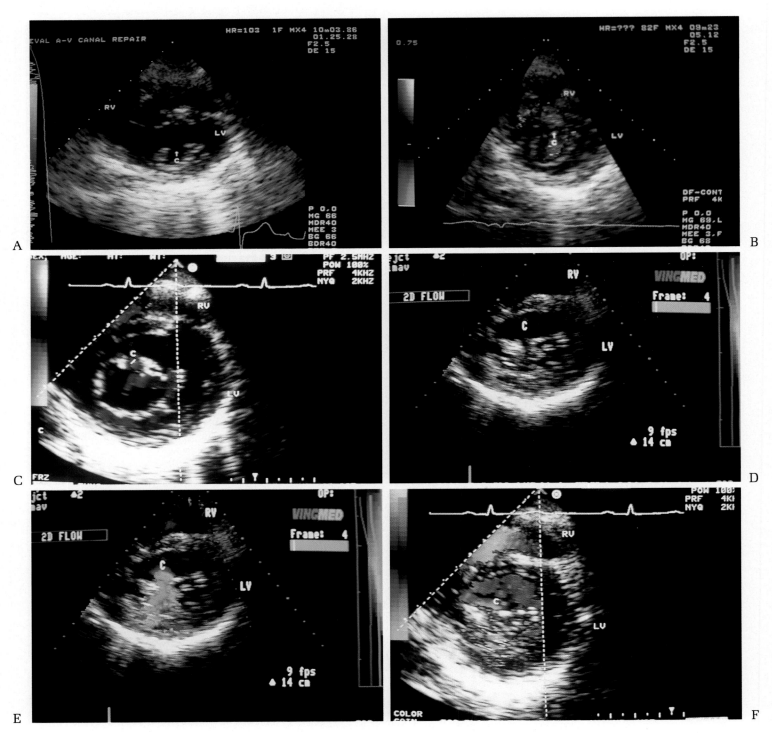

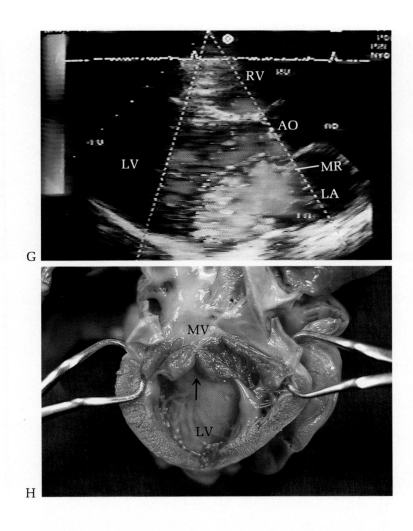

G

H

Figure CA-17   Ostium primum atrial septal defect with mitral regurgitation into the right atrium. (A,B) Apical 4-chamber view demonstrates blue signals originating from the MV and moving through the defect into the right atrial cavity.

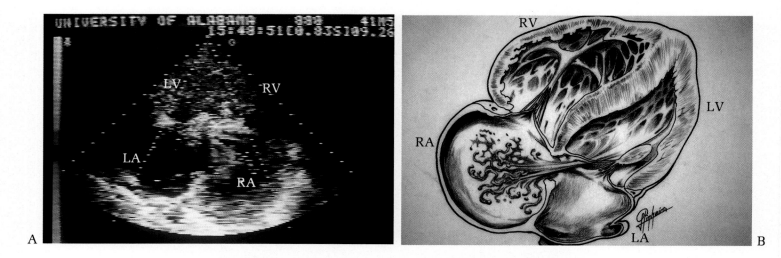

Figure CA-18   Ostium primum atrial septal defect: Residual mitral regurgitation. Mild residual MR is noted in an adult patient in whom the cleft in the anterior mitral leaflet was surgically repaired.

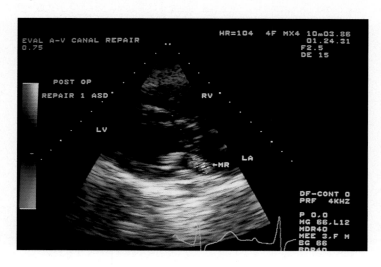

Figure ·CA-19 **Sinus venosus atrial septal defect.** (A) Right parasternal examination in a 5-year-old child shows prominent blood flow signals (red) moving from the LA into the RA through an ASD located at the entrance of the SVC into the RA. B is an autopsy specimen from another patient showing a large sinus venosus ASD (arrow). Note its location at the entrance of the SVC into the RA. RAA = right atrial appendage.

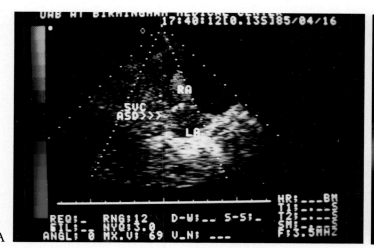
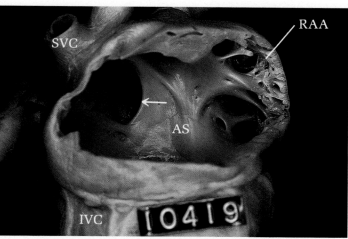

A   B

Figure CA-20 **Sinus venosus atrial septal defect.** A large flow jet (J) was consistently noted entering the RA in the vicinity of the aortic root imaged in short axis in a 74-year-old female. No ASD, however, could be visualized from any of the parasternal or apical transducer positions, and the right parasternal examination was not successful because of a very small cardiac window. Because all of the AS except the portion near the SVC could be well imaged in this patient and was intact, the possibility that this was a sinus venosus defect was raised, and was subsequently confirmed at cardiac catheterization and surgery.

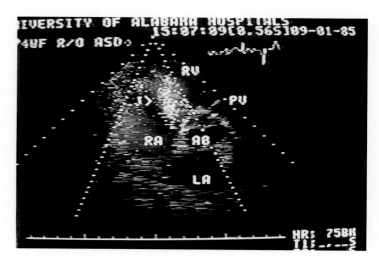

Figure CA-21 **Pulmonary artery flow in a patient with atrial septal defect.** Color M-mode of the PV shows a mosaic pattern of colors during systole, indicating increased flow through the PV.

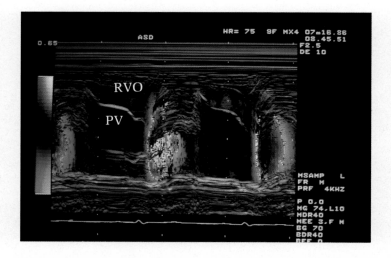

Figure CA-22 **Tricuspid valve in atrial septal defect.** M-mode recording of the TV shows high-frequency diastolic fluttering in a patient with a large secundum defect.

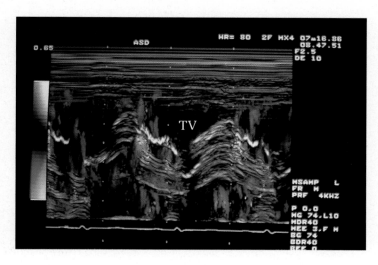

SECTION 10 CONGENITAL HEART DISEASE

Figure CA-23 **Partial anomalous pulmonary venous drainage.** An 11-year-old girl was thought to have an ASD by cardiac catheterization done at another hospital. Parasternal 4-chamber views (A,B,C,D) using two different brands of color Doppler equipment demonstrate a large discontinuity in the AS, suggesting a secundum defect (D). During color Doppler examination, an isolated systolic frame showed apparent continuity of blood flow signals between the two atria, further supporting the presence of an ASD (D). This was not seen, however, during diastole and right parasternal examination (E,F,G), which showed a completely intact AS with no evidence of shunting by color Doppler. Both the SVC and IVC flow streams were well visualized. Examination of the SVC (H) revealed a mosaic pattern of flow signals, indicating turbulence, and pulse Doppler interrogation (I,J) also demonstrated disturbed flow throughout the cardiac cycle. This finding suggested the presence of anomalous pulmonary venous drainage into the SVC. Further examination using right parasternal and suprasternal approaches demonstrated abnormal flow signals entering the SVC from another channel (K,L,M,N). Thus we were able to make a confident diagnosis of an anomalous PV entering the SVC. A second channel with flow directed superiorly and adjacent to the first channel was also visualized (O,P) but we could not delineate its termination. Right parasternal examination of the LA demonstrated two discrete streams originating from the "posterior" LA wall and directed anteriorly consistent with normal left-sided pulmonary venous connection. No streaming of blood flow was noted originating from the "anterior" LA wall. Pulse Doppler interrogation of both channels revealed flow patterns consistent with pulmonary venous flow (Q). Thus, despite cardiac catheterization findings, we were able to make a confident diagnosis of no ASD, one PV draining anomalously into the SVC, and another PV possibly draining into the SVC or innominate vein. Because of the discrepancy between echocardiographic and catheterization findings, the patient underwent repeat cardiac catheterization at our hospital. A left atrial angiogram (performed by passing a catheter into the LA through a patent foramen ovale) confirmed the absence of an ASD. Angiography also showed anomalous pulmonary venous drainage from the right upper lobe into the SVC and from the right middle lobe into the innominate vein. The remaining two PVs appeared to drain normally into the LA.

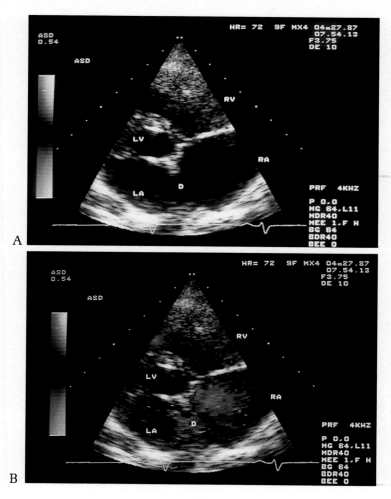

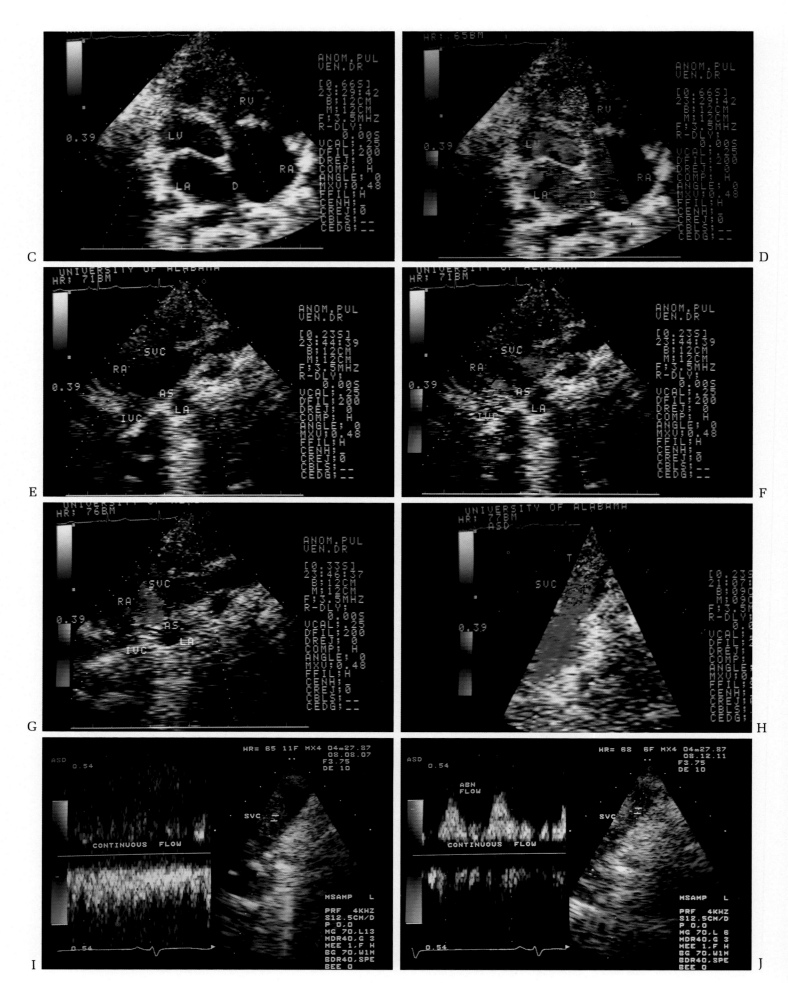

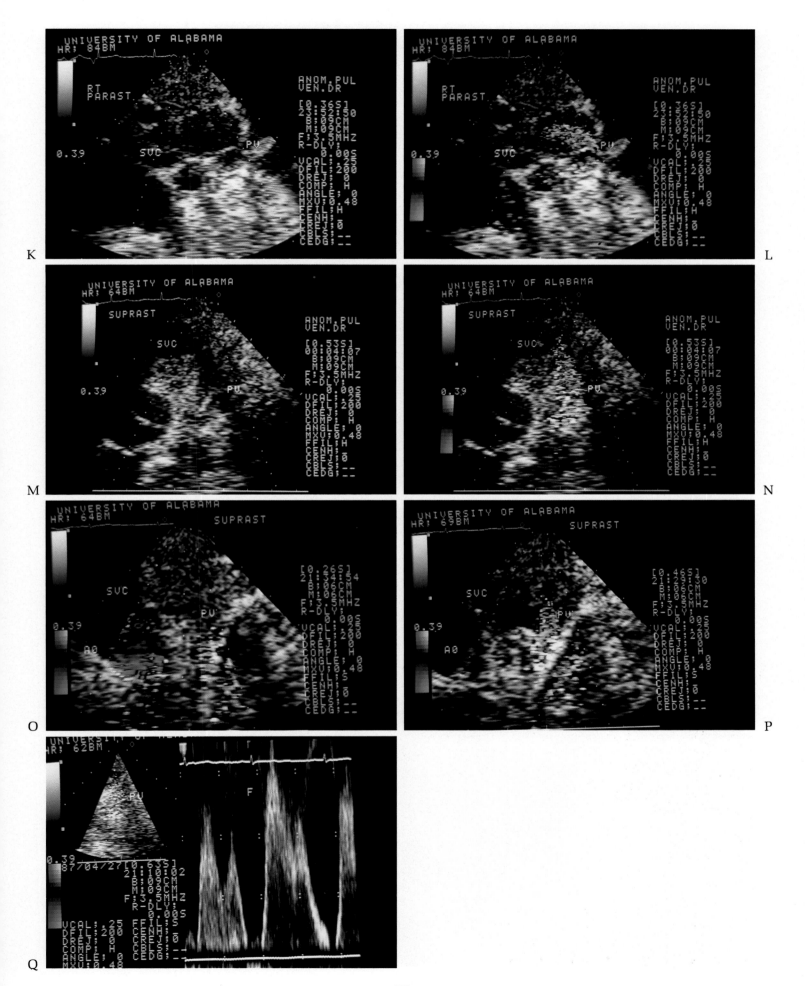

SECTION 10 CONGENITAL HEART DISEASE

Figure CA-24 **Total anomalous pulmonary venous return.** (A,B,C,D) Parasternal long and short axis and apical 4-chamber views in a pediatric patient show a large echo-free space behind the LA, consistent with a common pulmonary venous chamber (labeled ?). Prominent flow signals are visualized in the LA and in the common chamber (B). The large obligatory secundum ASD is noted in D. The common chamber communicated with the left innominate vein through a vertical vein. (Courtesy Dr. Rajendra Goyal, Bombay Hospital, Bombay, India.) E is an autopsy specimen from another patient showing a large common pulmonary venous chamber (CC) and a left vertical vein (LVV). PV = pulmonary vein.

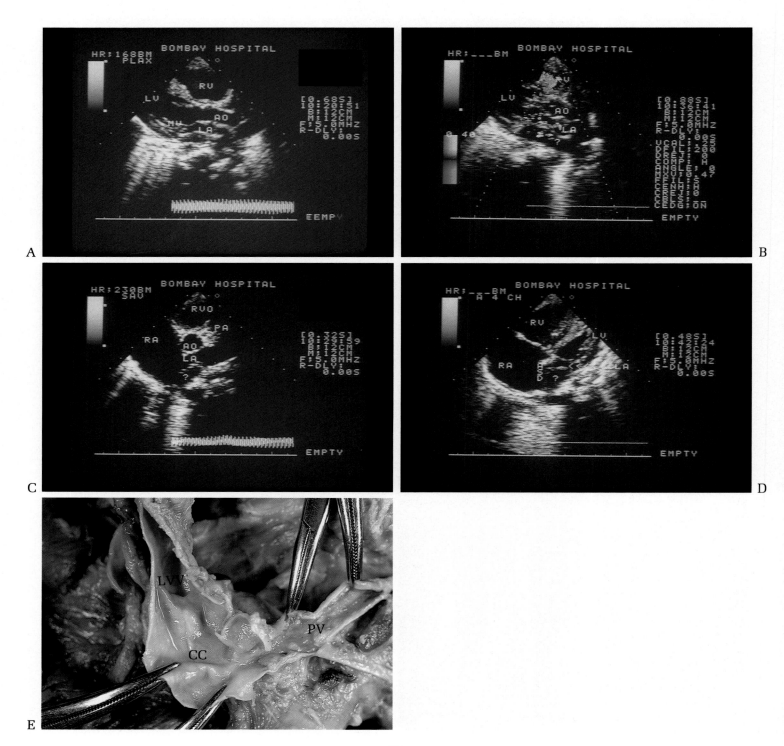

Figure CA-25 **Left-sided superior vena cava.** (A,B) Routine 2D echocardiographic study demonstrates a large CS imaged in the long axis and modified short axis views in a 24-year-old man with scleroderma. THV = thebesian valve. Because of this finding and the absence of right heart enlargement, the transducer was placed in the left supraclavicular region to look for the presence of a left-sided SVC. Initially, no channel could be visualized, but when the examination was performed with the color flow turned on, prominent inferiorly directed flow could be easily noted (C). Further angling in this area (D and E) resulted in clear demonstration of the abnormal channel. Pulse Doppler interrogation of this channel (F) revealed flow patterns typical of vena caval flow. Right supraclavicular examination (G) showed the presence of a normal right-sided SVC. LSVC = left-sided superior vena cava.

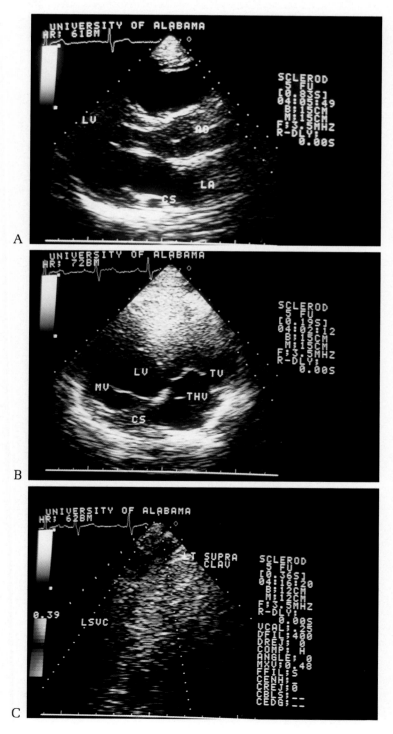

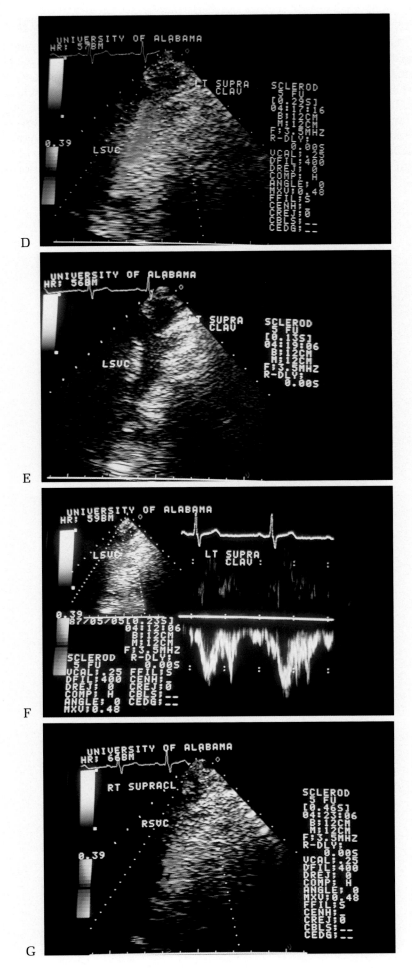

D

E

F

G

Figure CV-1 **Large ventricular septal defect.** (A) Schematic. (B) Long axis view in an adult shows flow signals moving from the LV into the RV through a large proximal VSD (arrows) during systole. The blue signals contained within the red signals are due to aliasing.

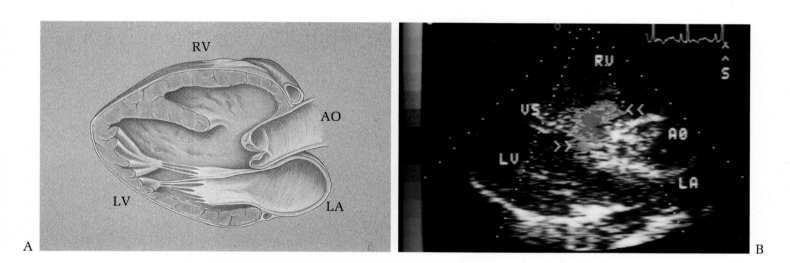

A   B

Figure CV-2 **Perimembranous ventricular septal defect with inlet extension.** (A,B) Short axis views at the level of the high LVOT and aortic root show a defect adjacent to the origin of the septal leaflet of the TV, indicating a perimembranous defect. Mosaic-colored flow signals moving along the septal leaflet of the TV in early systole indicate inlet extension.

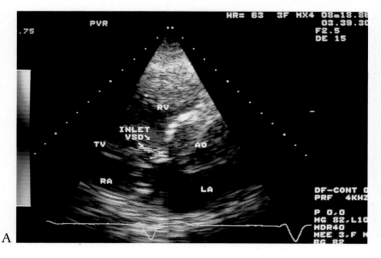

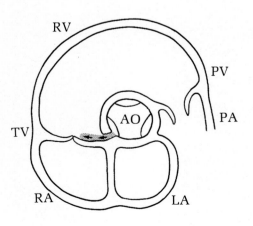

A   B

Figure CV-3   **Perimembranous ventricular septal defect with inlet extension.** Short axis view at the level of the high LVOT shows flow signals in the RV at the origin of the septal leaflet of the TV and moving along it, indicating perimembranous VSD with inlet extension. The small VSD was not evident on 2D echocardiographic examination.

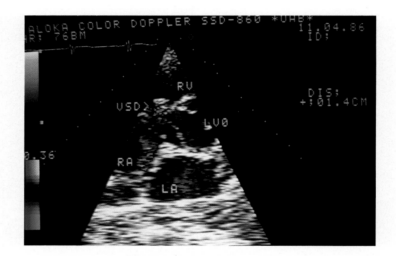

Figure CV-4   **Perimembranous ventricular septal defect with inlet extension.** (A) Short axis view at the level of the high LVOT shows a small defect adjacent to the origin of the septal leaflet of the TV with flow (downward-pointing arrow) moving along it, indicating a perimembranous defect with inlet extension. In addition, mosaic-colored flow signals (upward-pointing arrow) are seen in the RA behind the TV consistent with minimal TR. Fenestrations in the septal tricuspid leaflet are known to occur in some patients with this type of defect, resulting in flow moving from the LV through the VSD into the RV and RA. (B) Color M-mode examination shows systolic mosaic-colored signals due to TR on the atrial aspect. It is not clear in this patient whether the right atrial signals are due to associated minimal TR or whether the VSD jet found its way into the RA through a small fenestration in the TV. The TR may also be secondary to minimal damage or deformity of the TV produced by impaction of the high velocity VSD jet.

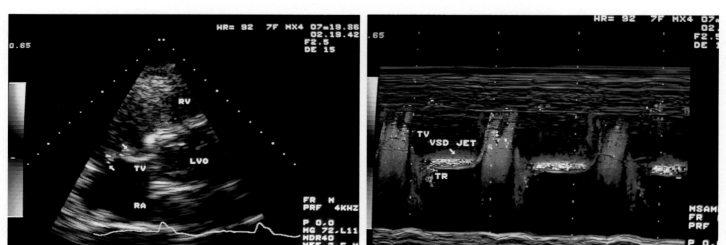

SECTION 10 CONGENITAL HEART DISEASE

Figure CV-5 **Shunting into right atrium in perimembranous ventricular septal defect with inlet extension.** (A) In a pediatric patient with a perimembranous ventricular septal defect with inlet extension, short axis view at the level of the high LVOT shows a discrete jet (arrow) moving into the RA in the region of the origin of the septal tricuspid leaflet. This represents a high velocity VSD jet moving into the RA through a fenestration in the septal leaflet of the TV, which is known to occur in a proportion of patients with this type of VSD (LV-to-RV-to-RA shunt). (B) Autopsy specimen shows a perimembranous VSD with inlet extension (arrow). The septal leaflet of the TV and its attachment are visualized through the defect.

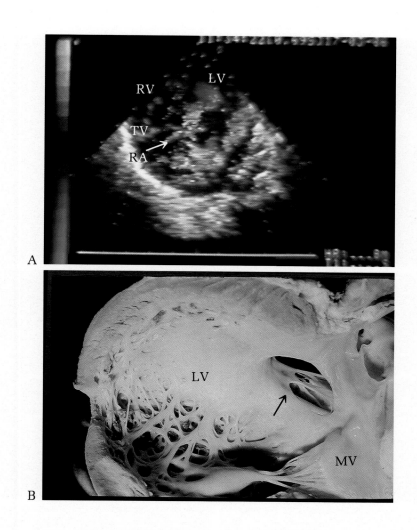

SECTION 10 CONGENITAL HEART DISEASE

Figure CV-6 **Perimembranous ventricular septal defect with inlet extension and aneurysm of the membranous septum.** (A,B) Short axis views at the level of the high LVOT and aortic root in an 8-year-old child show a defect adjacent to the origin of the septal leaflet of the TV and flow signals moving into the RV along the leaflet, indicating perimembranous VSD with inlet extension. The linear echo (arrowheads in A) surrounding the defect represents an aneurysm of the membranous septum. (C,D) Parasternal long axis and apical 4-chamber (E,F) views in another pediatric patient show systolic mosaic-colored signals moving into the RV through the VSD and a prominent aneurysm (AN) of the membranous septum. (Courtesy of Dr. Rajendra Goyal, Bombay Hospital, Bombay, India.)

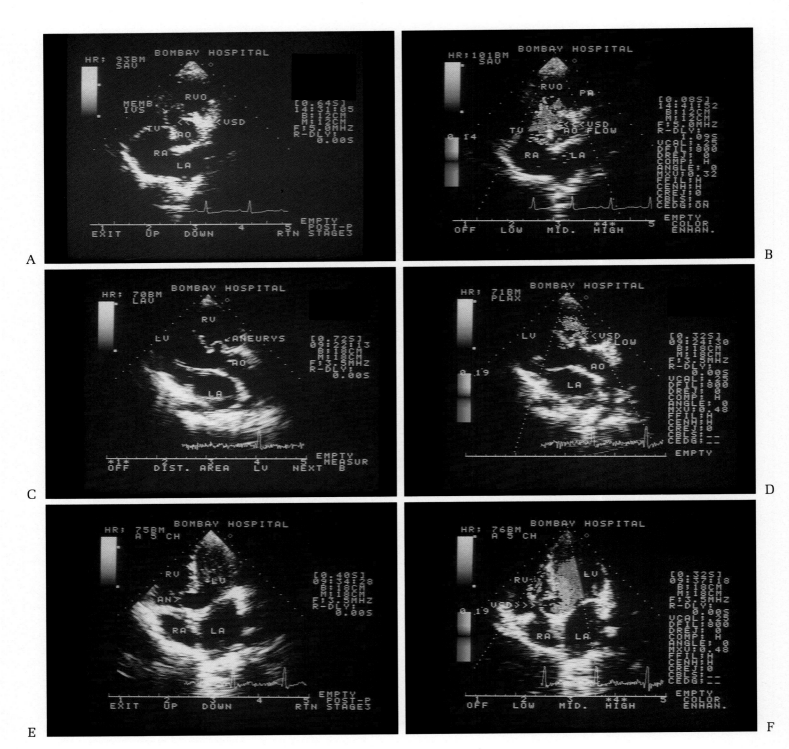

Figure CV-7 **Perimembranous ventricular septal defect with inlet extension.** (A) Modified long axis view (systole) in an adult shows the septal leaflet of the TV in close vicinity to the VS. (B) Color flow examination shows yellowish-colored signals (due to turbulence) between the septal leaflet of the TV and the VS, suggesting inlet extension.

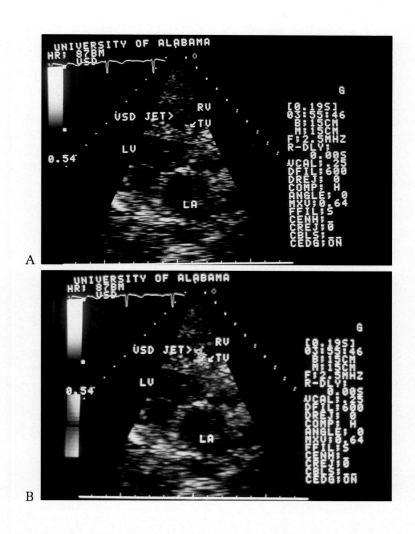

Figure CV-8 **Perimembranous ventricular septal defect with trabecular extension.** (A,B) Short axis views at the level of the high LVOT in a 13-year-old child show a large defect adjacent to the origin of the septal leaflet of the TV, indicating a perimembranous VSD. The mosaic-colored jet signals extend beyond the tip of the septal leaflet of the TV all the way to the lateral wall of the RV, consistent with trabecular extension. With inlet extension, the flow signals also move along the septal tricuspid leaflet but do not extend beyond its tip because the jet is directed medially rather than laterally after its initial appearance in front of the septal tricuspid leaflet. (C) Continuous wave Doppler cursor line placed along the flow signals records a high pressure gradient of 53 mm Hg. This suggests the absence of significant pulmonary hypertension in this patient. Assuming a systolic blood pressure of 100 mm Hg, the right ventricular systolic pressure can be estimated as 47 mm Hg (100 minus 53), which is only mildly elevated. (D) Flow acceleration in ventricular septal defect. Modified long axis view in the same patient shows a discrete area of relatively high velocity signals (arrow) on the left side of the VS, although no defect is visualized on 2D imaging. Mosaic-colored flow signals due to turbulence are not seen in the RV in this frame. Recognition of this discrete area of FA frequently alerts one to the presence of a small VSD and the transducer should then be moved and angled in multiple directions to scan the septum extensively to visualize the VSD jet in the RV. FA is usually visualized at the site of the defect or very close to it, and hence helps to pinpoint its exact site. In this patient, the defect is easily visualized in the short axis view taken at the level of the high LVOT (A,B). Presence of FA also helps to identify the left ventricular side of the defect in patients with serpiginous or irregular VSDs where the sites of communication between the two ventricles are at different levels. (E) Color M-mode examination shows the occurrence of FA (arrow) in both diastole and systole in the LVOT. Mosaic-colored signals in the RV represent the VSD jet. (F,G) Autopsy specimens show perimembranous VSD with trabecular extension (arrows).

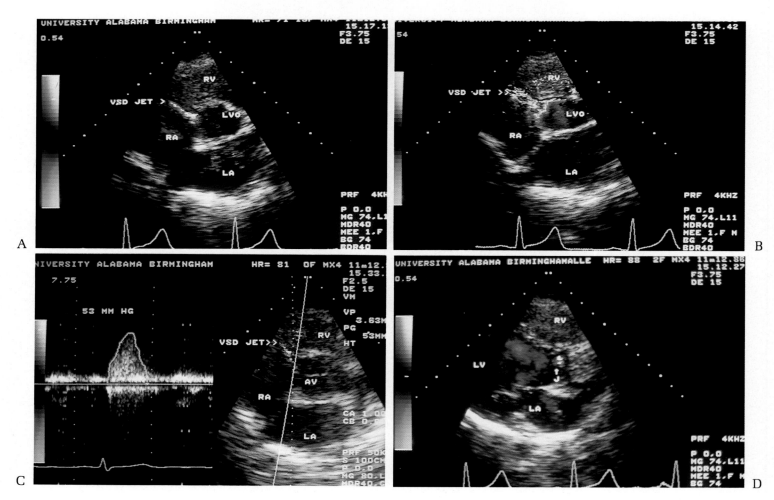

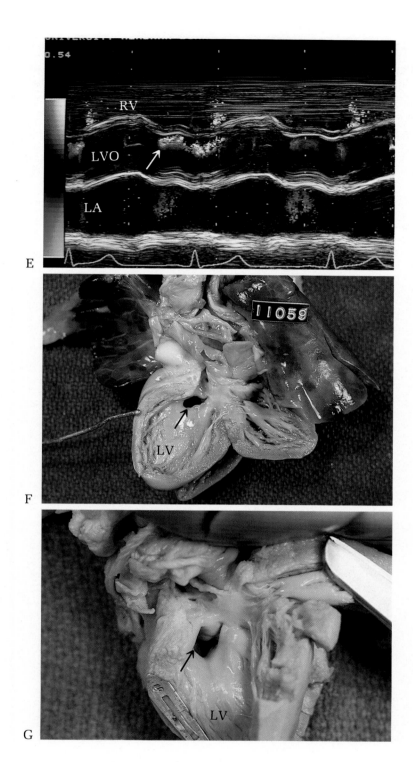

SECTION 10   CONGENITAL HEART DISEASE

Figure CV-9 **Perimembranous ventricular septal defect with both inlet and outlet extensions.** (A) Short axis view at the level of the LVOT and aortic root shows the VSD jet directed towards the RVOT and along the septal TV leaflet, consistent with both outlet and inlet extensions. Mild TR is also visualized. B is an autopsy specimen of a perimembranous VSD with outlet extension (arrow). The PV is visualized through the defect.

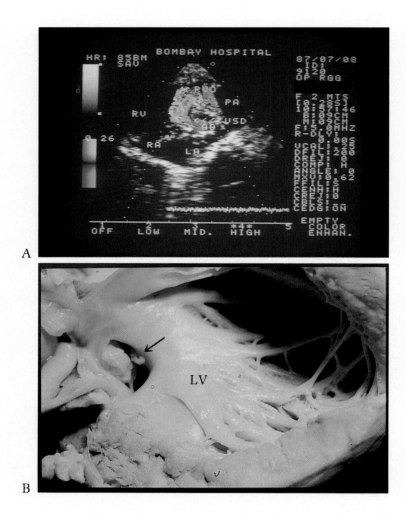

Figure CV-10 **Muscular inlet ventricular septal defect.** The long axis (A) and apical 4-chamber (B) views show a thin high-velocity jet (arrow) originating from the proximal VS and fanning out in the body of the RV. The flow signals are directed along the septal TV leaflet (STV) and along the VS, indicating an inlet defect. This small defect was not visualized on 2D examination. C is an autopsy specimen showing a muscular inlet (1) and a muscular outlet (2) VSD (near the AV). D shows a muscular inlet VSD (arrow) which has closed spontaneously.

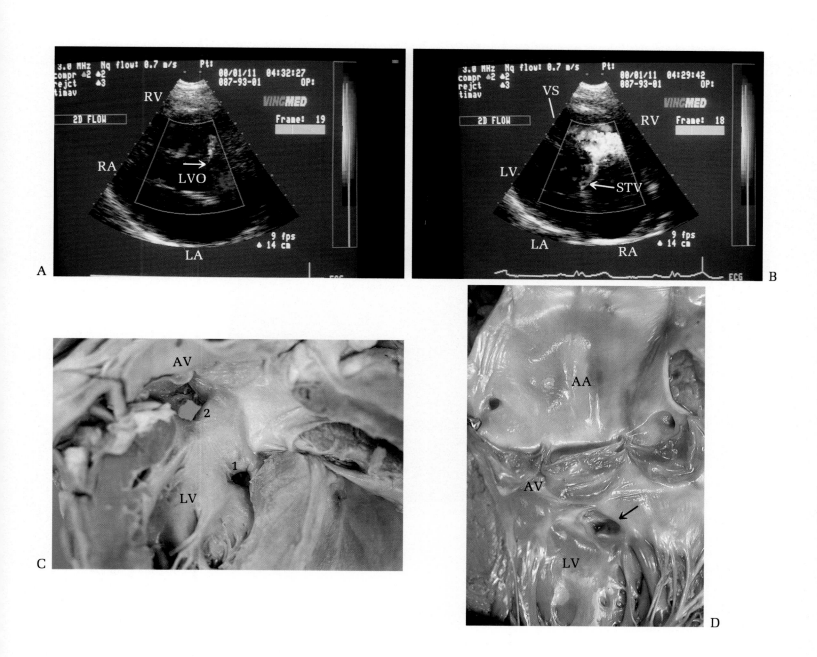

Figure CV-11   **Muscular trabecular ventricular septal defect.** (A) Long axis view in a 40-year-old woman shows mosaic-colored signals originating from the proximal muscular portion of the VS. Note intact septum between the origin of the flow signals and the aortic root. The shunt is from left to right. (B) Modified short axis view at the level of the high LVOT also shows intact septum between the septal tricuspid leaflet attachment and the VSD jet. The flow signals in this patient are directed toward the RV free wall, indicating a trabecular extension. In this patient, the defect is very small and is therefore not imaged by 2D echocardiography, but color Doppler clearly shows its location in the basal anterior muscular portion of the VS.

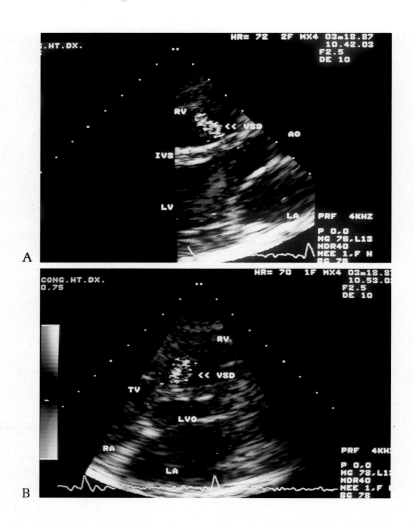

Figure CV-12 **Muscular trabecular ventricular septal defect.** (A,B) Long and short axis views in a 10-year-old child demonstrate left-to-right shunting through a VSD located in the proximal anterior muscular septum. Intact septum between the VSD and the septal TV leaflet attachment is clearly delineated. C represents a similar VSD in an 18-month-old child (Courtesy of Dr. Rajendra Goyal, Bombay Hospital, Bombay, India). D and E represent systolic parasternal long and short axis views in a 24-year-old man showing mosaic-colored signals moving from the LV into the RV through the proximal anterior muscular VS. Prominent flow acceleration (FA) is noted in the LV at the site of the defect (D). Laminar flow moving through the VSD (D) during diastole (F) clearly delineates its size, which is 3 to 4 mm. Because of markedly turbulent flow, it is difficult to assess the size of the VSD accurately in systole, but this is often easily accomplished in diastole because the relatively low pressure gradients between the LV and RV in this phase of the cardiac cycle result in laminar flow through the VSD. The width of the flow signals moving through the VS can then be measured and provides an accurate estimation of VSD size. In all three patients, the flow signals are directed laterally towards the RV free wall, indicating trabecular extension.

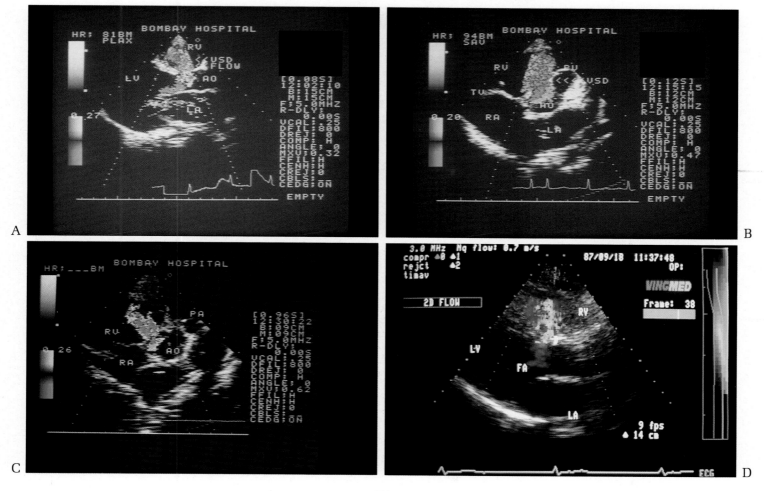

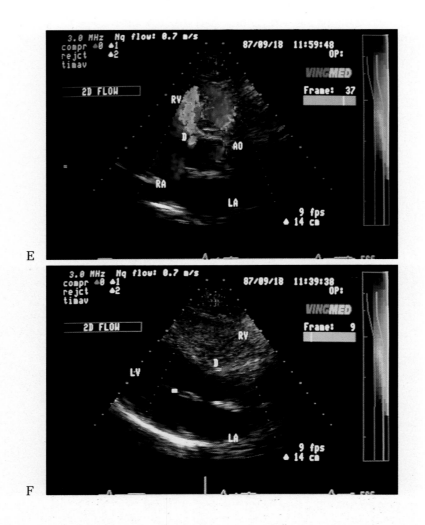

E

F

Figure CV-13 **Muscular ventricular septal defect.** A (schematic) and B show a VSD which is separated from the septal attachment of the TV by a small portion of intact septum. This defect is therefore not perimembranous but muscular in type. The flow jet bifurcates, one jet (J2) is directed towards the lateral wall of the RV and the other jet (J1) is directed towards the RVOT.

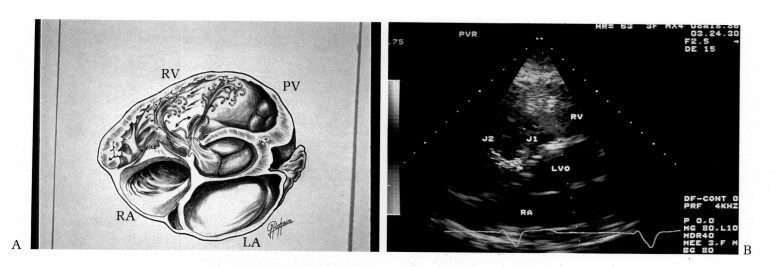

Figure CV-14 **Very small muscular ventricular septal defect.** (A, B) Parasternal long and short axis views. Very few mosaic-colored signals are seen in the proximal VS, consistent with a very small muscular defect. The defect itself was not visualized on 2D examination, but continuous wave Doppler examination revealed high velocities in this region. Unless a meticulous examination is performed, tiny VSDs can be missed by color Doppler examination. The paucity of the flow signals is most likely related to the nonparallel orientation of the ultrasonic beam with respect to the direction of the VSD jet.

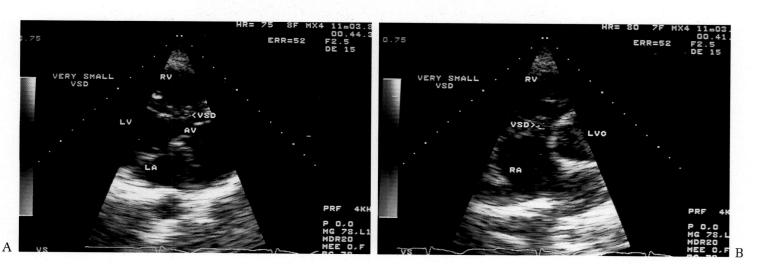

SECTION 10   CONGENITAL HEART DISEASE

Figure CV-15   **Small muscular outlet ventricular septal defect.** (A,B) Short axis views at the level of the high LVOT in a 43-year-old woman clearly show mosaic-colored signals moving through the proximal and anterior portion of the VS and directed towards the RVOT, indicating outlet extension. The narrow band of mosaic-colored signals on the left ventricular side of the defect represents FA. The defect was not visualized by 2D examination, but its site is indicated by a localized area of thickening in the VS (B).

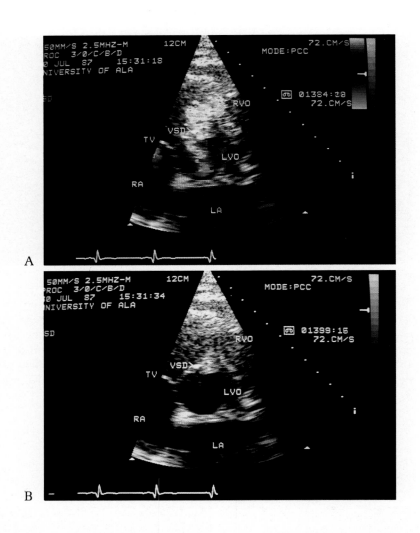

Figure CV-16 **Muscular trabecular ventricular septal defect (mid-septum).** (A, B, and C) Muscular VSD is shown in the long axis view in a woman. Note that the defect is separated from the aortic root by a large length of intact VS, and the flow is from left to right. The blue-colored signals within the red flow represent aliasing. Short axis view at the level of the MV (D) shows the defect in the anterior muscular septum.

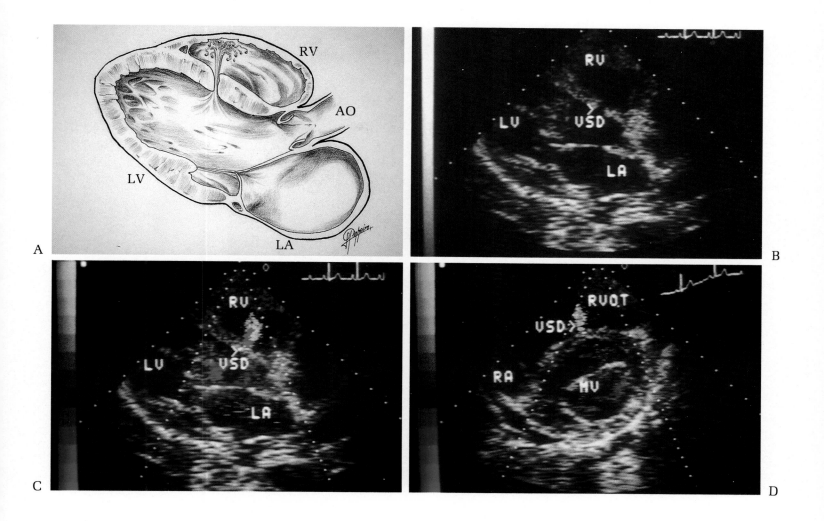

Figure CV-17 **Muscular trabecular ventricular septal defect.** Para-apical view in a pediatric patient shows mosaic-colored signals moving from the LV to the RV through the midportion of the VS. (Courtesy of Dr. Edward V. Colvin, Pediatric Cardiology Division).

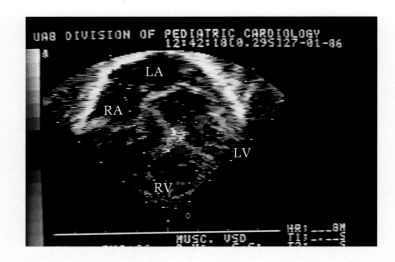

Figure CV-18   **Apical trabecular ventricular septal defect.** (A) A 4-year-old child with a pan-systolic murmur shows mosaic-colored signals originating from the apical portion of the VS imaged in oblique apical plane. Another apical view (B) shows the same high velocity VSD jet impacting on the closed TV. The continuous wave Doppler cursor line is placed parallel to the VSD jet signals (C) to obtain a peak pressure gradient of 59 mm Hg using the Bernoulli equation. The cuff systolic blood pressure is 100 mm Hg in this patient, and therefore the right ventricular pressure was calculated as 41 mm Hg.

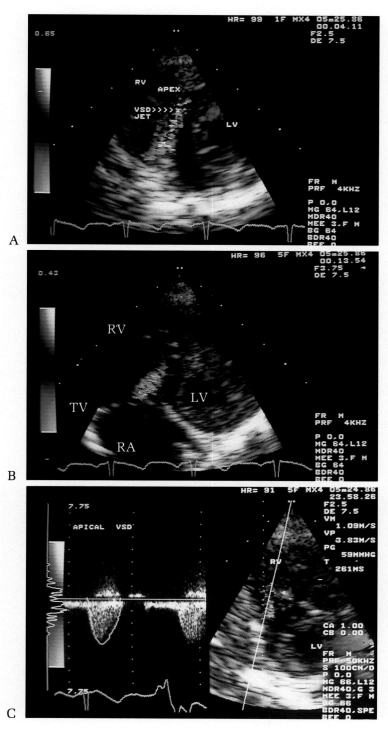

Figure CV-19 **Multiple ventricular septal defects.** Autopsy specimen shows multiple muscular VSD's (arrows), or "Swiss cheese" VS.

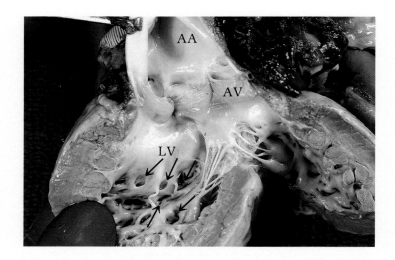

Figure CV-20 **Muscular outlet ventricular septal defect.** (A) Short axis view at the level of the aortic root and high LVOT shows flow signals originating from the muscular portion of the VS in close vicinity to the pulmonary valve (PV). Note the leftward direction of the VSD jet and the presence of a small length of intact septum between it and the PV. This small defect was not visualized on 2D imaging. The mosaic-colored signals seen in systole in front of the VS on the color M-mode study (left) represent the high velocity VSD jet. The CW Doppler cursor line (B) was placed through the VSD jet signals and a peak pressure gradient of 61 mm Hg was obtained. The systemic blood pressure was 110 mm Hg, and therefore the RV pressure was calculated as 49 mm Hg.

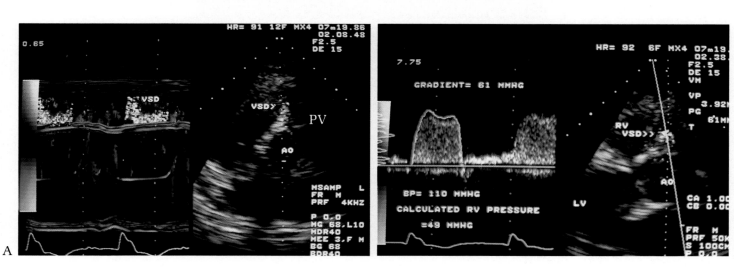

Figure CV-21   **Muscular outlet ventricular septal defect.** Short axis view (A) at the level of the high LVOT in a 21-year-old man shows blood flow moving from the LV into the RV (red signals) through a small VSD separated by a small rim of intact VS from the PV. This VSD is therefore of the muscular outlet type and not subarterial or perimembranous. The defect is also seen in the long axis view (B) and is located in the proximal part of the VS. An autopsy specimen (C) from another patient also shows a muscular outlet VSD. Note that the defect (arrow) is completely surrounded by muscle tissue. The PV is visualized through the defect.

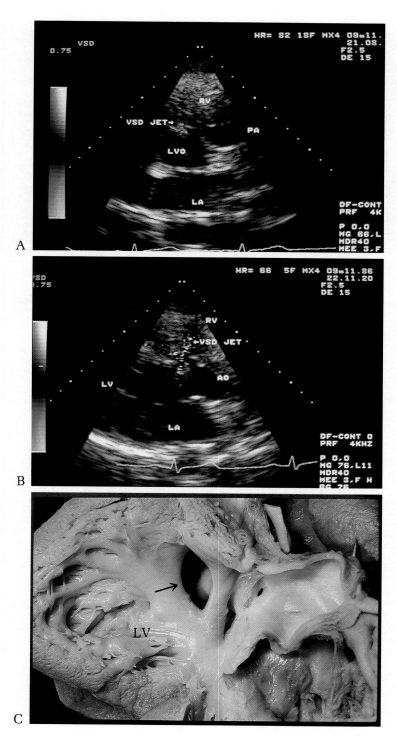

Figure CV-22 **Doubly committed ventricular septal defect.** (A,B) Short axis views in a pediatric patient show no evidence of intact VS between the defect (arrow) and the PV. (C) Autopsy specimen from another patient shows a doubly committed VSD (arrow) which is roofed by both the AV and PV.

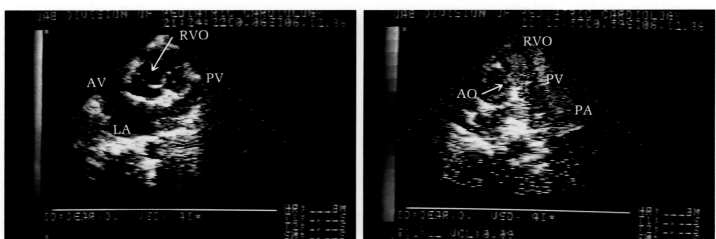

Figure CV-23 **Ventricular septal defect.** Short axis view at the level of the aorta shows mosaic-colored signals in the RVOT, indicating turbulent (T) and high-velocity flow. This finding often provides a clue to the presence of a VSD, which can be detected by meticulous scanning of the septum using various transducer positions and angulations.

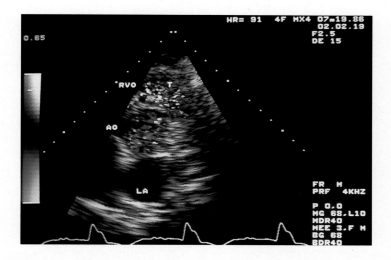

SECTION 10 CONGENITAL HEART DISEASE

Figure CV-24 **Large ventricular septal defect with pulmonary hypertension.** (A) Subcostal 4-chamber view shows a large proximal VSD (D) in a 28-year-old adult with Down's syndrome. (B) Color flow examination shows a large flow jet moving from the LV through the defect into the RV. Note the absence of TR or MR. (C) Another frame from this patient shows more clearly the large defect and the marked right ventricular hypertrophy due to pulmonary hypertension. (D) Color flow examination shows predominantly left-to-right shunting. The blue signals within the red signals represent aliasing. (E) The defect is also well visualized from the right parasternal transducer position. (F) In the short axis view at the level of the high LVOT and aorta, the flow signals from the large defect extend to the origin of the septal leaflet of the tricuspid valve (STV) and run parallel to it, indicating perimembranous VSD with inlet extension. These findings were confirmed on the angiogram, which also showed posterior extension of the defect toward the crux cordis (the so-called atrioventricular canal type of VSD). (G) The continuous wave Doppler cursor line is placed parallel to the flow signals and a peak gradient of only 7 mm Hg was obtained using the Bernoulli equation. Because the patient's systemic systolic blood pressure was 90 mm Hg, the RV and the PA systolic pressure is calculated as 83 mm Hg. RVH = right ventricular hypertrophy.

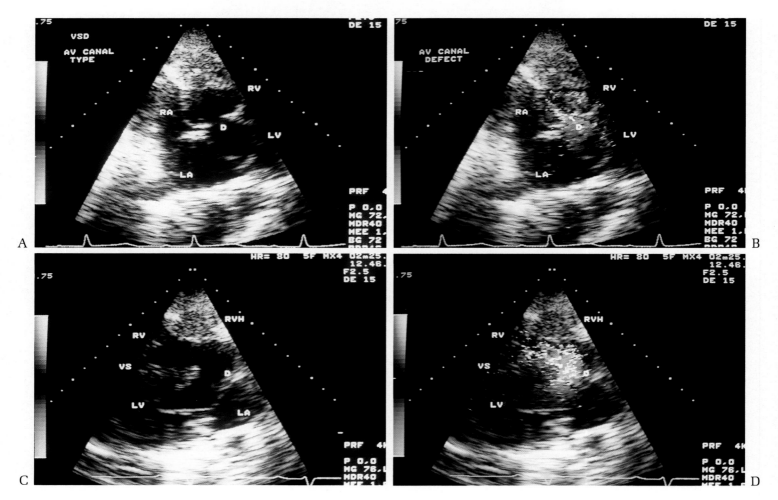

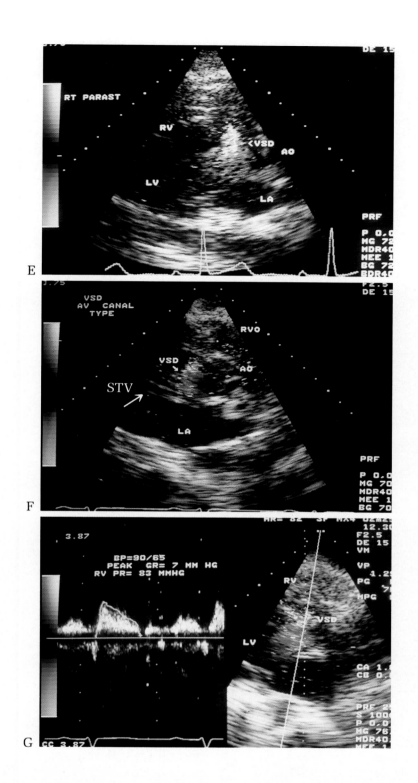

SECTION 10 CONGENITAL HEART DISEASE

Figure CV-25 **Large ventricular septal defect with systemic level pulmonary hypertension (Eisenmenger's complex).** (A) Long axis view shows left-to-right shunting (red signals) during diastole through a large proximal VSD (D) in a 33-year-old man with Eisenmenger's complex. (B) Schematic shows left-to-right shunting during diastole. (C) Systolic frame shows right-to-left shunting (blue signals) through the VSD. (D) Schematic shows right-to-left shunting during systole. (E) These frames have been gated using the ECG and show left-to-right shunting in early systole (left) and right-to-left shunting (right) in midsystole. (F,G) Color M-mode examination in the same patient shows left-to-right shunting in early systole and in mid and late diastole and right-to-left shunting during mid and late systole and in early diastole. Color M-mode examination is more accurate in timing the onset and duration of the shunt flows because the frame rates are much higher as compared to the color 2D examination. (H) Low parasternal 4-chamber view in the same patient shows the large VSD, with the color examination (I) demonstrating systolic right-to-left shunting.

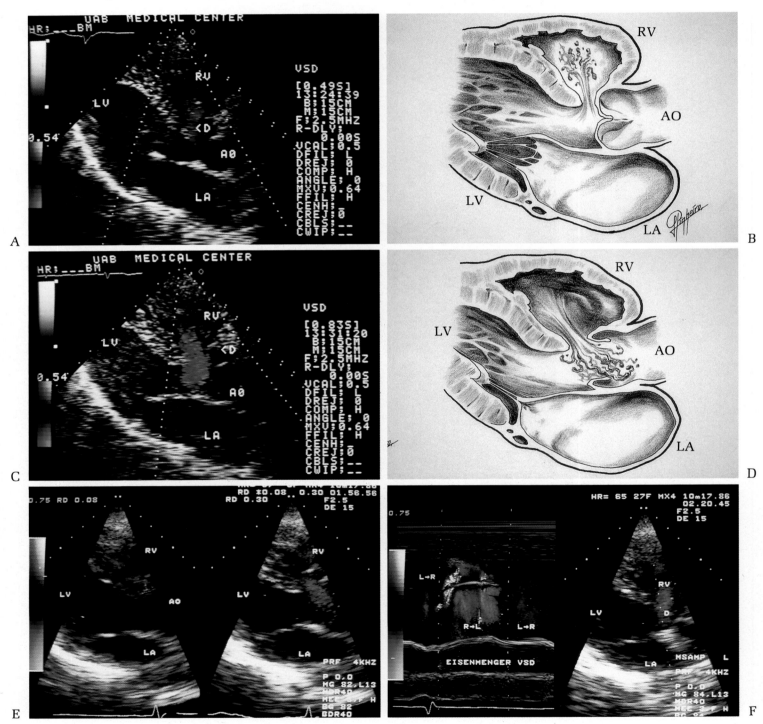

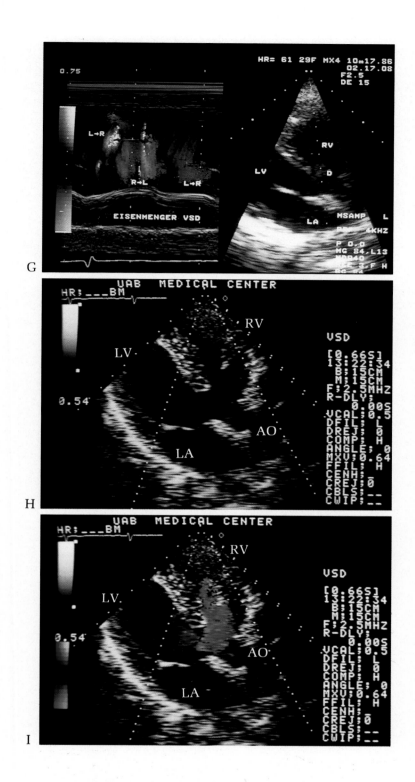

Figure CV-26 **Large muscular inlet ventricular septal defect with systemic level pulmonary hypertension.** Short axis view at the level of the MV in a 22-year-old woman shows prominent right-to-left shunting through a large defect located in the posterior portion of the VS.

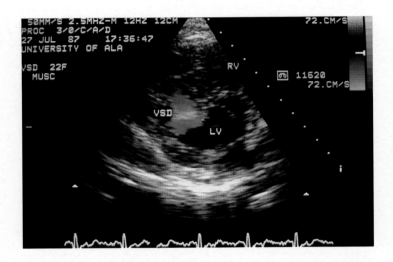

SECTION 10   CONGENITAL HEART DISEASE

Figure CV-27   **Ventricular septal defect associated with aneurysm of the ventricular septum.**
(A) Long axis view in a 17-year-old boy shows left-to-right shunting through a defect in the
proximal part of the VS and a ventricular septal aneurysm (AN). The defect does not appear to be
related to the aneurysm. (B) Apical 4-chamber view shows the defect in the proximal septum,
while the aneurysm involves its midportion. (C) Power mode imaging shows flow signals in the
aneurysm (arrow). (D) The transducer has been rotated to obtain a short axis cut through the
ventricular septal aneurysm (arrow). This patient is asymptomatic and the VSD is small, so no
surgical intervention is planned.

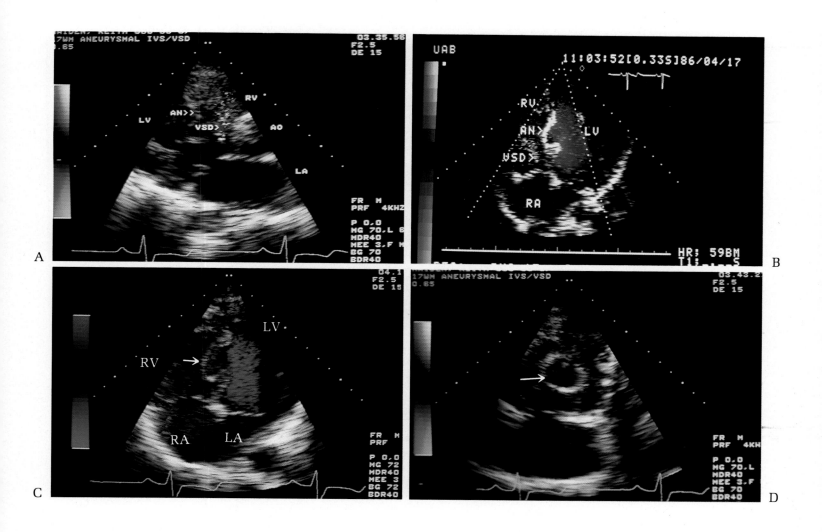

Figure CV-28   **Residual VSD mimicking prosthetic pulmonary valve obstruction.** (A) CW Doppler interrogation of the RVO and porcine PV prosthesis in a 29-year-old woman demonstrates a high velocity of 5.53 m/sec (peak pressure gradient 122 mm Hg) from a residual VSD. 2D echo examination showed normally moving porcine valve leaflets. Short axis view at the level of the LVOT (B) in the same patient shows VSD flow signals originating adjacent to septal tricuspid leaflet insertion and directed toward the RVO (perimembranous VSD with outlet extension). PVR = pulmonary valve replacement.

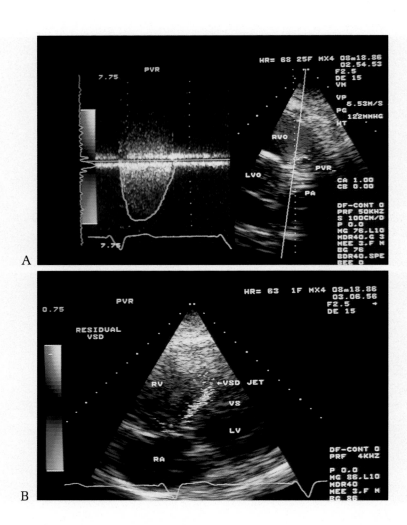

Figure CV-29   **Multiple residual ventricular septal defects following surgical repair.** Modified parasternal 4-chamber view in a 48-year-old woman after patch repair of a large VSD shows systolic mosaic-colored signals in the RV originating from a residual defect (A). Careful angling of the transducer reveals 3 separate VSD jets (B,C,D,E) originating in the area of the patch (P), which is highly echogenic. Circumscribed aliased red flow signals in the LV opposite VSD jet 3 represent flow acceleration, which helps to pinpoint the exact site of the VSD opening on the left side.

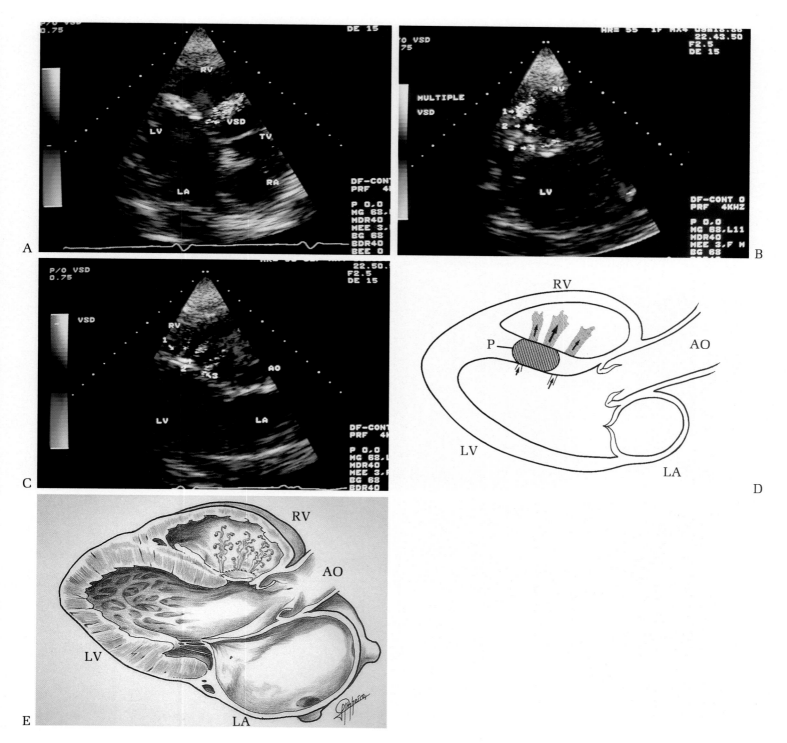

SECTION 10   CONGENITAL HEART DISEASE

Figure CV-30 **Multiple residual ventricular septal defects following surgical repair.** (A) Three discrete residual VSD jets (J1, J2, and J3) were identified only in diastole (right-to-left shunting) in a 28-year-old man who had patch (P) repair of a large VSD, and RV-to-PA conduit for PV atresia. Careful angling of the transducer was required from the apical position to detect these three small residual defects. Systolic frames (B,C) suggest the presence of only one residual communication between the two ventricles. Thus the area of the VSD repair must be meticulously scanned in both systole and diastole to localize all residual leaks. F = VSD flow. Color-guided CW Doppler examination (D) demonstrates a high velocity of 3.5 m/sec (peak pressure gradient of 49 mm Hg) across the defect, implying absence of severe pulmonary hypertension. Color M-mode examination (E) shows right-to-left shunting in diastole and left-to-right shunting in systole.

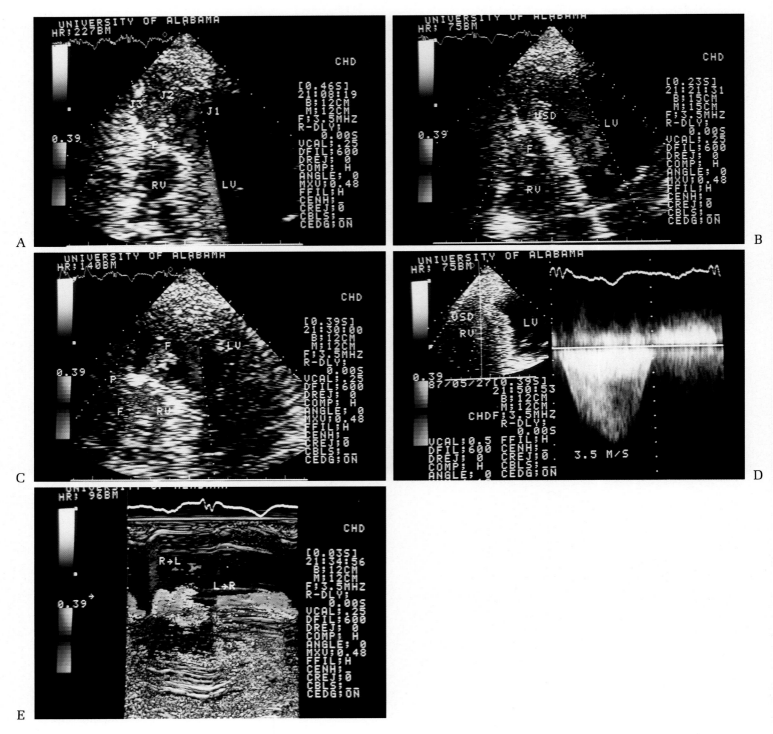

SECTION 10 CONGENITAL HEART DISEASE
C. PATENT DUCTUS ARTERIOSUS
AND ABNORMAL CORONARY
ARTERY COMMUNICATIONS

Figure CP-1 **Patent ductus arteriosus.** (A) High left parasternal echo examination in an 8-year-old child clearly delineates the ductal communication (arrow) between the PA and DA. (B) Color Doppler study shows mosaic-colored flow signals moving through the wide but short ductus into a dilated PA along its lateral wall. The red and green signals in the DA near the ductal opening represent FA and the blue signals in the DA and LPA represent normal flow patterns. Pulse Doppler (C) and color M-mode (D) interrogation of the ductal region show high-velocity continuous flow throughout the cardiac cycle. Higher velocity and turbulence in late systole (arrows), denoted by the appearance of mosaic-colored signals in D, correspond to the late systolic accentuation of the continuous murmur on clinical examination in this patient. Increasing the PRF from 4 (C) to 8 KHz (D) raised the Nyquist limit from 0.54 m/sec to 1.08 m/per, enabling better identification of the higher-flow velocity in late systole. Aortic short axis view (E) in the same patient shows a thin band of reddish-green signals along the lateral wall of the PA, representing ductal flow moving anteriorly towards the PV, while the more medially placed blue signals represent ductal flow moving posteriorly in an opposite direction. This phenomenon is related to ductal flow swirling around in the dilated PA during diastole. The ductus (DU) in this patient was also easily identified from the suprasternal approach (F) because it "lighted up" during diastole due to clearly visible higher-velocity flow in its lumen and less conspicuous lower-velocity flows in the much larger adjacent PA and DA. Schematics show PDA viewed from suprasternal and high parasternal transducer position (G), and ductal flow moving along the lateral aspect (H) and in the middle (I) of the PA lumen. An autopsy specimen (J) shows a large curved PDA (arrow) in a newborn.

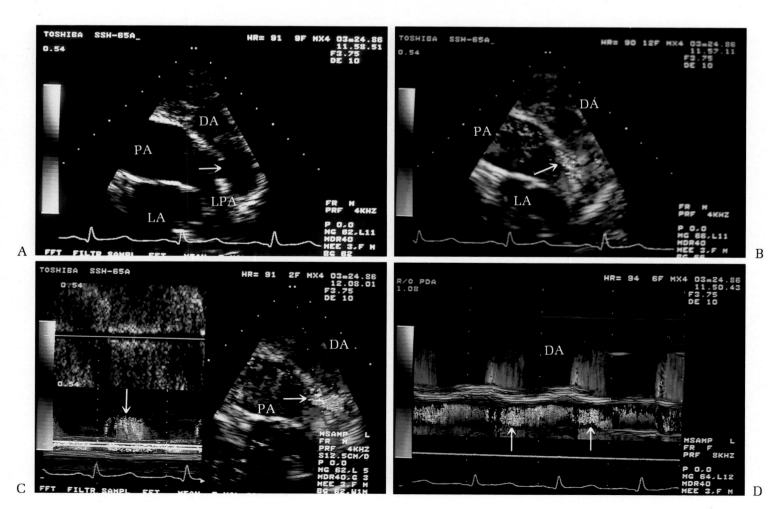

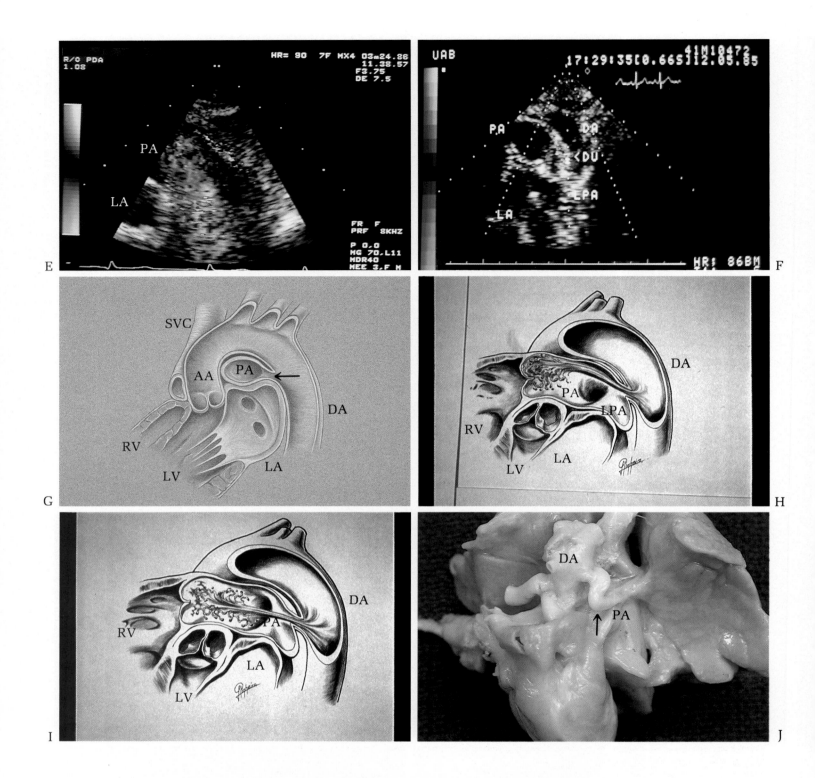

Figure CP-2   **Patent ductus arteriosus.** Aortic short axis view in a 7-year-old child shows continuity of flow between the DA and PA (arrow). The jet bifurcates and is directed both laterally and medially, and the mosaic pattern of colors is due to variance and high velocity. The blue signals in the middle of the PA represent flow velocities below the Nyquist limit.

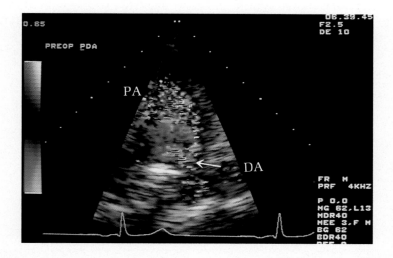

Figure CP-3   **Patent ductus arteriosus.** Aortic short axis view in a 5-month-old baby shows mosaic-colored signals (DF) moving from the DA into the PA through a wide ductus (arrowheads). The blue signals medially represent ductal flow swirling around and moving posteriorly in the PA.

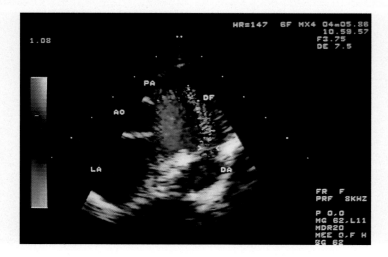

SECTION 10   CONGENITAL HEART DISEASE

Figure CP-4   **Patent ductus arteriosus.** (A) Aortic short axis view in a 22-year-old man shows an area of discontinuity between the DA and the PA consistent with PDA. Color Doppler examination (B) shows mosaic-colored signals due to turbulent flow in the PA laterally and lower velocity signals (blue with some red in it due to aliasing) medially, typical of PDA. Other frames (C through H) show continuity of flow between the DA and the PA through the PDA. D shows mosaic-colored signals filling the distal PA completely. The prominent red and mosaic-colored signals in the DA represent anteriorly directed turbulent flow acceleration, which often helps to pinpoint the site of PDA origin during patient examination. Color M-mode examination (I,J,K) shows the presence of turbulent flow (mosaic-colored signals) throughout the cardiac cycle. K also shows prominent coarse diastolic fluttering of the PV related to diastolic impaction of the PDA flow. L,M,N, and O represent postoperative studies following PDA ligation and show absence of turbulent flow in the PA and no evidence of discontinuity between the DA and PA. Blue and red signals seen in early and middle systole in PA (M,N) represent aliased antegrade flow, while the red signals in late systole and early diastole (N,O) represent retrograde or back flow (BF) due to a swirling effect. These flow patterns result from PA dilatation and are not specific for any particular etiology. P is an autopsy specimen from another patient showing a large, wide PDA. DESC AO = Descending thoracic aorta; FA = flow acceleration.

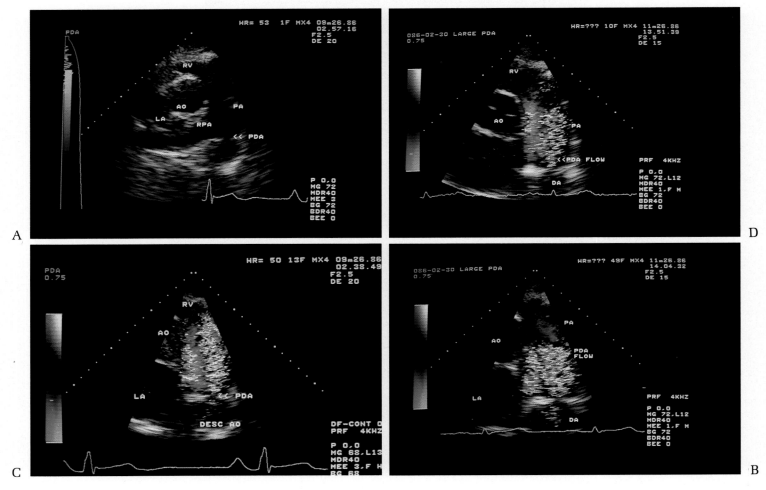

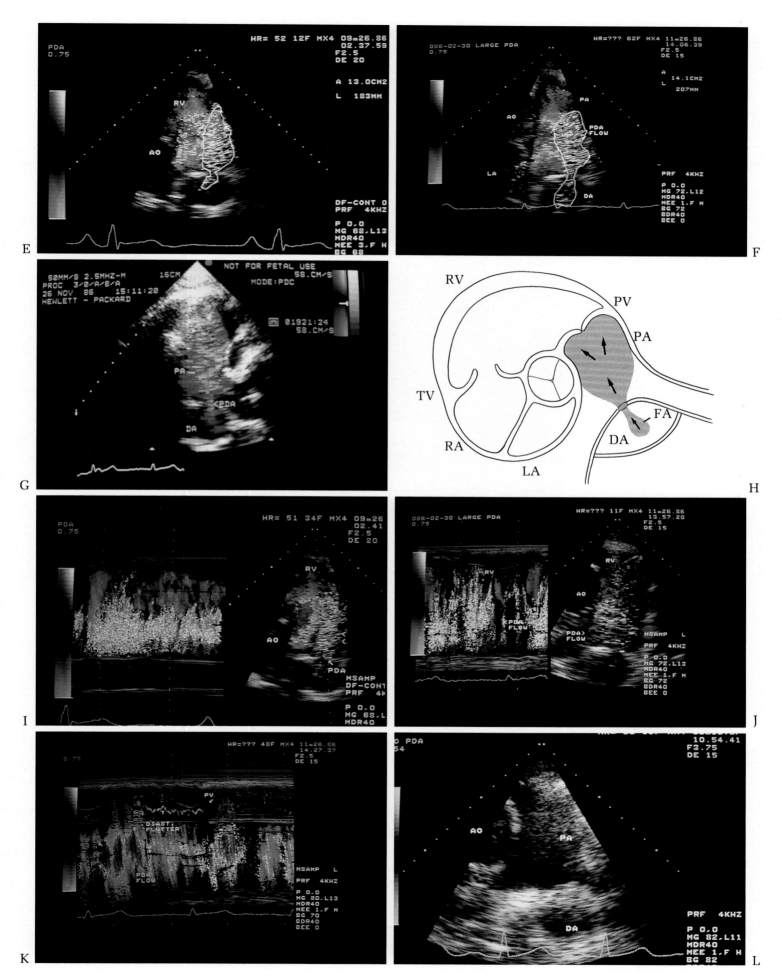

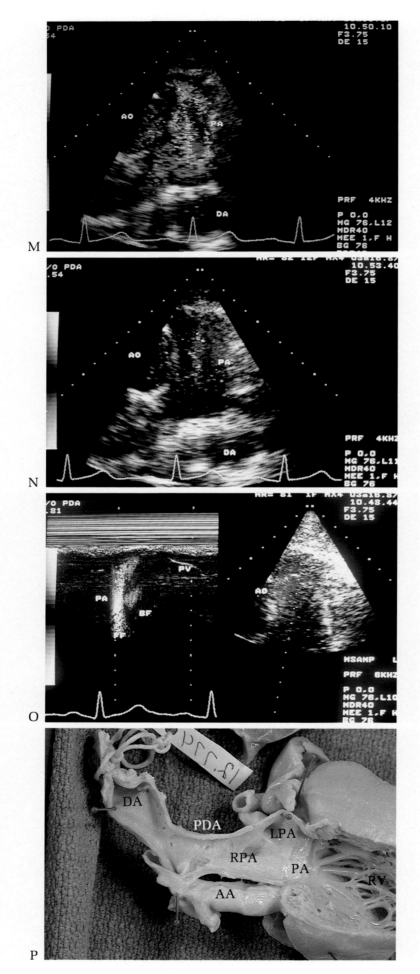

Figure CP-5 **Patent ductus arteriosus.** (A) Detection of mosaic-colored signals (due to turbulence) in the PA imaged from the suprasternal approach provided the first clue that this 55-year-old woman with MV prolapse may also have a PDA. The PA was not well visualized from the parasternal transducer position. (B) Color M-mode showed continuous flow in the PA. Careful transducer manipulation (C,D,E,F) demonstrated an 8 mm wide ductus with mosaic-colored signals moving through it into the PA along its superior wall. Color M-mode (G,H) and pulse Doppler (I) interrogation of the ductus show flow signals throughout the cardiac cycle.

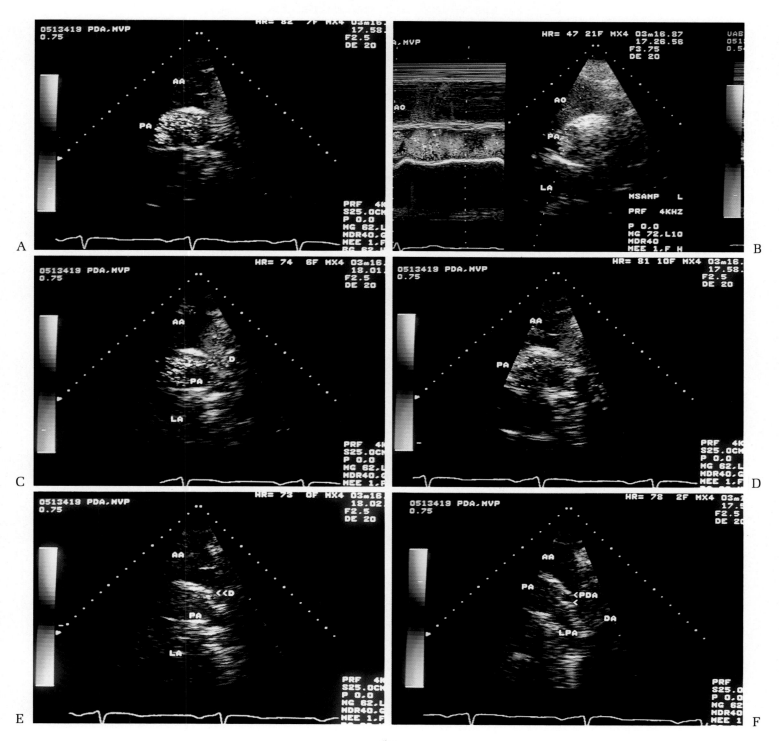

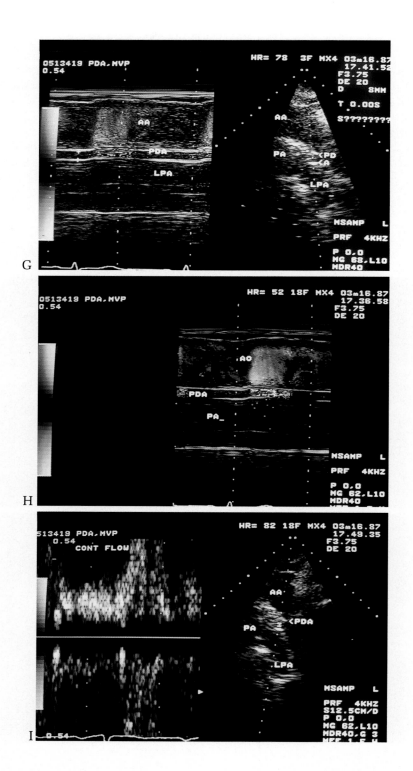

SECTION 10 CONGENITAL HEART DISEASE

Figure CP-6 **Patent ductus arteriosus.** (A) Aortic short axis view shows mosaic-colored signals in the PA during systole in this 48-year-old woman clinically suspected to have MV prolapse and MR. Pulse Doppler interrogation of this region (B) revealed continuous flow (CF) throughout the cardiac cycle, alerting us to the presence of PDA. Other frames (C,D) showed flow signals (F) moving posteriorly during diastole in both the RVOT and PA.

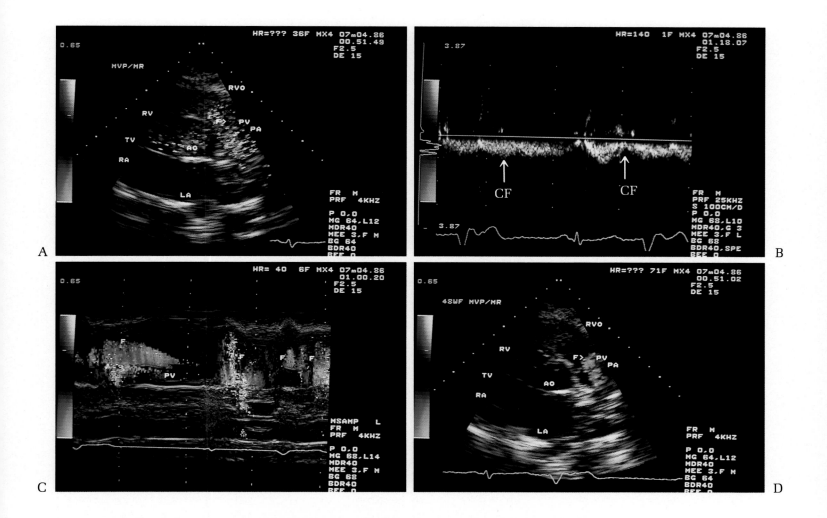

SECTION 10 CONGENITAL HEART DISEASE

Figure CP-7 **Patent ductus arteriosus associated with atrial septal defect.** (A,B) Suprasternal examination in a 17-year-old girl with PV atresia (who underwent Brock's procedure at age 3) shows flow signals moving from the DA into the PA through a large PDA. Short-axis views (C,D,E,F) taken at the level of the aortic root and high LVO show a large secundum ASD (D) with both left-to-right (red) and right-to-left (blue) shunting.

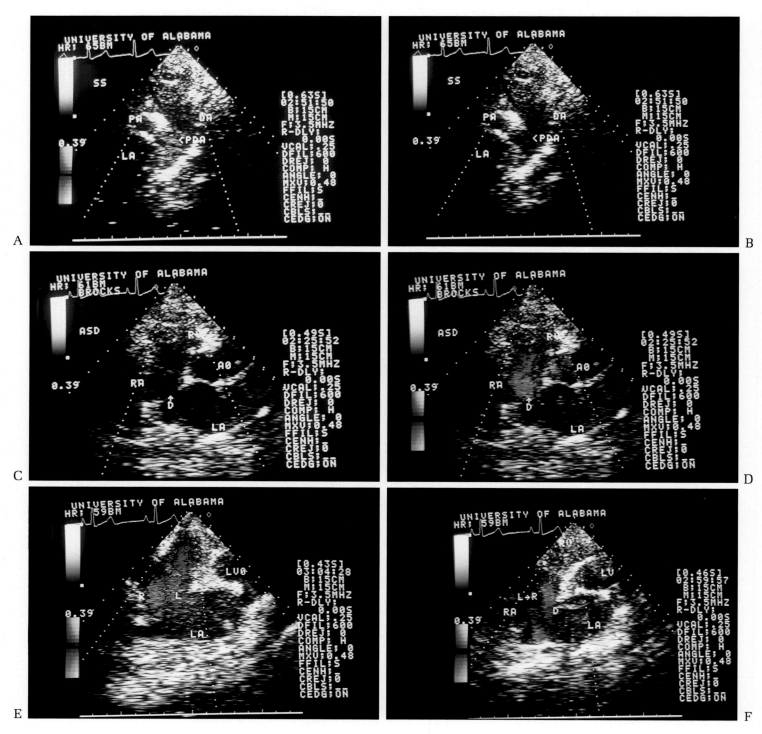

Figure CP-8 **Demonstration of the ductal ampulla.** (A,B) Suprasternal examination in an adult with a dilated aorta shows a prominent notch in the aortic wall opposite the origin of brachio-cephalic branches (BB) representing the ductal ampulla (A). This diverticulum often persists after natural closure of the PDA in the neonatal period.

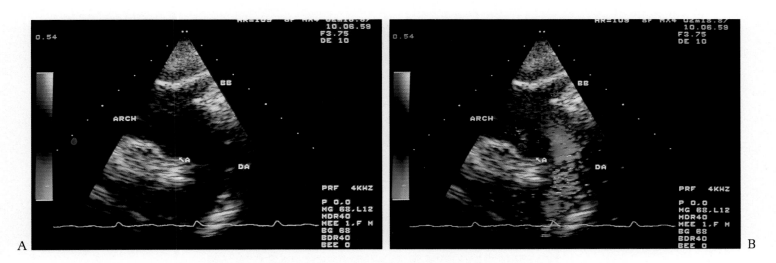

A
B

Figure CP-9 **Anomalous origin of the right coronary artery from the PA.** Aortic short axis view in a 66-year-old woman presenting with acute myocardial infarction shows prominent flow signals (blue) streaming from the anomalous right coronary artery (RCA) into the PA during diastole.

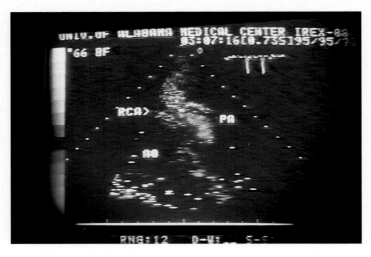

Figure CP-10 **Left coronary artery – right ventricular fistula.** (A,B) Aortic short axis views in a 38-year-old man presenting with chest pain shows mosaic-colored signals indicating turbulence in the markedly enlarged left main coronary artery (LCA). (C) RV inflow plane shows mosaic-colored signals (F) moving from the aneurysmal left coronary artery into the RV approximately 3 cm distal to the TV, diagnostic of a fistulous communication. This finding has been confirmed by angiography in this patient. (Courtesy of Ming Hsiung, M.D., Tri-Service General Hospital, Taipei, Taiwan).

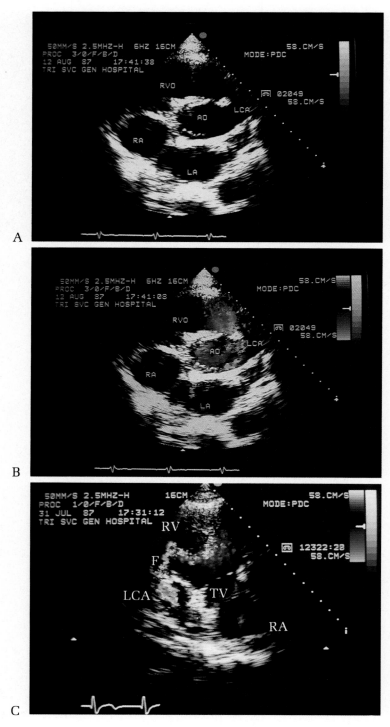

SECTION 10   CONGENITAL HEART DISEASE
D. OBSTRUCTIVE LESIONS

Figure CO-1   Cor-Triatriatum. (A) Apical view in a 45-year-old man presenting with atrial fibrillation and clinically suspected to have MV disease. The MV appears to be structurally normal, but an abnormal linear echo consistent with a membrane (M) is noted in the LA. Color Doppler examination (B,C,D,E,F) shows mosaic-colored signals (due to turbulence) in the LA which originate from the membrane and move through the open MV into the LV. Note that the velocity decreases to below the Nyquist limit of 0.75 m/sec in the region of the MV and LV. Color-guided continuous wave Doppler examination (G) demonstrates a peak pressure gradient of 15 mm Hg across the membrane (peak velocity 1.94 m/sec). Color M-mode and standard Doppler examination (H,I,J) shows mosaic-colored signals in both systole and diastole, indicating continuous flow (F) through the obstructing membrane. This feature serves to differentiate cor-triatriatum from an obstructing supravalvular membrane which, because of its location near the MV, demonstrates flow through it mainly during diastole. On the other hand, in cor-triatriatum the obstruction is near the entrance of the pulmonary veins, and the flow is therefore both systolic and diastolic. M-mode examination (K) also shows high-frequency diastolic flutter (arrow) of the MV resulting from turbulent flow. The patient underwent successful surgical resection of the membrane and his rhythm converted to sinus. Apical long axis views (L,M) in a 68-year-old man presenting with congestive cardiac failure show a linear echo (arrow) in the LA with mosaic-colored signals originating from it medially during diastole. Color-guided continuous wave examination (not shown) revealed a peak pressure gradient of 16 mm Hg. A few red signals in the LVO originating from the AV in diastole represent associated mild AR in this patient. Angiocardiography was diagnostic of cor-triatriatum, and the patient is awaiting surgery (courtesy Ming Hsiung, M.D., Tri-Service General Hospital, Taipai, Taiwan). Autopsy specimen of cor-triatriatum (N) shows the thick muscular partition with a hole (arrow) in it and pulmonary veins opening proximal to it. Another autopsy specimen of cor-triatriatum (O) shows the obstructing membrane (M) and pulmonary veins (PV) draining into a common chamber (CC) behind it.

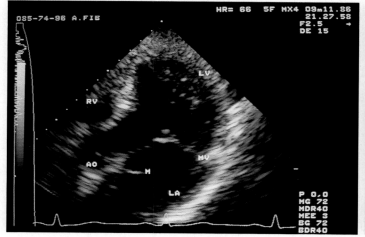

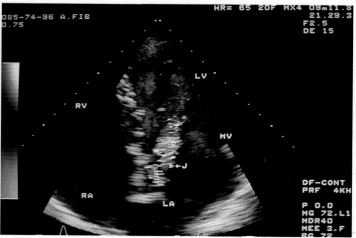

A   B

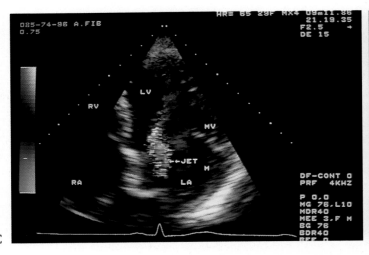

C

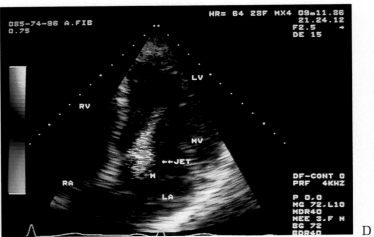

D

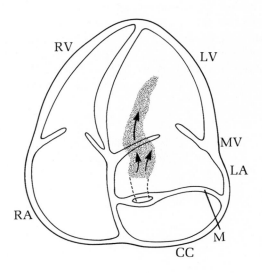

E

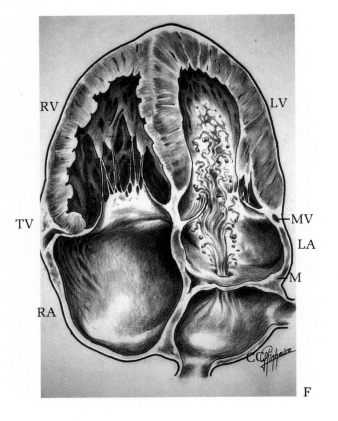

F

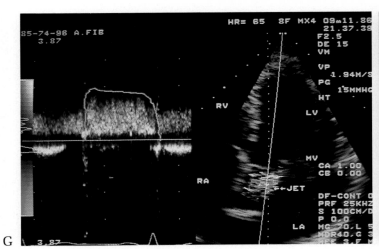

G

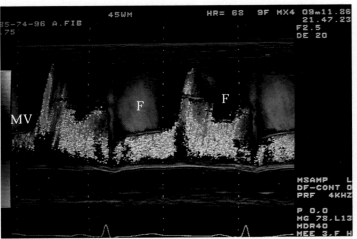

H

468

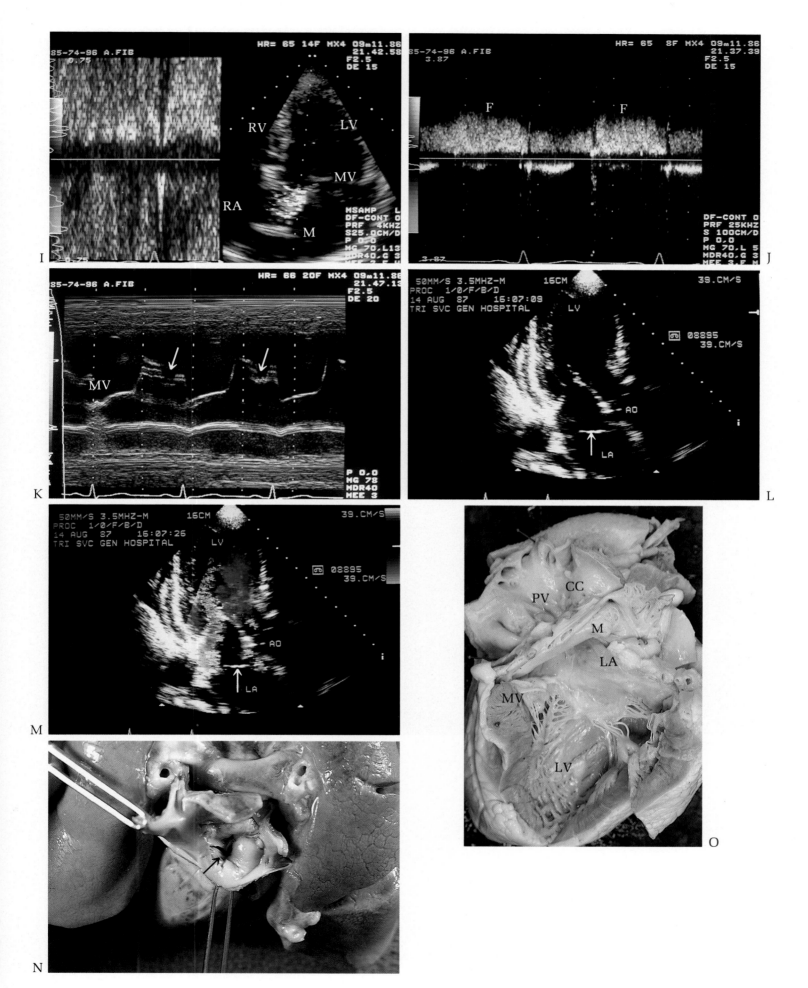

Figure CO-2 **Supravalvar mitral membrane.** (A,B) Parasternal long axis views in a 15-year-old boy show a linear echo in the LA which almost reaches into the mitral orifice. This is consistent with a supravalvular membrane which, in this patient, did not produce significant obstruction to mitral inflow, but resulted in considerable MR. C and D represent apical 4-chamber views, which also demonstrate the membrane and MR. Minimal TR is also present. (Courtesy of Dr. Goyal, Bombay Hospital, Bombay, India.)

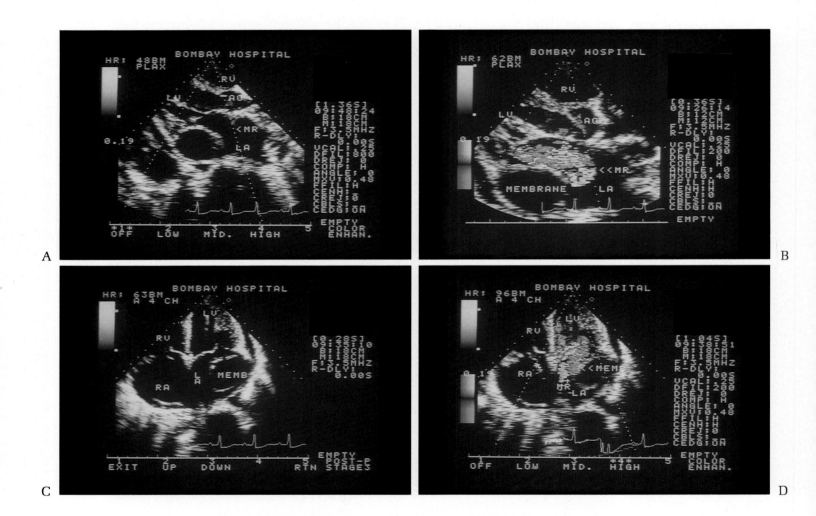

SECTION 10   CONGENITAL HEART DISEASE

Figure CO-3   **Congenital mitral stenosis.** Apical 4-chamber view shows thickened mitral leaflets and a peak velocity of 1.7 m/sec, obtained by placing the CW Doppler cursor line parallel to the stenotic flow signals. Associated subaortic stenosis and coarctation of the aorta were also present in this 7-year-old child with mild MS.

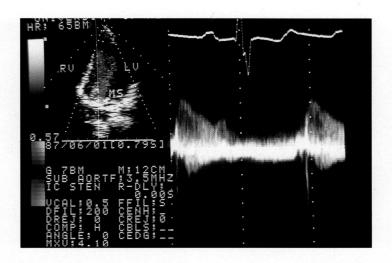

SECTION 10 CONGENITAL HEART DISEASE

Figure CO-4 **Parachute mitral valve.** (A,B) Long axis and apical views in a 66-year-old man show a posteriorly placed prominent papillary muscle (PM) and mildly thickened MV leaflets and chordae (C). (C,D) Color Doppler examination during systole shows mosaic-colored signals filling a large portion of the LA, consistent with severe MR. The bluish-white and mosaic-colored signals on the ventricular aspect of the MV and diametrically opposite the MR jet represent flow acceleration. Color-guided CW Doppler examination (E) demonstrates a peak pressure gradient of 9 mm Hg (peak velocity 1.5 m/sec), consistent with only mild mitral inflow obstruction. At surgery, two papillary muscles were found, one larger than the other; this represents a part of the wide spectrum of findings seen in this entity. The patient has done well after successful mitral annuloplasty. F represents an autopsy specimen from another patient showing classical features of parachute MV: thickened and fused MV leaflets with chordae from both leaflets inserted into a single papillary muscle.

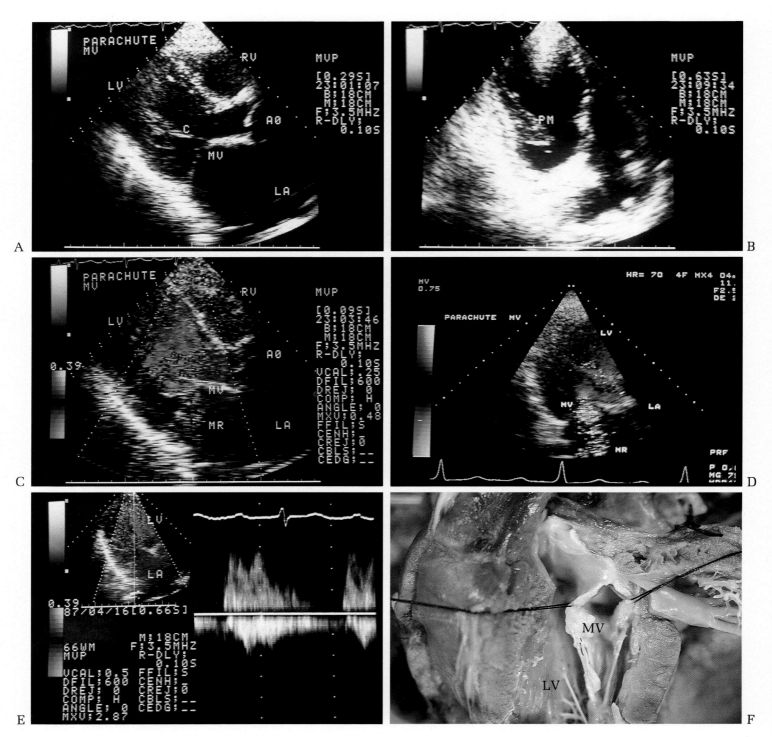

SECTION 10 CONGENITAL HEART DISEASE

Figure CO-5 **Discrete subaortic membranous stenosis.** (A) Long axis view in a 7-year-old child with subaortic stenosis shows mosaic-colored signals in the LVOT, indicating turbulent (T) flow. The AV was structurally normal. B and C are schematics. The arrows point to the subaortic membrane. Color M-mode examination of the AA (D) from the right parasternal approach in another patient with subaortic stenosis shows systolic mosaic-colored flow (F) signals due to turbulence in the AA. The AV was normal in this patient also. Diastolic long axis frames (E,F,G,H) in an 8-year-old child show mosaic-colored signals originating from the AV and moving into the LV due to AR, as well as a linear echo (M, arrow) protruding into the LVOT, representing a subaortic membrane in this patient. Autopsy specimen (I) from another patient shows subaortic membranous stenosis (arrow).

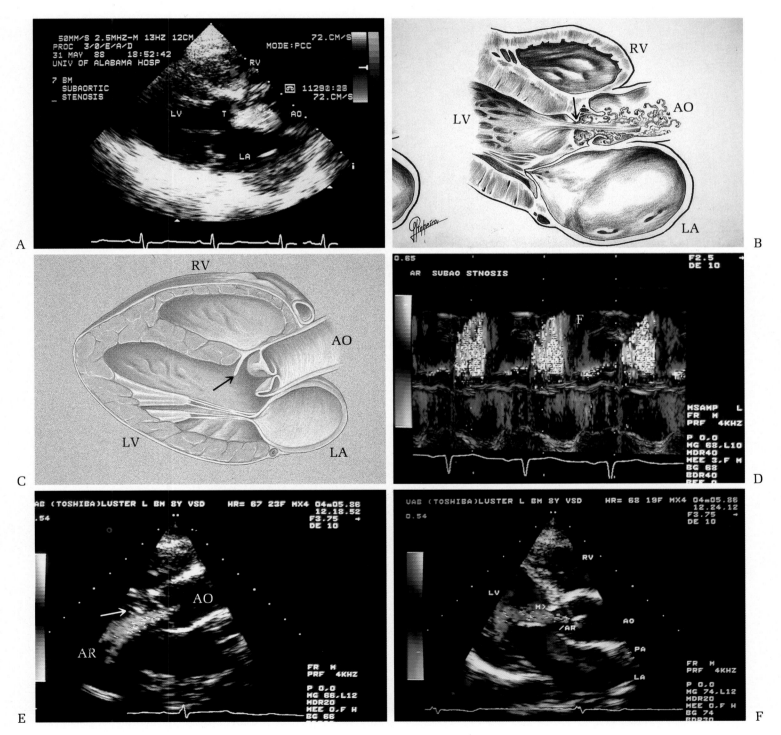

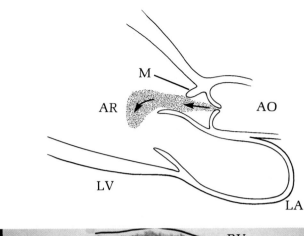

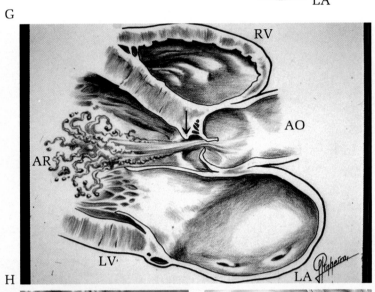

G

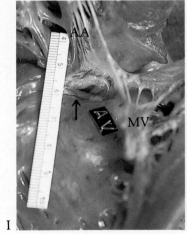
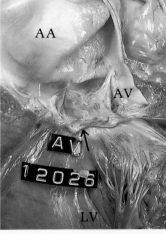

H

I

474

SECTION 10 CONGENITAL HEART DISEASE

Figure CO-6 **Discrete subaortic membranous stenosis.** (A,B) Apical long axis views in a 61-year-old woman presenting with syncope show a linear echo (M) projecting into the LVOT. The AV was structurally normal in this patient. (C) M-mode examination shows the typical early systolic preclosure (P) of the AV. Systolic frames (D,E,F) show mosaic-colored signals in the LVOT due to turbulence produced by the membrane. Bluish-green and red signals in the LV proximal to the membrane (M) represent flow acceleration (FA). Color-guided CW Doppler examination (G) reveals a peak pressure gradient of 78.5 mm Hg and a mean gradient of 48 mm Hg across the membrane. The diastolic frame (H) shows mosaic-colored signals originating from the AV in diastole and filling about 70% of the proximal LVOT indicating severe AR. The blue signals in the LV in this frame indicate normal flow directed toward the aortic root in late diastole.

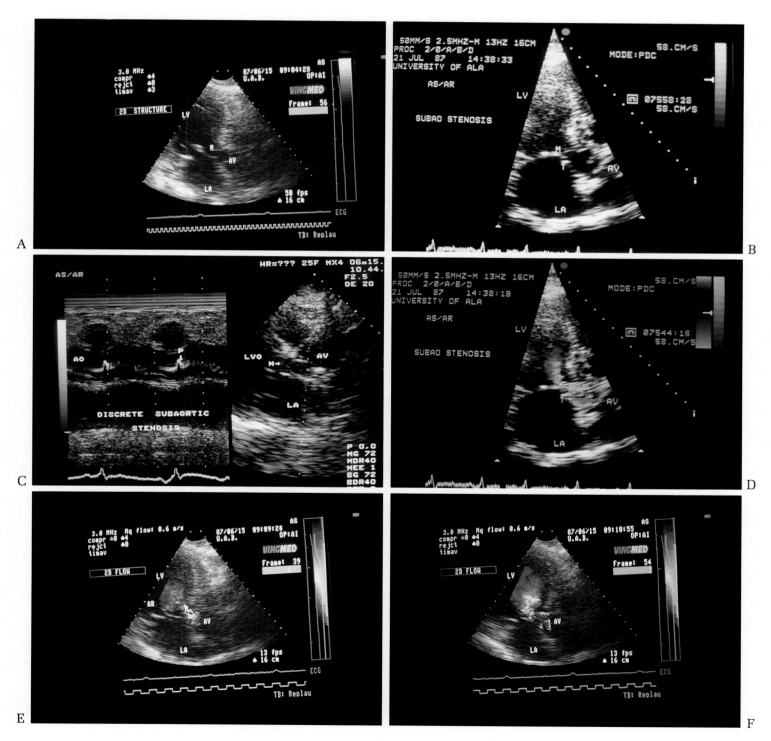

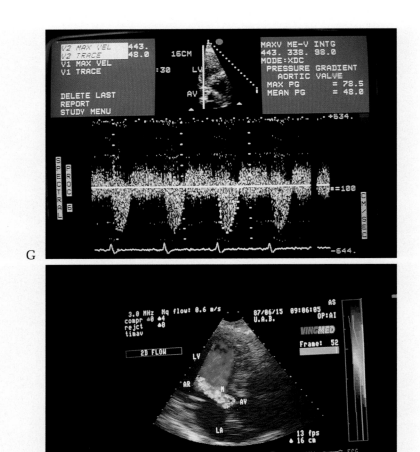

G

H

Figure CO-7 **Congenital aortic valve stenosis.** (A) Long axis view in a 4-year-old child shows a narrow band of mosaic-colored signals moving through a domed AV during systole, typical of congenital AS. Short axis views (B,C) show the classical "circle within a circle" appearance. (Courtesy of Dr. Rajendra Goyal, Bombay Hospital, Bombay, India). Autopsy specimen (D) from another patient shows a thickened, dysplastic AV.

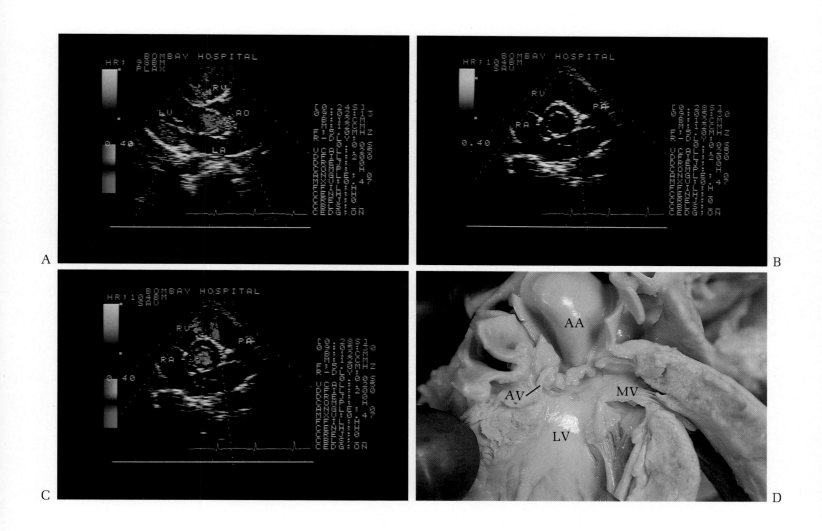

Figure CO-8   **Biscuspid aortic valve.** (A,B,C) Aortic short axis views in a 36-year-old man clinically presenting with AR shows a bicuspid AV with two equal-sized leaflets, a horizontal line of closure, and two discrete jets of AR. Autopsy specimen (D) from another patient with a bicuspid AV also shows a horizontally oriented commissure and two equal-sized leaflets.

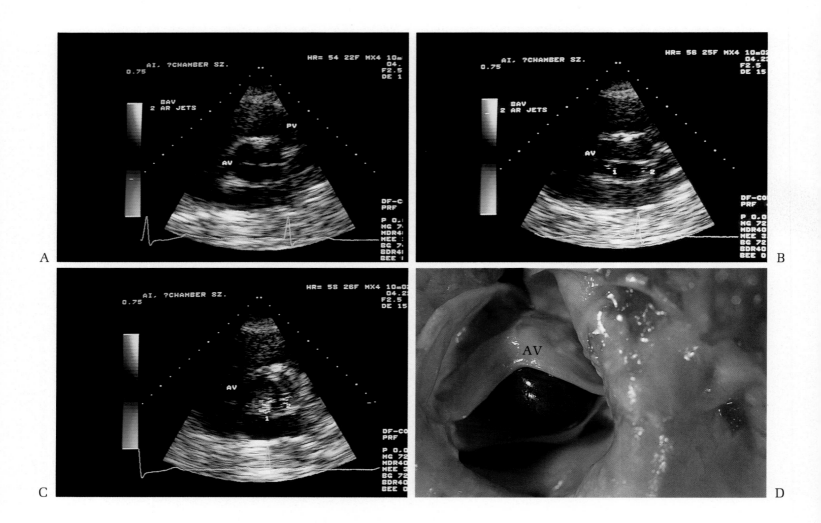

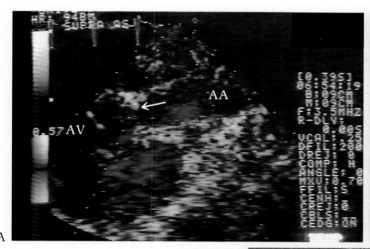

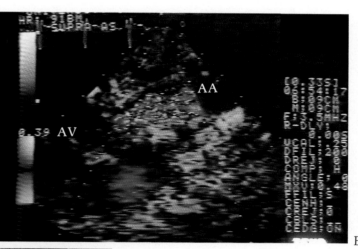

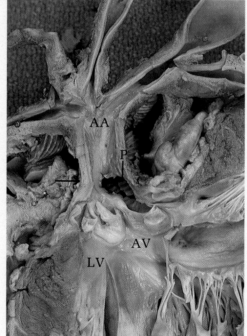

SECTION 10 CONGENITAL HEART DISEASE

Figure CO-10 **Coarctation of aorta.** (A,B,C) High left parasternal examination in a newborn shows marked tubular narrowing of the aortic arch and poststenotic dilatation of the DA. Red flow signals in the AA represent normal antegrade systolic flow, while the blue signals in the coarcted segment (arrow) represent aliasing due to high-flow velocity.

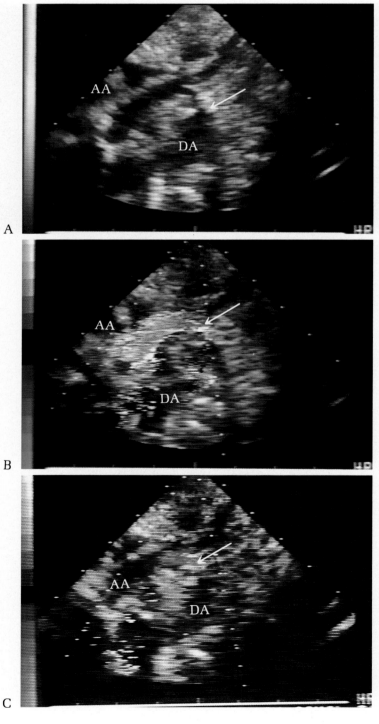

Figure CO-11   **Coarctation of aorta.** (A,B) Suprasternal examination in an 18-year-old man shows discrete coarctation (CO) of the aorta and poststenotic dilatation (PSD) of the DA. (C,D,E) Color Doppler examination shows a thin band of mosaic-colored signals in the coarcted segment and dilated aorta beyond, indicating turbulence and high blood flow velocity. The CW Doppler cursor line was placed parallel to the flow signals in the coarcted segment to initially obtain a peak pressure gradient of 48 mm Hg (F). The transducer was then angled minimally to interrogate the "core" of the coarctation jet to obtain a higher peak pressure gradient of 72 mm Hg (G). Schematic (H) and autopsy specimens (I,J,K) demonstrate aortic coarctation (arrow).

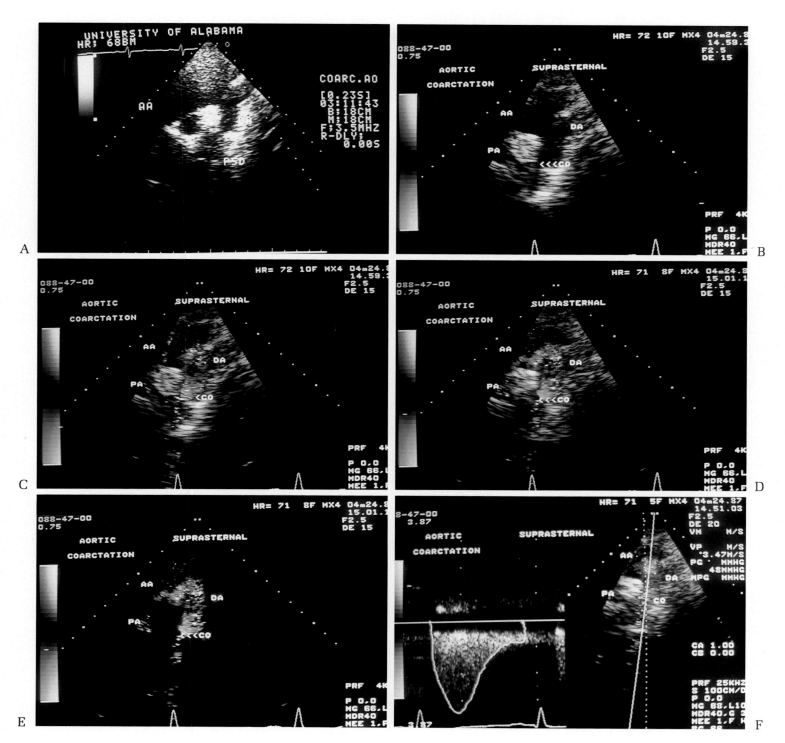

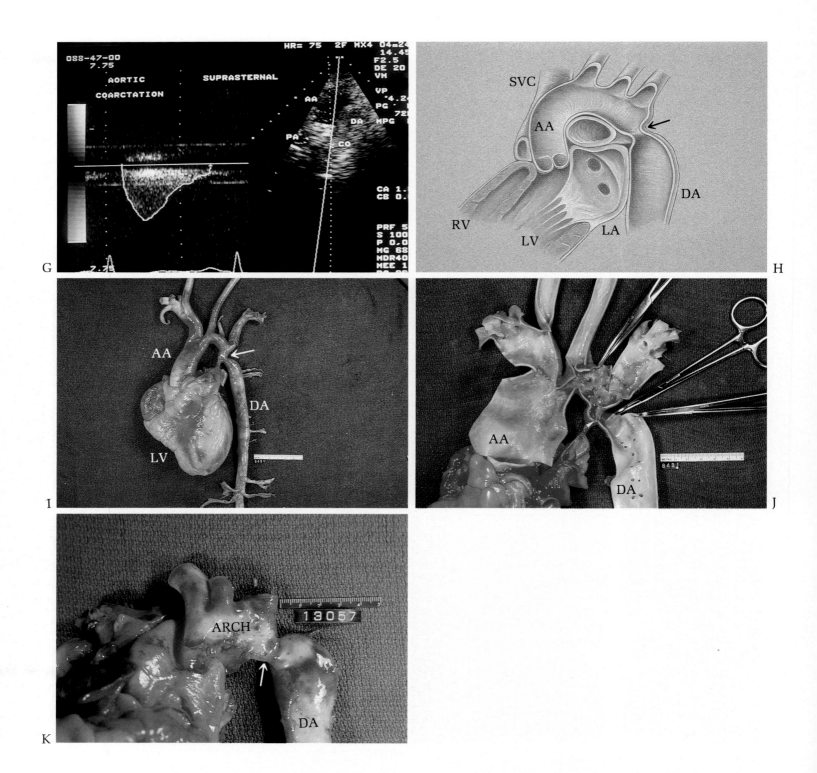

G

H

I

J

K

Figure CO-12 **Coarctation of aorta status post-repair.** (A) Suprasternal color Doppler examination in a man shows aliased but relatively wide signals in the DA, indicating absence of severe coarctation. The innominate artery (IA) is enlarged. Color-guided CW Doppler examination (B) demonstrates a residual peak pressure gradient of 35 mm Hg. C and D are suprasternal views in a 36-year-old woman with previous surgery for coarctation of the aorta, resection of subaortic membranous stenosis, and left ventricular–aortic conduit, showing a long segment of hypoplastic proximal descending thoracic aorta (DA), but there was no evidence of obstruction by color-guided continuous wave Doppler. The innominate artery (IA) is enlarged.

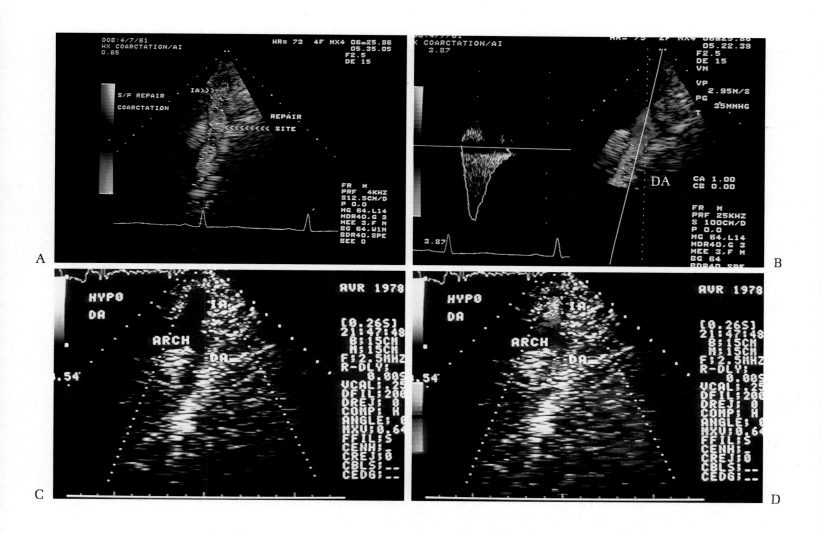

SECTION 10 CONGENITAL HEART DISEASE

Figure CO-13 **Infundibular stenosis.** Although short axis view (A) taken at the level of the high LVOT does not appear to show significant RVO narrowing, color Doppler examination (B) shows tubular narrowing and aliasing (blue, arrowheads) of the systolic RV flow signals in the infundibular region. The diastolic frames (C,D) show a thin yellowish jet originating from the PV, consistent with mild PR. Careful inspection of the RV body and RA, however, demonstrates a broad band of blue signals in continuity with the yellowish signals and extending all the way down to the TV, revealing the presence of severe PR. Late diastolic TR (DTR) results from transient reversal of RV–RA pressure gradient across a partially closed TV due to severe PR, producing marked elevation of RV end diastolic pressure. Narrowing of the PR jet produced by some degree of infundibular stenosis resulted in underestimation of the severity of PR in the initial stages of the color Doppler examination in this 24-year-old man, status post pulmonary valvotomy and closure of secundum ASD. Autopsy specimen (E) from another patient shows infundibular stenosis (arrows).

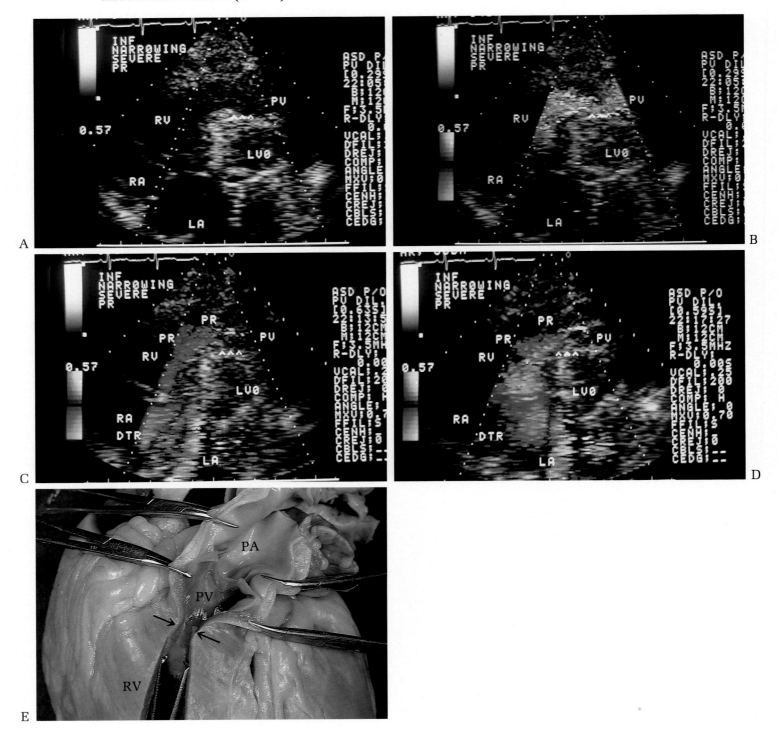

Figure CO-14 **Pulmonary valve stenosis.** (A) Aortic short axis view in a 25-year-old woman with PV stenosis shows mosaic-colored signals in the PA during systole, indicating turbulence and high velocity blood flow. CW Doppler cursor line (B) placed parallel to the PS jet signals shows a peak pressure gradient of 24 mm Hg, consistent with mild PS. The transducer was then angled for an optimal view of the markedly dilated PA (C,D,E,F). Color 2D and M-mode examination demonstrate prominent swirling of blood flow with mosaic and blue-colored signals directed posteriorly along the lateral wall of the PA, and anteriorly directed red signals present more medially near the aortic root. G is a schematic showing PS. H is an autopsy specimen from another patient, showing a markedly thickened, domed PV (arrows), RV hypertrophy, and dilatation of pulmonary arteries.

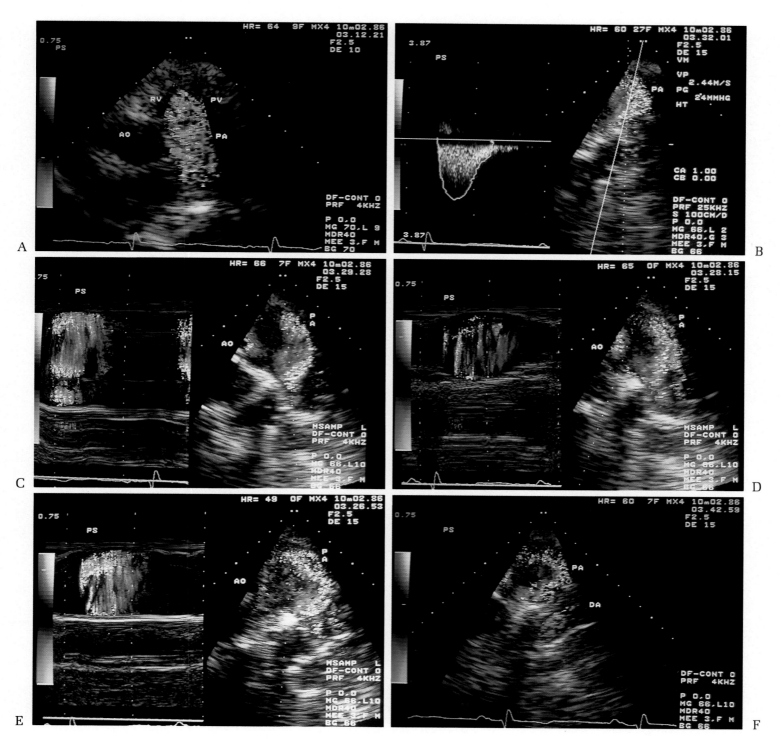

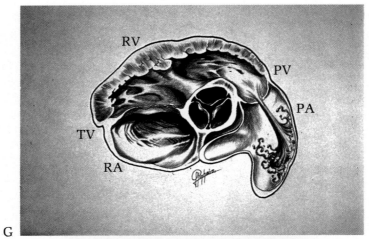

G

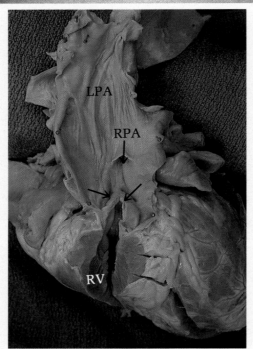

H

SECTION 10   CONGENITAL HEART DISEASE

Figure CO-15 **Pulmonary valve stenosis.** (A,B) Aortic short axis views in a 25-year-old man. The CW Doppler cursor line is placed parallel to the mosaic-colored signals in the PA to obtain a peak pressure gradient of 40 mm Hg. Note the associated presence of PR (C). Color M-mode studies (D,E) in the para-apical 4-chamber view in another patient (45-year-old woman) with PV stenosis (peak gradient by color-guided continuous wave Doppler and cardiac catheterization of 36 mm Hg) shows right-to-left shunting (blue) during early systole and left-to-right shunting (red) during most of diastole across a patent foramen ovale (D). Increase in the area of blue signals (right-to-left shunting) was noted with the Valsalva maneuver. AS = atrial septum.

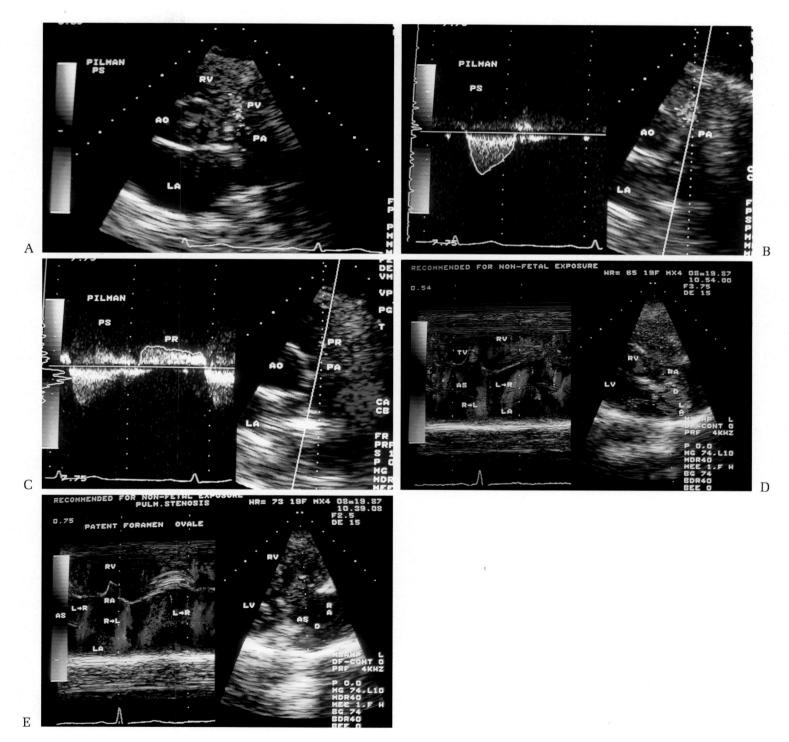

Figure CO-16   **Pulmonary valve replacement.** Left ventricular pulmonic plane in a 33-year-old man with tetralogy of Fallot who has had PV replacement for PS and AV replacement for AR. The CW cursor line is placed parallel to the flow signals in the region of the pulmonic prosthesis (P) to obtain a peak pressure gradient of 15 mm Hg, excluding the presence of prosthetic obstruction in this patient. The diastolic Doppler signals above the spectral baseline represent PR.

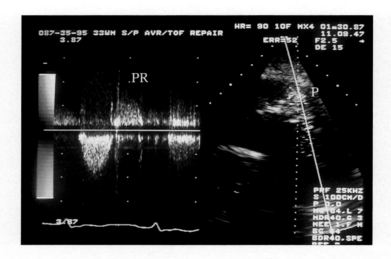

E. COMPLICATED LESIONS

Figure CC-1   **Complete atrio-ventricular canal defect (atrio-ventricular septal defect).** (A) Apical 4-chamber view in a 1-month-old infant shows flow signals moving from the LV into the RV (blue) and from the LA into the RA (blue) through ventricular (V) and atrial (A) components of the canal defect. Flow signals are also seen moving from the LA into the RA through a secundum (S) ASD. B and C are schematics. The secundum ASD is not drawn in C. D is an autopsy specimen from another patient showing a large defect (D) and the common atrio-ventricular valve (CAVV).

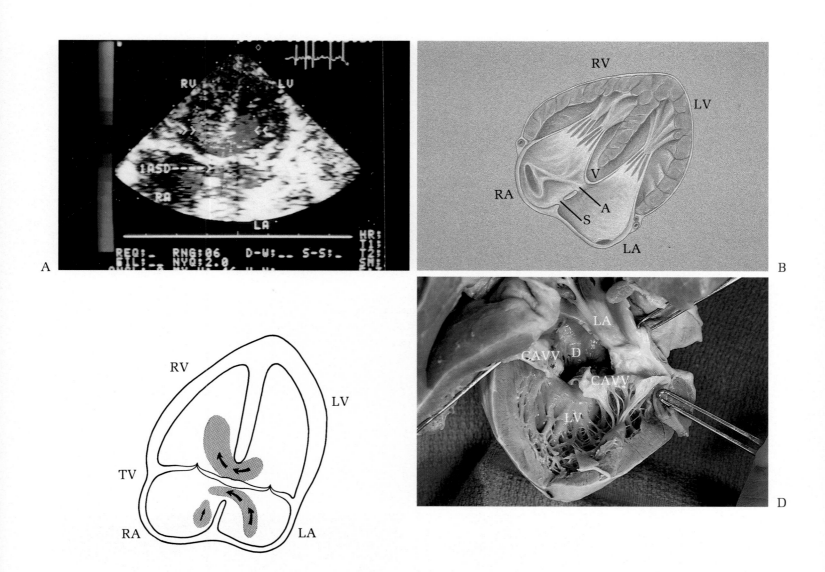

Figure CC-2   **Complete atrio-ventricular canal defect.** Para-apical 4-chamber view in another pediatric patient shows blood flow signals moving from the LV into the RV (red) and from the LA into the RA (red) through the AV canal defect. (Courtesy of Dr. Edward V. Colvin, UAB Pediatric Cardiology Division.)

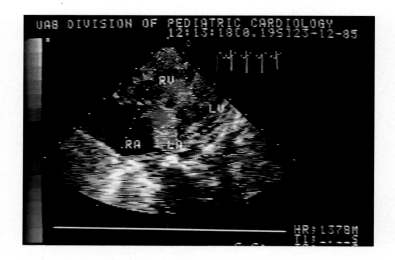

Figure CC-3   **Complete atrio-ventricular canal defect.** (A,B) Apical 4-chamber views in a 27-year-old woman demonstrate shunting through the ventricular and atrial components of the AV canal defect. (Courtesy of Dr. Rajendra Goyal, Bombay Hospital, Bombay, India.)

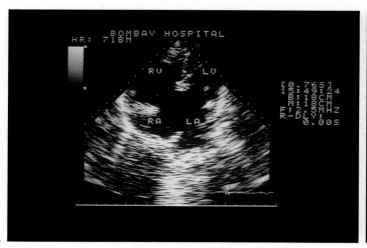
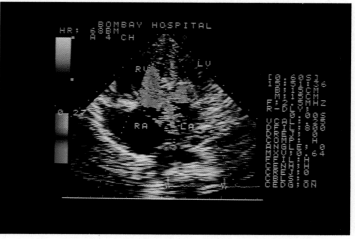

A

B

Figure CC-4   **AV valve regurgitation in complete AV canal defect.** (A) Apical 4-chamber view in a pediatric patient shows mosaic-colored signals filling more than 40% of the RA during systole, consistent with severe TR. A small band of systolic blue signals in the LA originating from the MV indicates the presence of mild MR in this patient. Another frame from the same patient (B) demonstrates right-to-left shunting through the ventricular component.

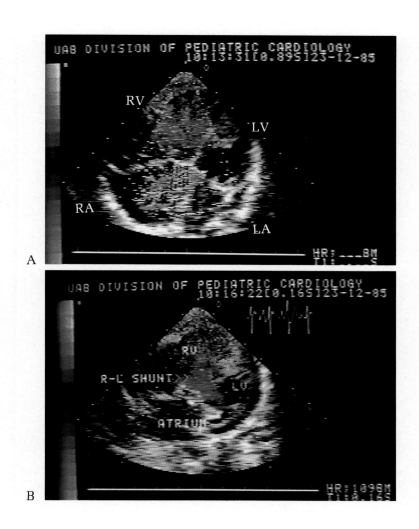

SECTION 10 CONGENITAL HEART DISEASE

Figure CC-5 Complete atrioventricular canal defect with pulmonary hypertension (Eisenmenger syndrome). (A) Long axis view in an adult shows a large VSD. The VS and the right ventricular wall are hypertrophied, suggesting the presence of significant pulmonary hypertension. (B,C) Late diastolic frames show flow signals (red) moving from the LA through the MV into the LV and then through the defect into the RV. (D) This frame is taken slightly earlier in diastole than the previous ones and shows predominantly right-to-left shunting, observed as blue signals moving from the RV through the defect into the LV and the aorta. The bidirectional shunting in this patient is related to the presence of pulmonary hypertension.

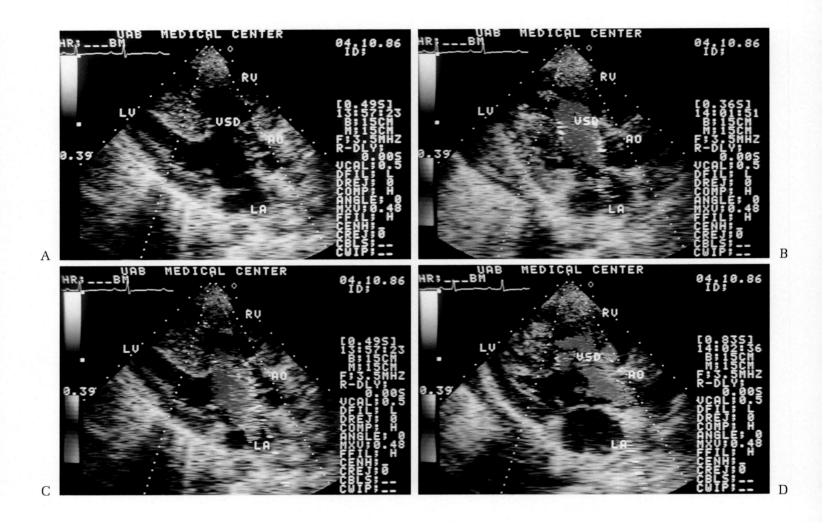

Figure CC-6 **Complete AV canal defect following surgical repair.** (A,B) Modified 4-chamber views show a bright linear echo from the patch (P) closing the ventricular component of the canal defect and mild residual TR and MR. (C) Color M-mode examination also shows bright echoes from the patch with no residual shunting from the LV into the RV during systole. Aliased signals during diastole represent tricuspid inflow. (D,E) Autopsy specimens from another patient show a pericardial patch (P) closing the atrial component (AP) and a synthetic patch closing the ventricular component (VP) of the AV canal defect. A second synthetic patch (arrow, surrounded by pledgets) closes a muscular VSD. Suture repair of the cleft (C) anterior MV leaflet is also seen (D).

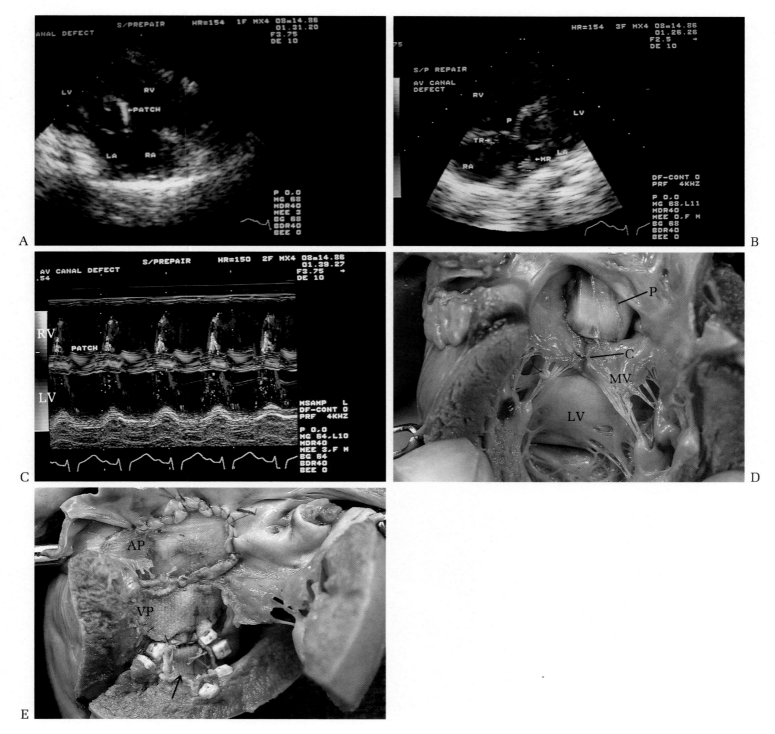

SECTION 10   CONGENITAL HEART DISEASE

Figure CC-7   **Tetralogy of Fallot.** (A) Long axis view shows aortic overriding and a large VSD (arrow) in a 24-year-old man. (B) Color flow examination shows predominantly left-to-right shunting in late diastole with blue and yellow areas within the red representing aliasing and turbulence. (C) Somewhat earlier in diastole, the shunt is right-to-left with the blue signals representing blood flow moving from the RV into the LV and aorta. (D) Color M-mode examination done by passing an M-line cursor through the flow signals demonstrates left-to-right shunting confined to the isovolumic contraction period and predominantly right-to-left shunting during the remainder of the cardiac cycle. E is an autopsy specimen from another patient showing a large portion of the aorta arising from the RV (RV–AO connection has been opened). F shows a large perimembranous VSD (D) with outlet extension in tetralogy of Fallot. IS = infundibular septum; TS = trabecular septum; RCC = right coronary cusp, NCC = noncoronary cusp; AL = anterior tricuspid leaflet; SL = septal tricuspid leaflet.

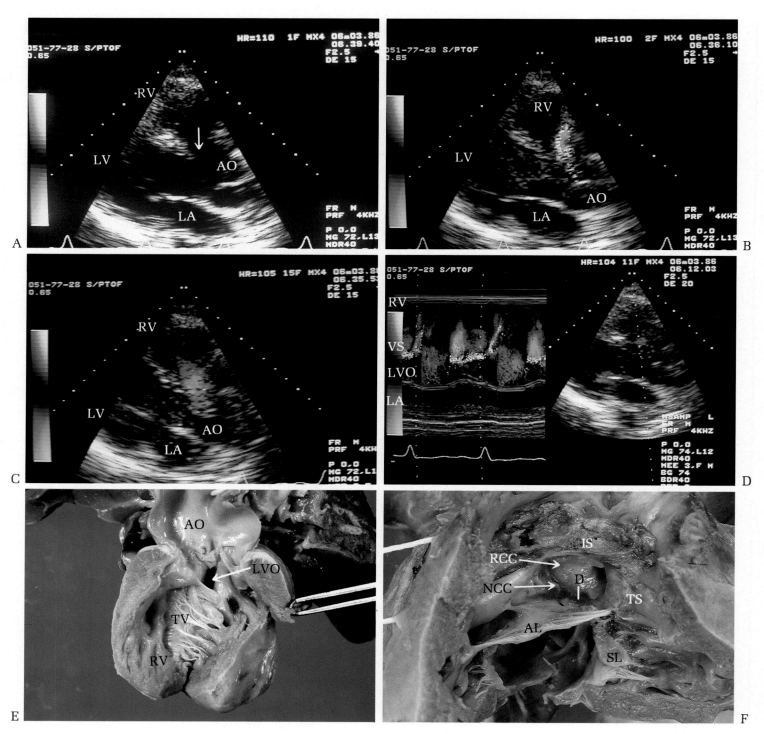

SECTION 10   CONGENITAL HEART DISEASE

Figure CC-8 **Tetralogy of Fallot with aortic regurgitation.** (A) Long axis view in a 38-year-old cyanotic woman shows marked aortic overriding and blood flow signals (red) moving from the LV into the RV in diastole through a large defect. (B) Another frame shows both left-to-right shunting (red) and right-to-left shunting (blue) occurring at the same time (arrow) through different portions of the defect. Both the AV and MV are in the closed position (isovolumic contraction period). (C) Another diastolic frame shows turbulent flow (mosaic-colored signals) along the right side of the VS due to AR and shunting from the LV into the RV (red signals) through the VSD. (D) Long axis view clearly shows the mosaic pattern of color signals arising from the AV and moving into the RV along the right side of the VS due to AR. (E) This shows AR into the RV and prolapse of the right coronary cusp of the aortic valve (AVP) into the defect. (F) Another frame in the same patient shows bluish and mosaic-colored signals due to AR moving along both the right and left sides of the VS. Right-to-left shunting is also noted here. Thus the AR in this patient is directed into both ventricles. (G) Color M-mode examination shows left-to-right shunting during middle diastole and right-to-left shunting in early diastole. D = VSD. (H) Color M-mode examination shows mosaic-colored signals of AR in front of the right side of the VS.

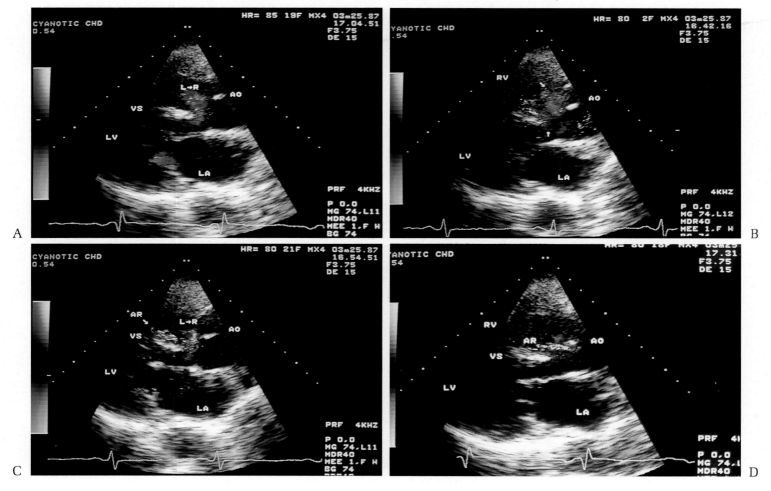

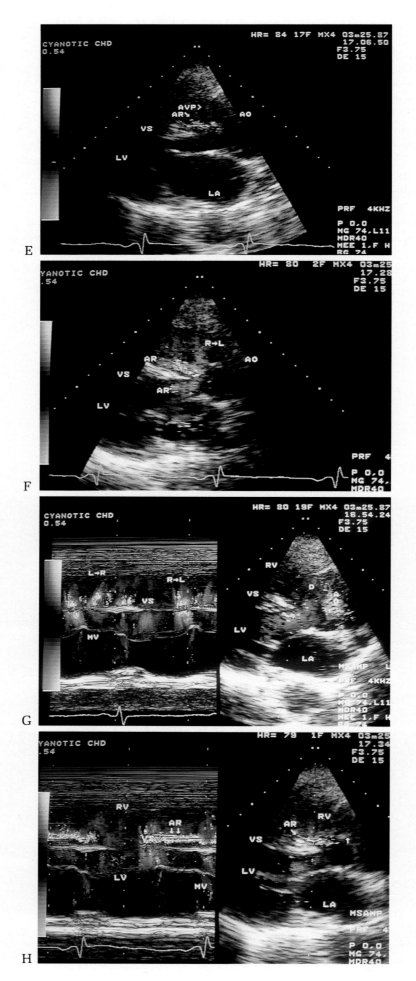

Figure CC-9 **Tetralogy of Fallot after surgical repair.** (A) 2D echo shows mild residual infundibular stenosis (N) and a normal-appearing PV in a 23-year-old man who underwent patch (P) repair of his VSD and resection of infundibular stenosis. (B) Color Doppler examination shows mosaic-colored signals moving through the narrowed infundibulum and high-velocity aliased signals in the RVO just proximal to the narrowing, representing a residual VSD jet. Color-guided continuous wave Doppler examination showed a high velocity of 3.96 m/sec (peak pressure gradient 63 mm Hg) in the RVO (C) and a much lower velocity of 2.0 m/sec (peak pressure gradient 17 mm Hg) in the narrowed infundibular region (D). At cardiac catheterization, a gradient of 23 mm Hg was found across the infundibulum. Great care should be taken not to mistake the high gradient across very small residual VSDs for significant infundibular stenosis. Small residual VSDs after surgical repair are easily detected by CW and color Doppler, even though they may not be evident on cardiac catheterization and angiography. Color M-mode examination (E) shows systolic mosaic-colored flow signals (F) in the RVO and PA, indicating turbulent flow and three discrete flow jets (red) in diastole due to significant PV incompetence. F is a schematic showing the close proximity of a VSD (D) to infundibular stenosis (arrow). G is an autopsy specimen from another patient with tetralogy of Fallot, showing patch (P) repair of VSD. AO = aorta.

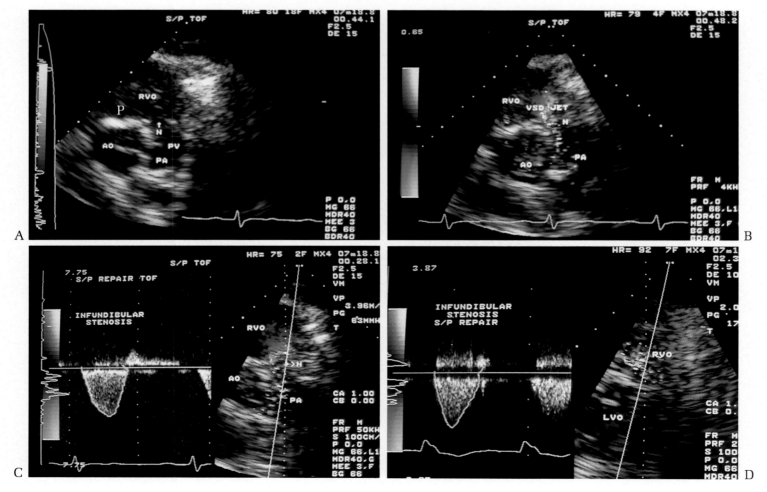

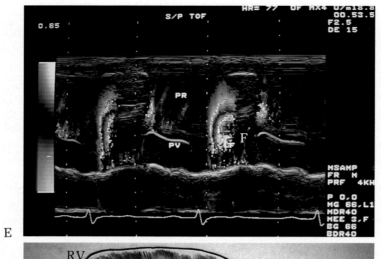

E

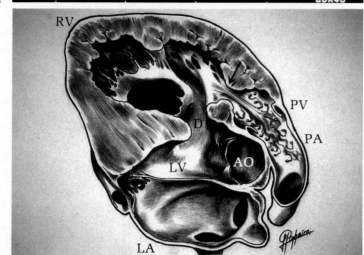

F

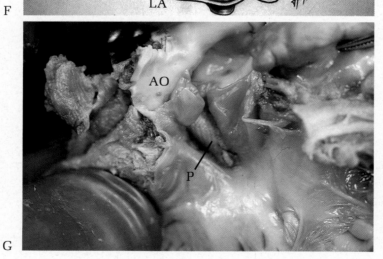

G

SECTION 10   CONGENITAL HEART DISEASE

Figure CC-10   **Double outlet right ventricle.** (A) Parasternal examination in a 6-year-old child shows both great vessels (GV1, GV2) arising from the RV. AV1 and AV2 represent the MV and TV respectively. The anterior great vessel (GV2, aorta) is larger and located directly anterior in relation to the posterior great vessel (GV1, PA), consistent with transposition of the great vessels (B). Apical 4-chamber views (C,D,E) show the large VSD with bidirectional shunting (LV to RV in D and RV to LV in E). (Courtesy of Dr. Rajendra Goyal, Bombay Hospital, Bombay, India). F is an autopsy specimen from another patient showing both great vessels arising from the RV and a subpulmonic VSD (D).

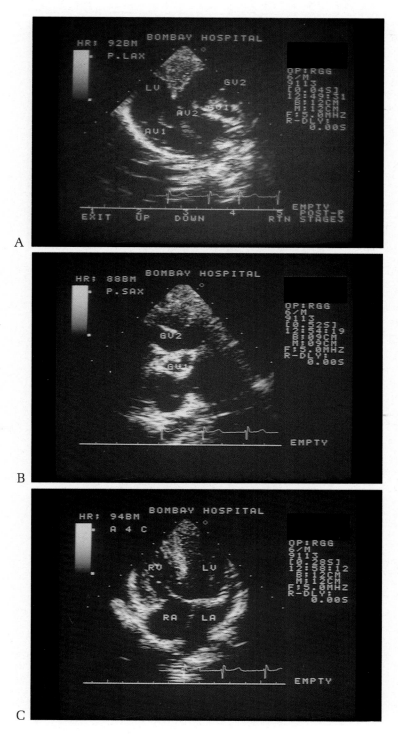

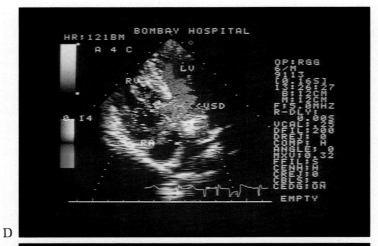

D

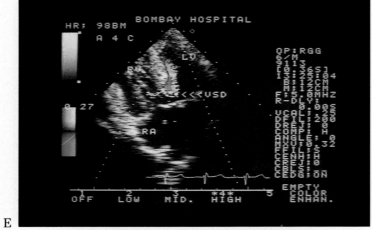

E

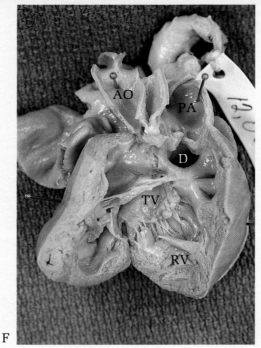

F

500

SECTION 10   CONGENITAL HEART DISEASE

Figure CC-11   **Single ventricle.** Subcostal 4-chamber (A) and parasternal short axis (B) views in a 6-year-old child show two atrioventricular valves (AV1 and AV2) communicating with a single ventricle. Apical 4-chamber views (C,D) show blood flow signals moving through both AV valves into the single ventricular chamber. Apical 4-chamber views (E,F) in another pediatric patient show diastolic flow signals moving from both atria into a single ventricular chamber (SV). (Courtesy of Dr. Rajendra Goyal, Bombay Hospital, Bombay, India.) G is an autopsy specimen from another patient with single ventricle showing univentricular AV connection to the LV and discordant ventriculo-arterial connection. The rudimentary RV and the VSD are shown. H shows univentricular AV connection to a ventricle of indeterminate type. Note multiple prominent papillary muscles and trabeculations in the single ventricle (SV). AVV = large atrioventricular valve. A = atrium.

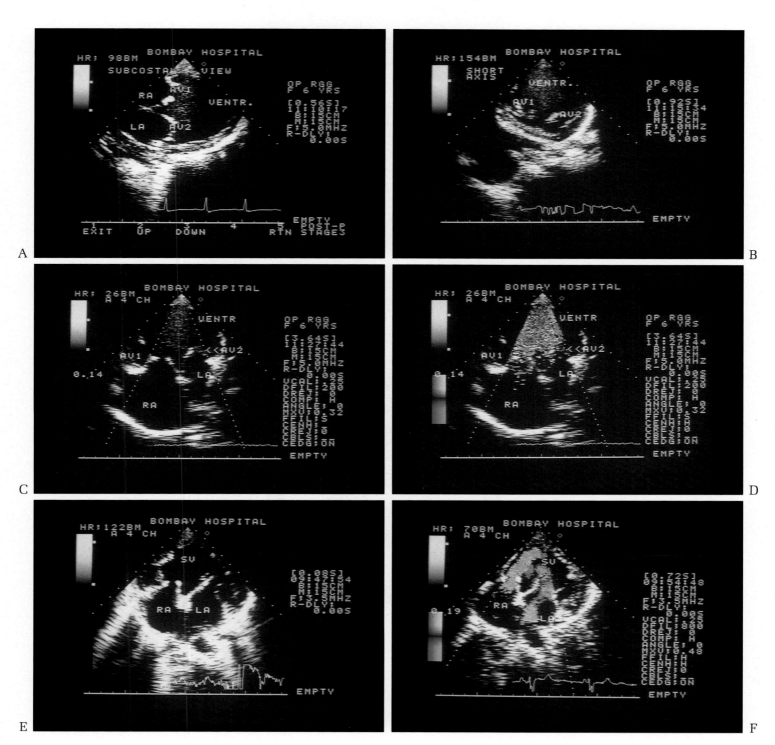

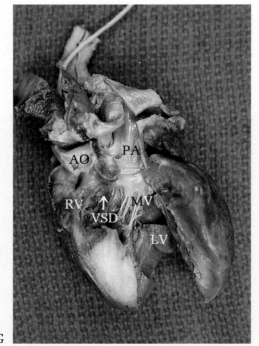

G

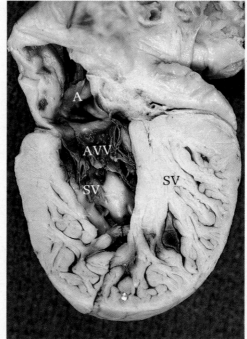

H

Figure CC-12   **Single ventricle.** Short axis view at the level of the great vessels in a 9-year-old child shows the anterior vessel (aorta) located to the right of the posterior vessel (PA), typical of dextro-transposition of the great vessels.

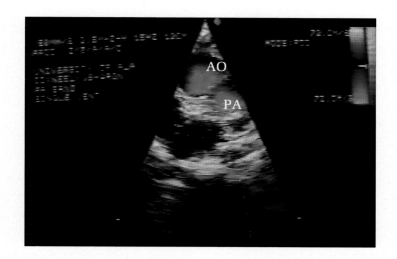

Figure CC-13   **Truncus arteriosus after valved conduit repair.** In this adult patient, the color-guided CW Doppler cursor line is placed within the flow signals in the conduit (CON) near the porcine valve (V, imaged from a high left parasternal approach) to obtain a peak pressure gradient of 14 mm Hg, excluding significant obstruction to blood flow.

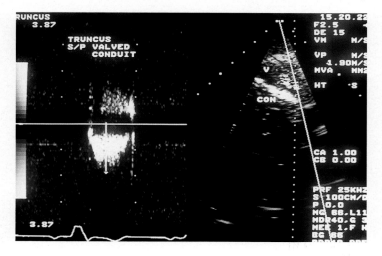

SECTION 10   CONGENITAL HEART DISEASE

Figure CC-14   **Dextro-transposition of the great vessels.** (A,B) Short axis views at the level of the great vessels in a 23-year-old woman who has undergone the Mustard procedure show the anterior vessel located to the right of the posterior vessel, diagnostic of dextro-transposition of the great vessels. The baffle (B) is visualized as a linear echo posteriorly. A = atria. (C,D) Para-apical views demonstrate prominent flow signals (red with blue due to aliasing) moving from the pulmonary venous atrium into the RV through the open TV. Flow signals are also observed in the systemic venous atrium, which is separated from the pulmonary venous atrium by the baffle. AT = atrium. Parasternal view (E) shows relatively low-velocity signals moving from the IVC into the systemic venous atrium (SAT), excluding presence of any obstruction to blood flow in the region of the IVC opening by the adjacent baffle. Aliased flow signals (red plus blue) are noted in the pulmonary venous atrium (PAT) near the TV level. Autopsy specimens (F,G,H) from another patient with dextro-transposition of the great vessels show the aorta arising from the RV, which has been opened to show the crista supraventricularis (CR) and the PA arising from the LV. The left anterior descending coronary artery (LAD) is also shown demarcating the two ventricles.

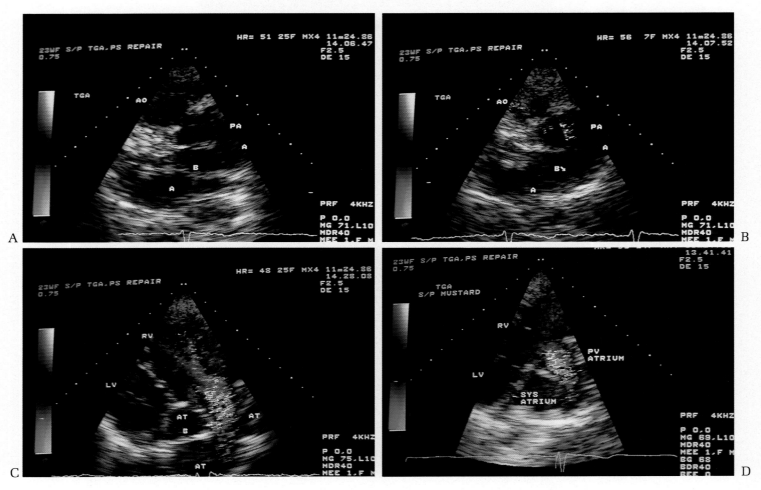

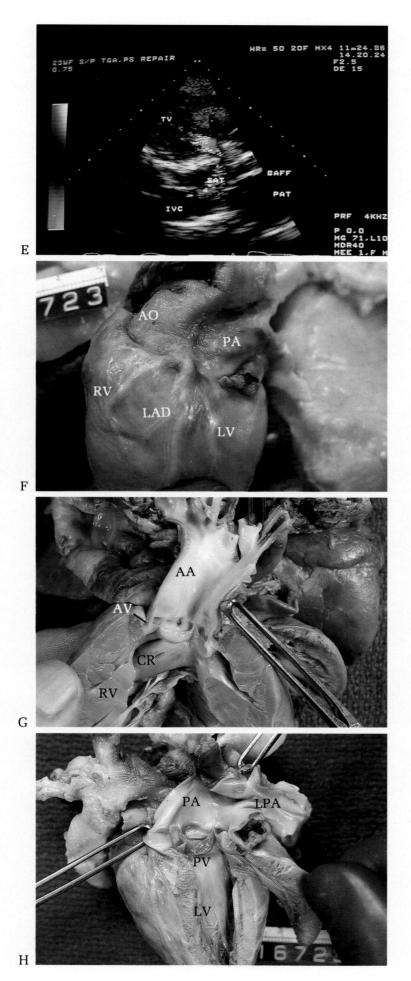

Figure CC-15 **Corrected transposition of the great vessels.** Left parasternal examination in a 40-year-old man shows the anterior vessel located to the left of the posterior vessel (A), but the posterior vessel, unlike the normally situated aorta, courses posteriorly (B), suggesting that it is the PA. These findings are typical of corrected or levo-transposition of the great vessels. C shows residual left-to-right shunting through a defect (D) in the patch (P) used to repair an associated VSD in this patient. D, E, and F are autopsy specimens from another patient with corrected transposition of the great vessels. D shows the RV in inverted position with the outflow tract oriented toward the right. In E, the MV and PV are in continuity and the LVO is oriented toward the left. F shows an associated perimembranous VSD (D) located adjacent to the TV. CR = crista supraventricularis.

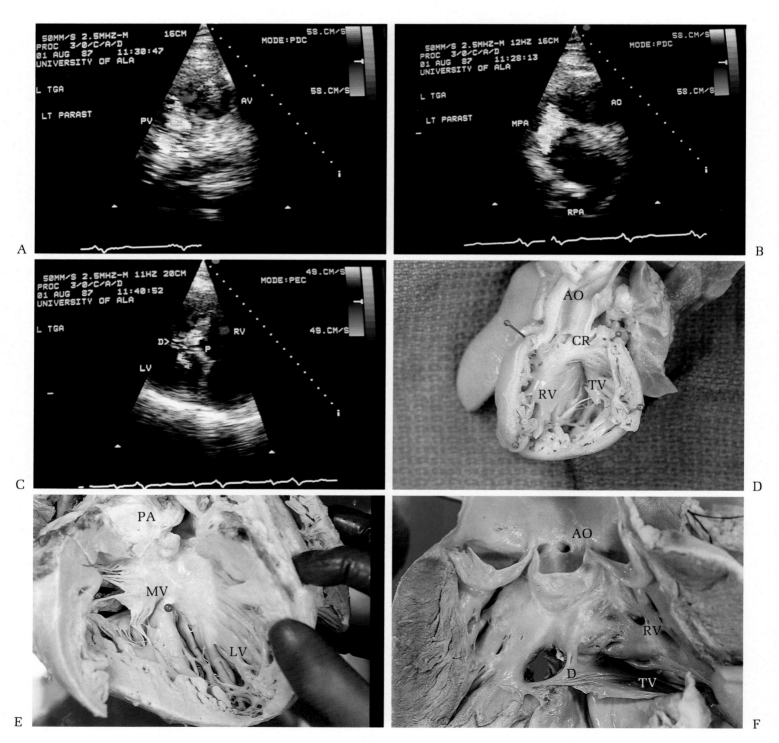

Figure CC-16   **Corrected transposition of the great vessels.** Long axis view in a 24-year-old man shows a thin band of mosaic-colored and blue signals originating from the closed PV due to minimal PR. VE = ventricle. OV = outflow vessel. REG = regurgitation.

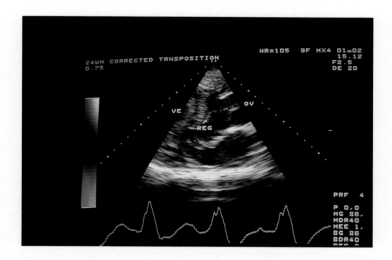

Figure CC-17   **Tricuspid atresia.** (A) Diastolic apical frame in a 9-year-old child shows normal flow signals moving through the open MV, but no flow signals are seen moving through the thickened, atretic TV (ATV). (B) Systolic frame in the same patient shows a small area of mosaic-colored signals in the LA originating from the MV, indicating mild MR. (C) Apical 4-chamber view in an 18-year-old man with tricuspid atresia shows prominent flow signals moving into the LV through the open mitral leaflets, but no flow moving into the RV through the thickened and atretic TV. (D) Systolic frame in the same patient as C, who has undergone a Fontan procedure, shows the presence of mild MR (arrow) and no flow across the surgically closed ASD. (E) Schematic shows a thickened atretic TV, hypoplastic RV, VSD (D), and flow (arrow) moving through the ASD into the LA and LV. F is an autopsy specimen from another patient showing the atretic TV (arrow) and pericardial patch (P) repair of the secundum ASD.

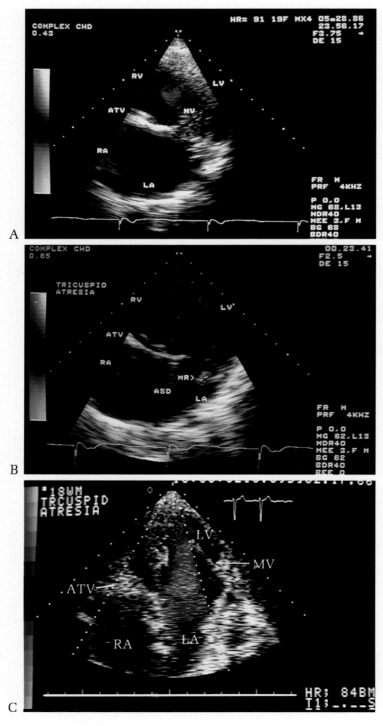

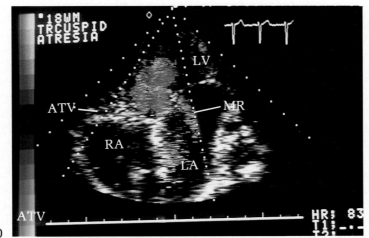

D

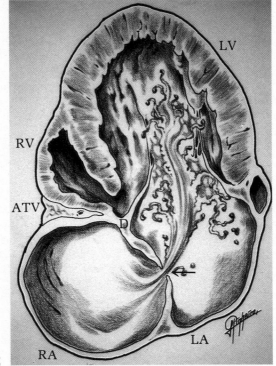

E

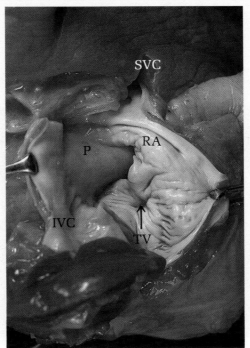

F

Figure CC-18   **Tricuspid atresia.** (A) Apical view in a 22-year-old man with tricuspid atresia, dextro-transposition of the great vessels, and subpulmonic membranous stenosis shows an atretic TV (ATV), hypoplastic and thickened RV, and a large ASD (D). The MV is structurally normal and the LV is enlarged. (B) Color Doppler examination shows blood flow signals moving from the RA through the ASD (D) into the LA cavity. A VSD is also noted and turbulent flow visualized in the LVOT. The transducer was slightly rotated to show the pulmonary veins (PV) draining into the LA (C,D) and blood flow signals moving from the RA through the ASD (D) into the LA and then into the LV through the open MV (E,F). Note absence of flow signals moving from the RA into the RV through the atretic TV (ATV). Apical view (G) shows a discrete membrane (M) below the PV which appears to be structurally normal. The diagnosis of dextro-transposition of the great vessels was made by noting the superior and rightward position of the anterior vessel (AV = aortic valve), the inferior and leftward position of the posterior vessel (PV = pulmonary valve, PA = main pulmonary artery), and the parallel orientation of the two great vessels. Color flow examination (H) shows flow signals (blue) moving from the LV into the RV through the large VSD. CW Doppler cursor line (I) placed in the mosaic-colored signals visualized in the subpulmonic area and PA reveals a peak pressure gradient of 56 mm Hg and a mean gradient of 35 mm Hg. Other apical views (J,K) show aneurysmal dilatation of the main PA. Predominantly bright blue signals (with some red areas in them due to aliasing) in the LV proximal to the membrane represent flow acceleration in K. Color M-mode examination (L,M) demonstrates mosaic-colored signals (T) due to turbulent flow in the subpulmonic area and PA and systolic fluttering of the PV. Long axis views (N,O) demonstrate the subpulmonic membrane (M) protruding into the LVO and mosaic-colored signals due to turbulence in that area. Aliased signals (red area surrounded by blue) just underneath the membrane represent flow acceleration. Para-apical views (P,Q) following a modified Fontan procedure demonstrate prominent flow signals in the RA at the site of the anastomosis (FON). R shows a thin band of mosaic-colored signals originating from the PV and directed toward the subpulmonic membrane (M), representing minimal PR seen postoperatively in the long axis view. Increased flow velocity in the RVO and aorta was also noticed after surgery due to improvement in cardiac output (S). Moderate MR seen before surgery persisted unchanged after the operation (T). U is a schematic showing dextro-transposition of the great vessels, a large VSD (D), and a subpulmonic fibrous ridge (R). Autopsy specimen (V) from another patient with dextro-transposition of the great vessels shows a subpulmonic fibrous ridge (R) and a subpulmonic VSD (D).

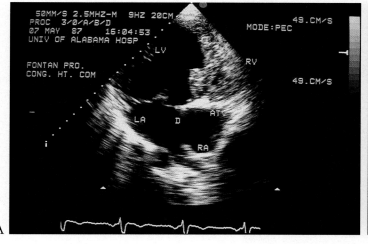

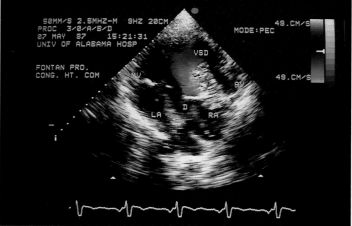

A   B

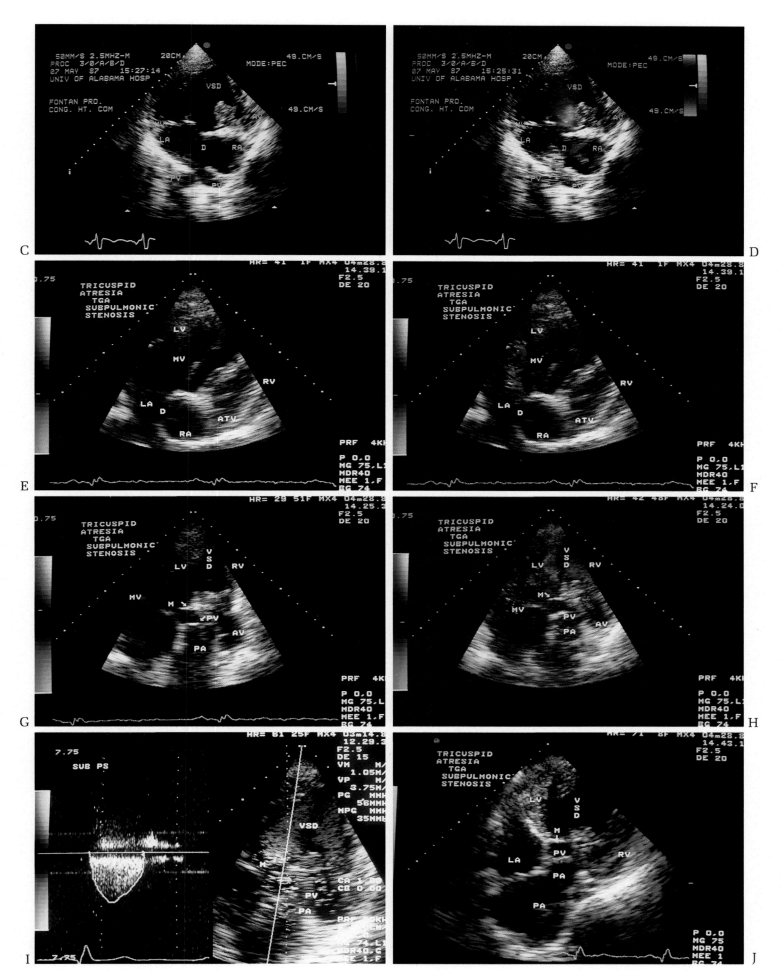

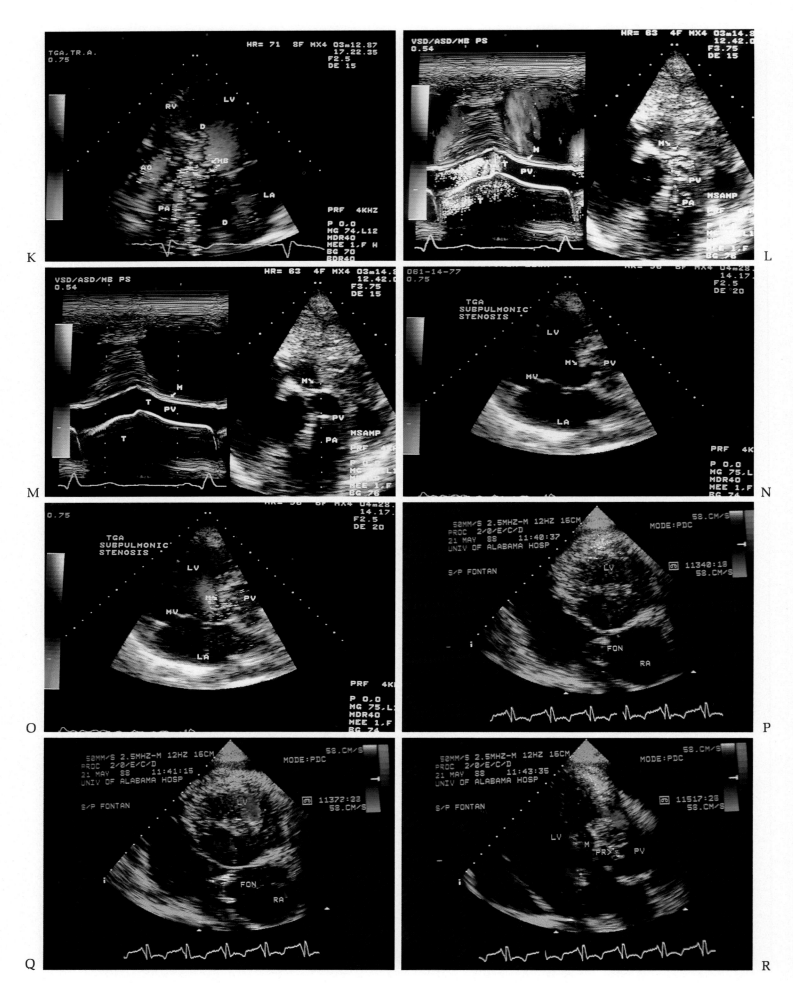

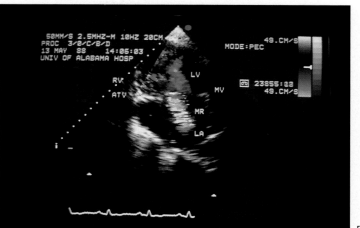

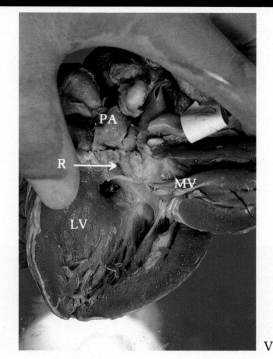

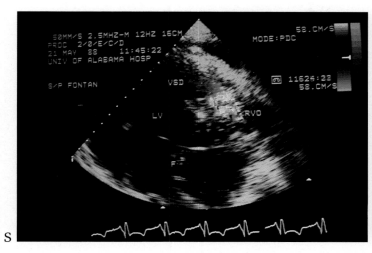

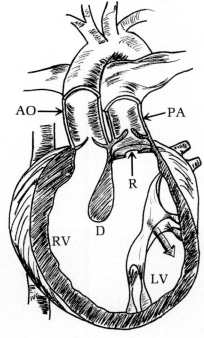

Figure CC-19 **Pulmonary atresia.** A 23-year-old woman with pulmonary atresia was found to have no pulmonary arteries when she underwent surgery for a possible Blalock shunt procedure at age 6. At that time, two large bronchial vessels were noted, one originating from the aorta and the other from the right subclavian artery, both draining into the hilum of the right lung. Short axis views (A,B,C) at the level of the high LVOT show septal discontinuity adjacent to the septal tricuspid leaflet attachment, diagnostic of perimembranous VSD and high velocity flow signals moving through the defect (D) towards the RVO, consistent with outlet extension. The linear echo (M) in the region of the VSD represents fibrous tissue. Tiny blue signals in the RA beneath the TV represent minimal TR. The long axis view (D) shows aortic overriding with right-to-left shunting through the VSD (D) in systole and left-to-right shunting in diastole. Suprasternal examination using a small sector angle (E) shows a dilated AA and two linear echo-free spaces beneath it, consistent with RPA and LA. Transducer angulation (E,F) reveals that the space labeled LA is in fact the DA. This finding led us to believe that the space initially labeled RPA could be the LA (G). Color M-mode and CW Doppler examination (H,I,J), however, demonstrated relatively high velocity and turbulent flow throughout the cardiac cycle in the space immediately beneath the aorta (AA). Subsequent correlation with the surgical findings indicated that this vessel was probably a large bronchial collateral vessel (arrow). In retrospect, the markedly dilated aorta and the large bronchial artery had probably displaced the LA so that it was not imaged from the suprasternal approach.

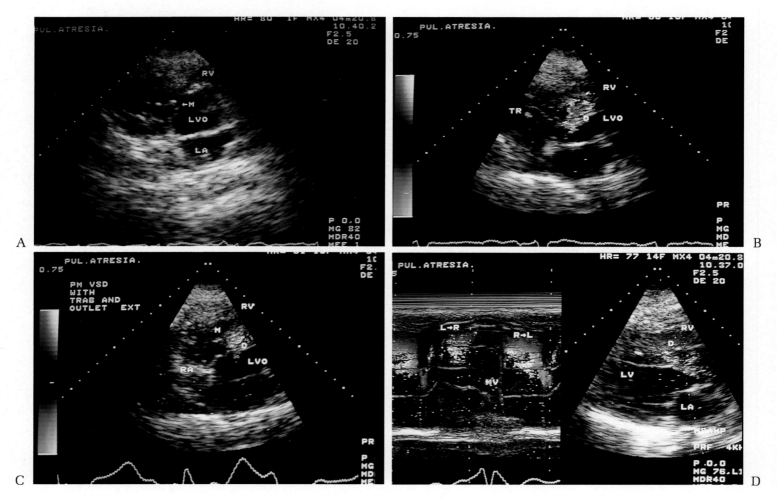

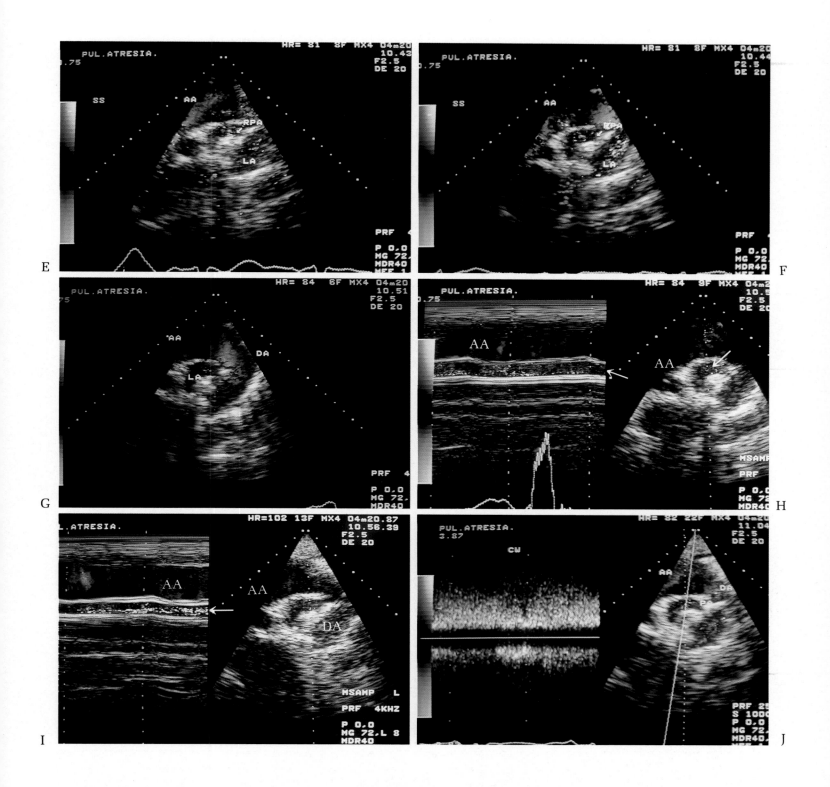

515

SECTION 10 CONGENITAL HEART DISEASE

Figure CC-20 **Hypoplastic pulmonary artery with Blalock-Taussig shunt.** A 31-year-old woman with complex congenital heart disease had bilateral Blalock-Taussig shunt at age 9 months. Recent cardiac catheterization showed tricuspid atresia, PV and main PA atresia with patent distal right and left pulmonary arteries, hypoplastic RV, secundum ASD, large VSD, and patent right- but occluded left-sided shunt. Short axis views (A,B,C) at the level of the great vessels show prominent flow signals in the large aorta (AO) and the much smaller, normally located PA. Note the prominent pulmonary venous (PV) flow into the LA. LAA = left atrial appendage. DA = descending thoracic aorta. Careful examination from the left infraclavicular transducer position demonstrates a small PV annulus and MPA viewed in long axis with the PV opening in systole (E) and closing in diastole (F), and flow signals moving antegrade (blue) in systole (G). The MPA, however, appeared to terminate distally, and no PA branching is visualized. Blue signals in LA (G) represent MR. Because of the discrepancy between color Doppler examination and angiography (which suggested both PV and MPA atresia), an NMR study was performed and corroborated the echocardiographic findings. The left infraclavicular/suprasternal examination (H through M) shows high-velocity blood flow signals moving from the innominate artery (IA) into the right subclavian artery (SA) and the right-sided Blalock-Taussig shunt (SH). AA = ascending aorta; PV = pulmonary venous flow; SP = spine. Pulse Doppler interrogation of the innominate artery (N) shows normal bifid pulsatile flow (PF) waveform in systole with evidence of turbulent flow in diastole. As the pulse Doppler sample volume is progressively moved into the shunt, turbulent flow is noted throughout the cardiac cycle (O,P). CF = continuous flow. Similar findings are also noted on the color M-mode study (Q).

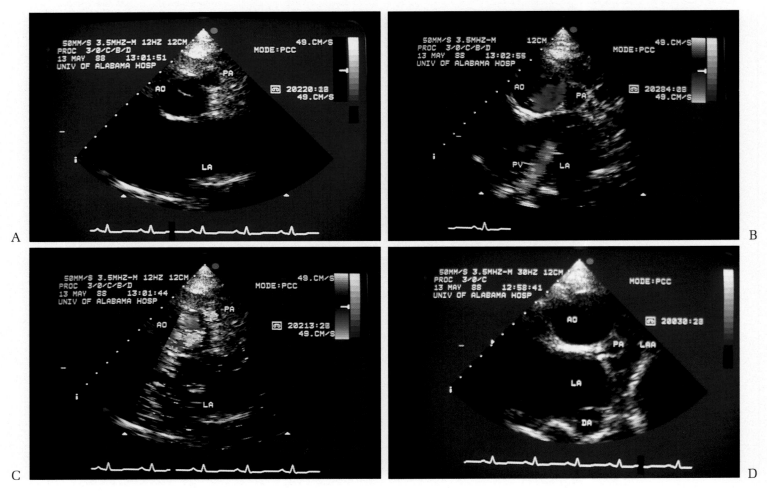

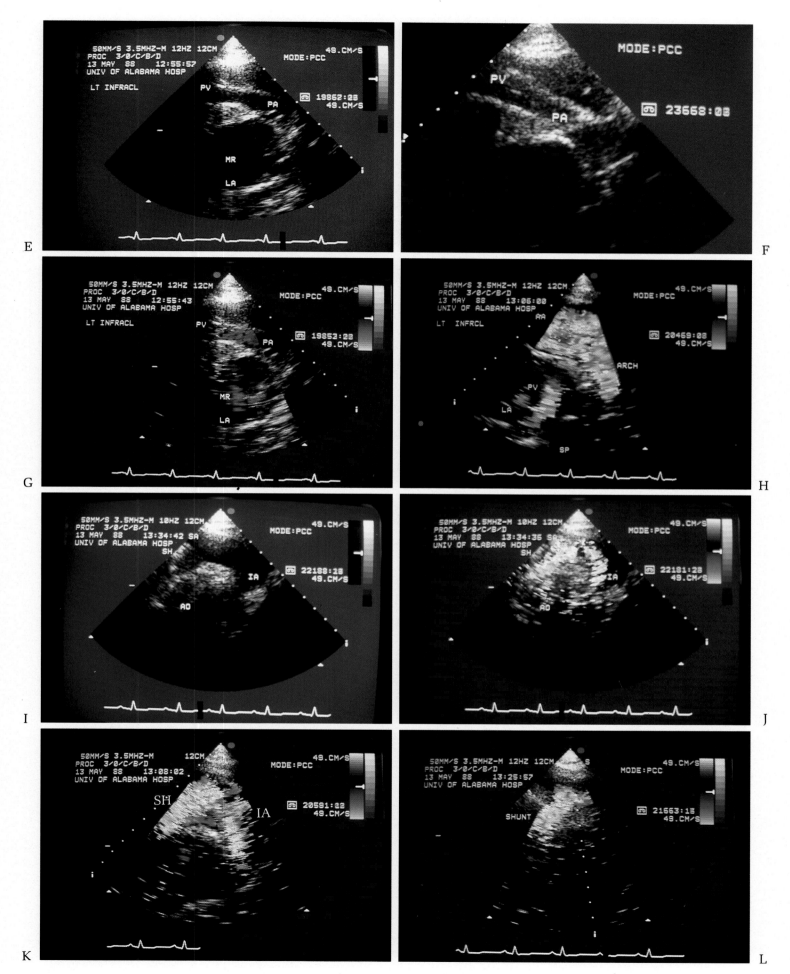

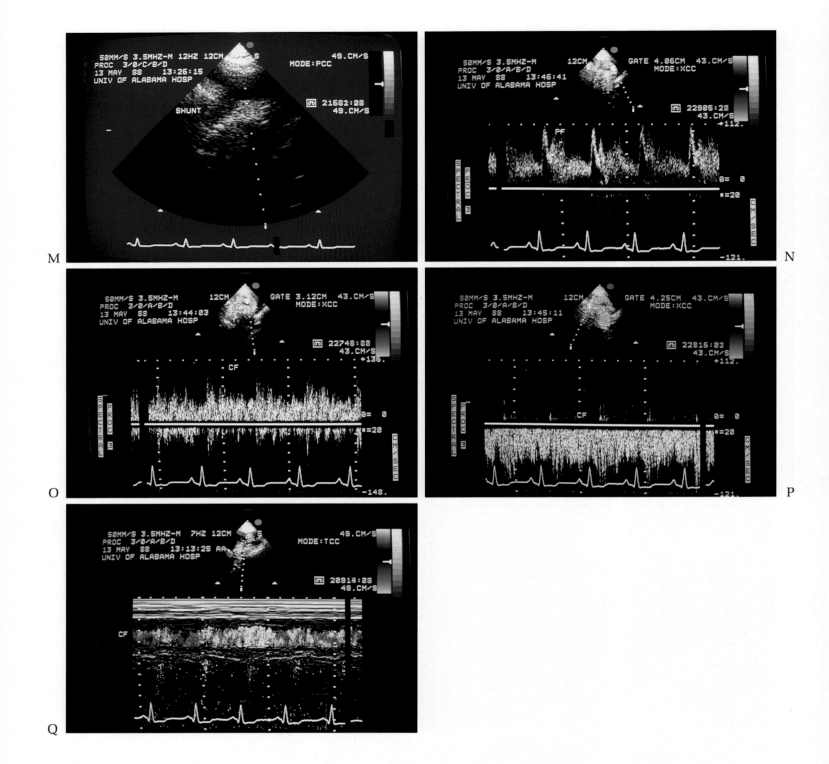

SECTION 10 CONGENITAL HEART DISEASE

Figure CC-21 **Pulmonary valve atresia.** A 21-year-old woman with PV atresia, hypoplastic main PA, and branch pulmonary stenosis had a Dacron transannular patch inserted 7 years ago. Parasternal examination (A) shows flow signals moving from the RVOT into the small main PA. No PV tissue was visualized. Color-guided CW Doppler examination (B) demonstrates forward flow into the PA during systole and retrograde flow (PR) into the RVO across the pulmonary ring in diastole. C,D, and E represent long axis views showing RV hypertrophy, aortic overriding, and bidirectional shunting across the VSD (D).

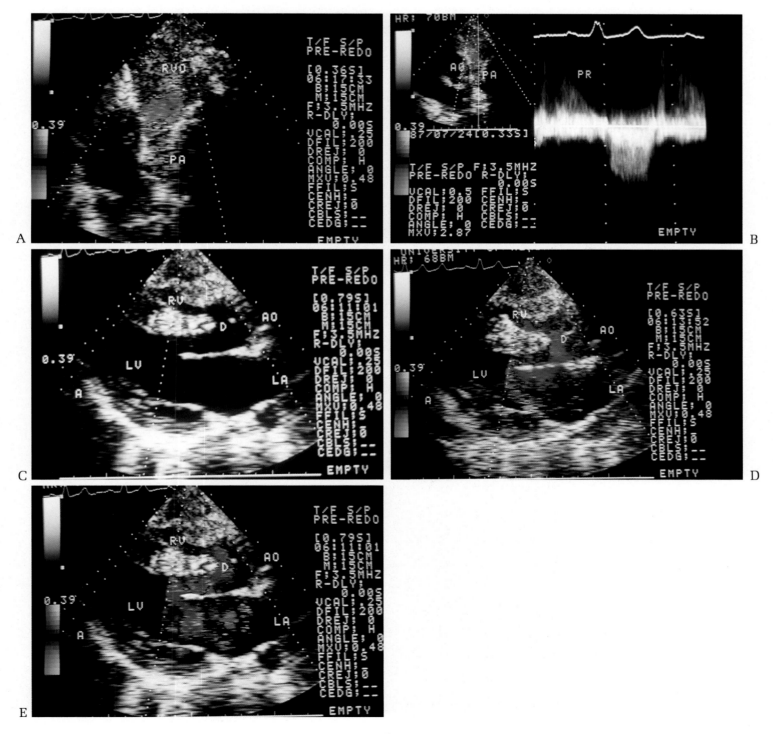

Figure CC-22 **Ebstein's anomaly.** (A) Apical 4-chamber view in a 21-year-old man shows marked apparent inferior displacement of the septal tricuspid leaflet (STV) attachment and an elongated anterior leaflet (ATV), typical of Ebstein's anomaly. (B) Schematic also shows an associated secundum ASD. TA = TV annulus. (C,D,E) Color Doppler examination shows mosaic-colored signals filling a large portion of the RA during systole, indicating severe TR. The arrow in E points to STV. LV short axis view at the level of the MV (F) shows marked enlargement of the right heart and mosaic-colored signals in the RA during systole, representing TR. Color-guided CW Doppler interrogation (G,H) demonstrates a peak systolic pressure gradient of 16 mm Hg across the TV, consistent with normal PA systolic pressure despite the presence of severe TR. Color M-mode study (I) shows delayed closure of the TV as compared to the MV, typical of Ebstein's anomaly. Autopsy specimen (J) from another patient with Ebstein's anomaly showing a markedly enlarged anterior TV leaflet (arrow). Another autopsy specimen (K) shows inferior displacement of the septal tricuspid leaflet (STV) attachment and an associated large fossa ovalis (secundum) ASD. TA = position of the tricuspid annulus.

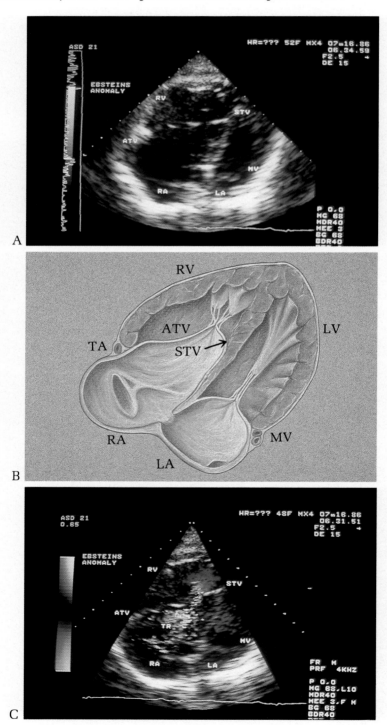

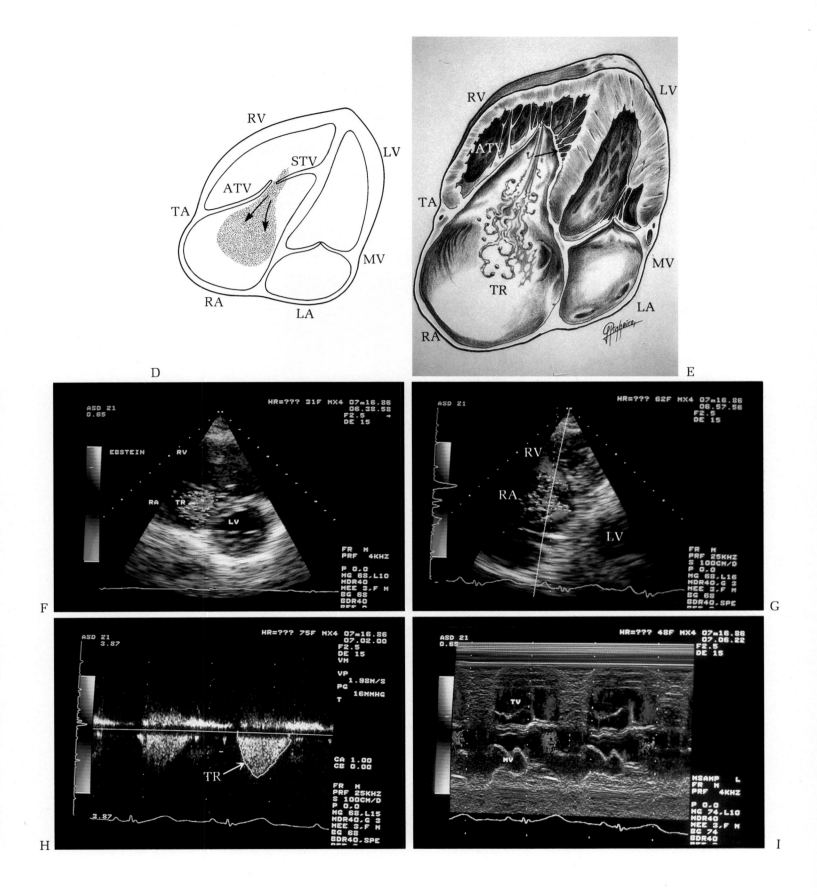

521

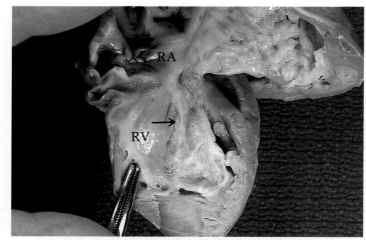

J

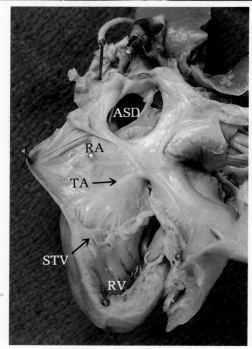

K

Figure CC-23   **Ebstein's anomaly associated with ventricular septal defect.** Long axis views in a 22-year-old man show flow signals (mainly red with some blue due to aliasing) moving from the LV into the RV through a large VSD (D) in systole (A) and mosaic-colored signals originating from the AV and filling most of the LVO during diastole, indicating severe AR (B). The abnormally enlongated anterior TV leaflet characteristic of Ebstein's anomaly is also shown (arrow). C shows the presence of prominent membrane-like fibrous tissue (M) in the defect, typical of perimembranous VSD. Mosaic-colored flow signals in the RA (D) originating from the septal TV leaflet insertion are consistent with LV-to-RV-to-RA shunt characteristic of inlet extension of perimembranous VSD. At surgery, the TV was completely closed and a modified Fontan procedure performed. Note absence of any diastolic flow signals moving into the RV through the TV, which appears echogenic (E).

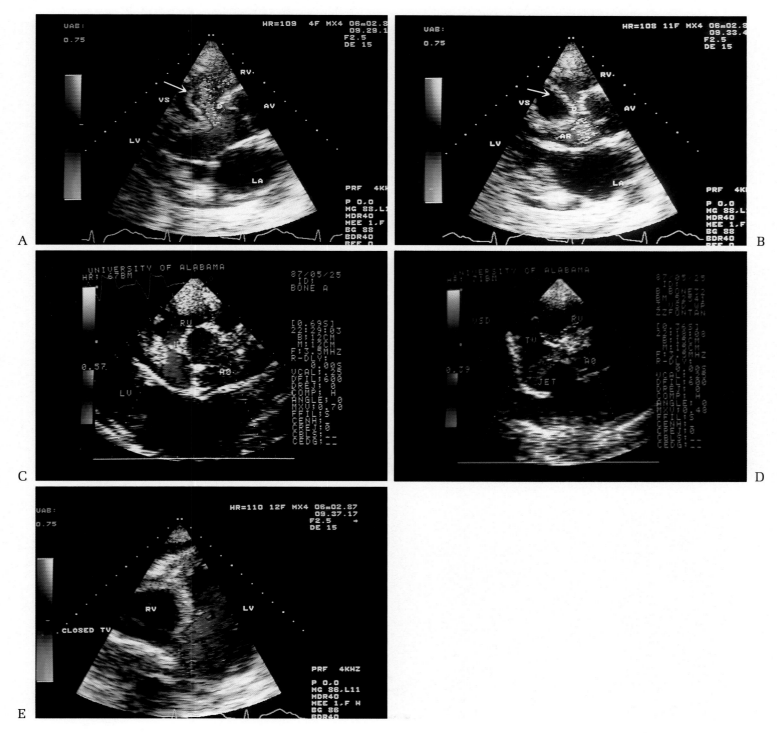

SECTION 10   CONGENITAL HEART DISEASE

Figure CC-24   **Sinus of Valsalva aneurysm.** (A,B) Modified parasternal long axis views in a 64-year-old male show a huge sac-like structure communicating with the aortic root and bulging into the RV, typical of right sinus of Valsalva aneurysm (SVA). Red and blue signals in the aneurysm (B) represent swirling of blood flow during diastole, but there is no evidence of rupture. Mosaic-colored signals filling the LVOT completely during diastole indicate associated severe AR (B,C). Short axis views (D,E,F) demonstrate turbulent flow (mosaic-colored signals) in the aortic root and LVOT but relatively undisturbed flow in the aneurysm. F also demonstrates noncoaptation of the AV cusps during diastole. R = right coronary cusp; L = left coronary cusp; N = noncoronary cusp. At surgery, the echocardiographic findings of a large unruptured aneurysm of the right sinus of Valsalva and severe AR were confirmed. The commissure between the right and noncoronary cusps had completely avulsed from the aortic wall and the aortic leaflets were thin but retracted. The patient underwent successful repair of the aneurysm and St. Jude AV replacement.

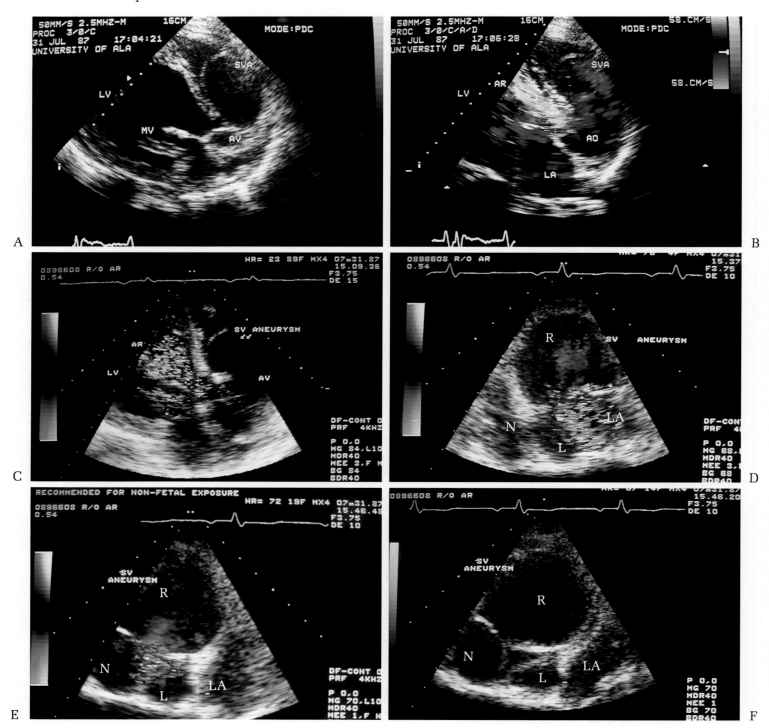

Figure CC-25   Ruptured sinus of Valsalva aneurysm (associated with doubly committed ventricular septal defect). (A,B,C,D) Parasternal long axis views in a 16-year-old boy demonstrate a tubular communication between the aortic root and the RVO, typical of ruptured right sinus of Valsalva aneurysm (S,SVR). Color Doppler examination (E through I) performed on 5 different systems shows mosaic-colored signals moving from the aortic root into the RVO through the ruptured aneurysm (S,SVA) in both systole and diastole. In G, diastolic mosaic-colored signals originating from the AV and directed into the LVO toward the base of the anterior mitral leaflet represent associated AR in this patient. Color-guided continuous wave Doppler interrogation (J) demonstrates both systolic and diastolic flow moving into the RVO through the aneurysm. Transducer angulation in the short axis view reveals an associated doubly committed VSD (K,L,M,N). Note absence of intact VS between the defect and the PV. D = VSD. These findings underline the importance of meticulous 2D and color Doppler examination in making a precise and comprehensive diagnosis of this lesion because an associated VSD may be present.

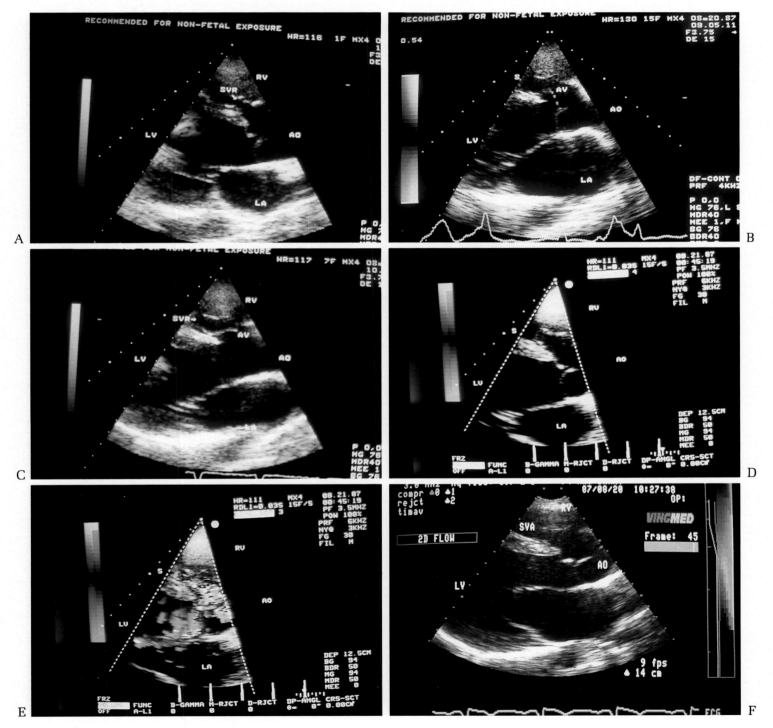

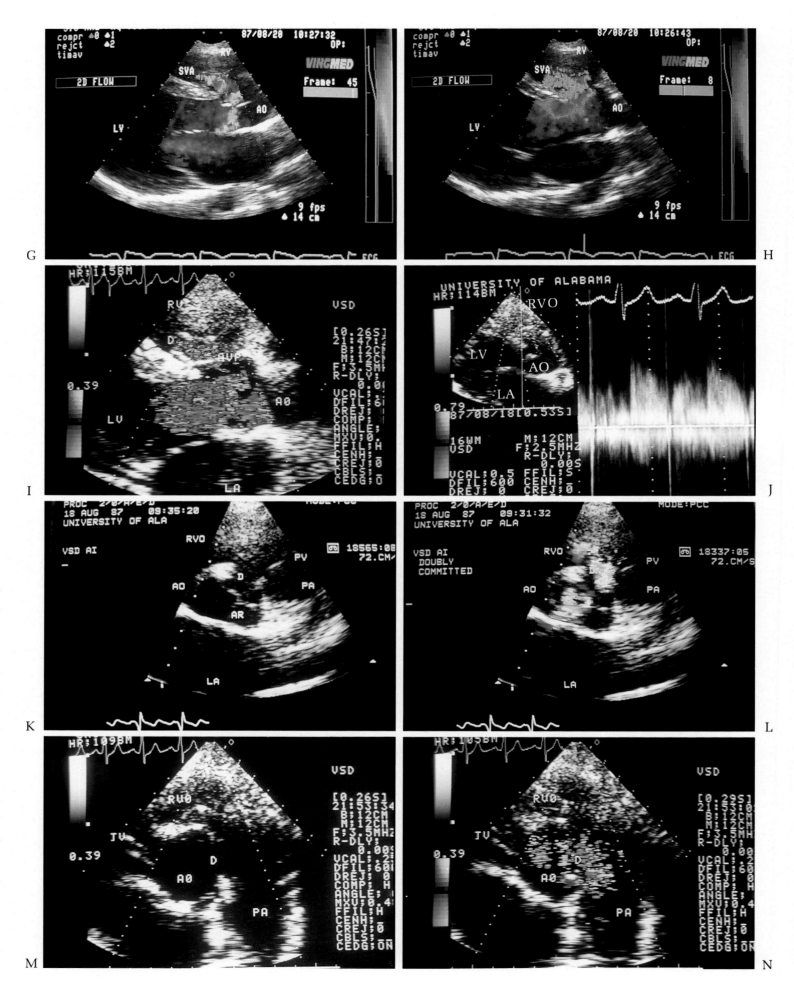

Figure CC-26   **Right coronary artery aneurysm.** (A,B) Aortic short axis views in a 54-year-old man show a large proximal right coronary artery (RCA) aneurysm with flow signals within it and in the aortic root (AO). Apical 4-chamber view (C) shows a few mosaic-colored signals in the LA during systole, indicating mild MR. The left coronary artery (LCA) in this patient was also dilated but not aneurysmal.

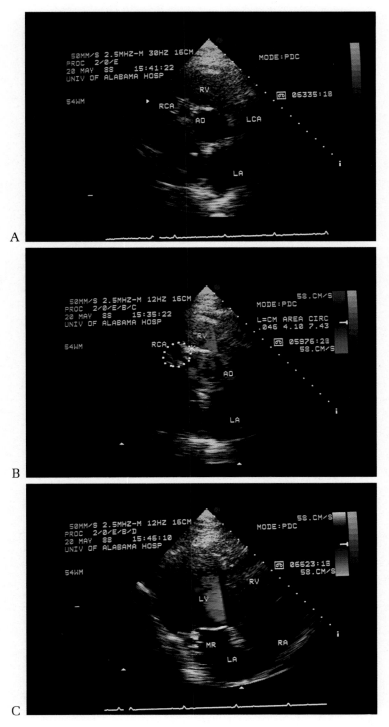

Figure CC-27   **Coronary sinus aneurysm.** (A,B,C) Aortic short axis and RV inflow views in a man show prominent mosaic-colored signals (indicating turbulence and high velocity) moving from an aneurysmally dilated coronary sinus (CS) into the RA during diastole. AN = aneurysm.

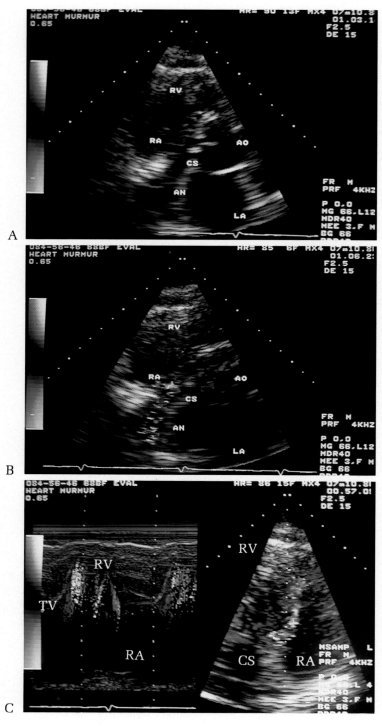

Figure CC-28. **Pulmonary artery aneurysm.** (A,B) Aortic short axis views in a 57-year-old woman show a markedly enlarged PA with the flow signals moving posteriorly near the lateral wall and then swirling back anteriorly (yellow with blue in it due to aliasing) near its medial wall. AN = aneurysm.

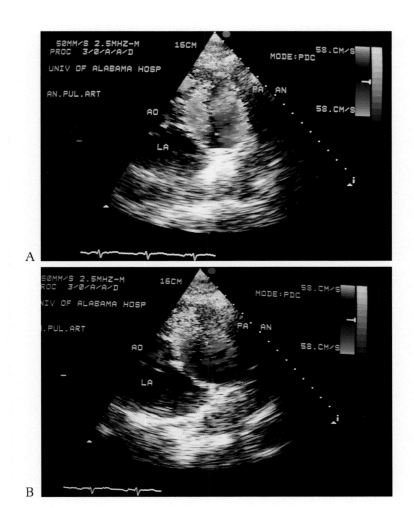

SECTION 11   MISCELLANEOUS

Various entities such as cardiac tumor masses and penetrating and nonpenetrating cardiac trauma are described in this section.

Figure M-1   **LV tumor.** Autopsy specimen shows multiple tumor masses (rhabdomyomas) in the LV.

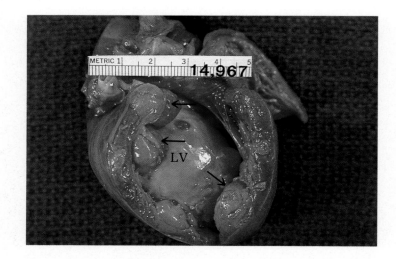

SECTION 11 MISCELLANEOUS

Figure M-2 **LV tumor.** (A,B,C,D) Subcostal 4-chamber views in an elderly patient with osteogenic sarcoma show a mobile metastatic mass (M) in the LV, which takes up color artifactually because of rapid movement. Red represents movement toward the transducer, blue away from it. In a patient with suboptimal acoustic window, this color artifact helps in the accurate delineation of the tumor boundary.

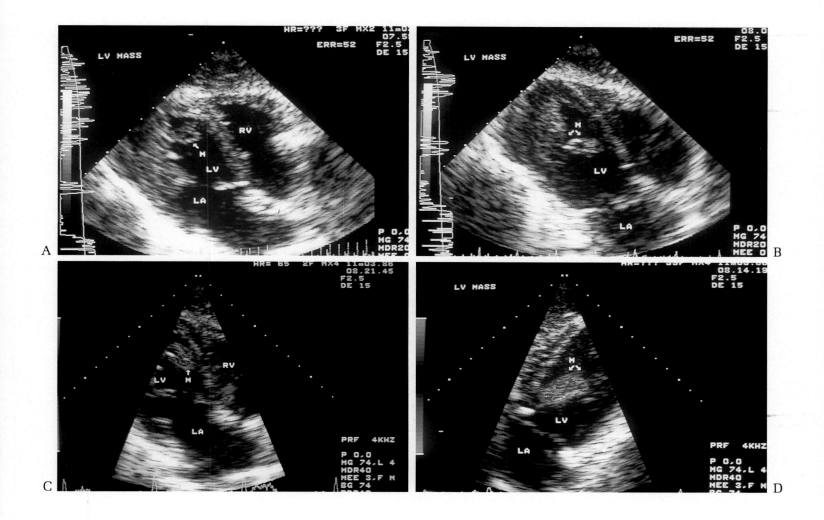

SECTION 11 MISCELLANEOUS

Figure M-3 **Malignant melanoma with cardiac metastasis.** Apical (A,B) and long axis (C) views in a 35-year-old man with malignant melanoma show marked thickening of the LV and LA posterior walls due to tumor infiltration, but the flow patterns are essentially normal, excluding significant obstruction to blood flow. The multiple echo densities in the cardiac walls are also related to tumor involvement. Examination from the right parasternal approach (D,E) shows normal flow signals moving into the RA from the IVC, indicating unobstructed blood flow. The opening of the SVC into the RA is also not narrowed. A large loculated pericardial effusion (PE) is present anteriorly.

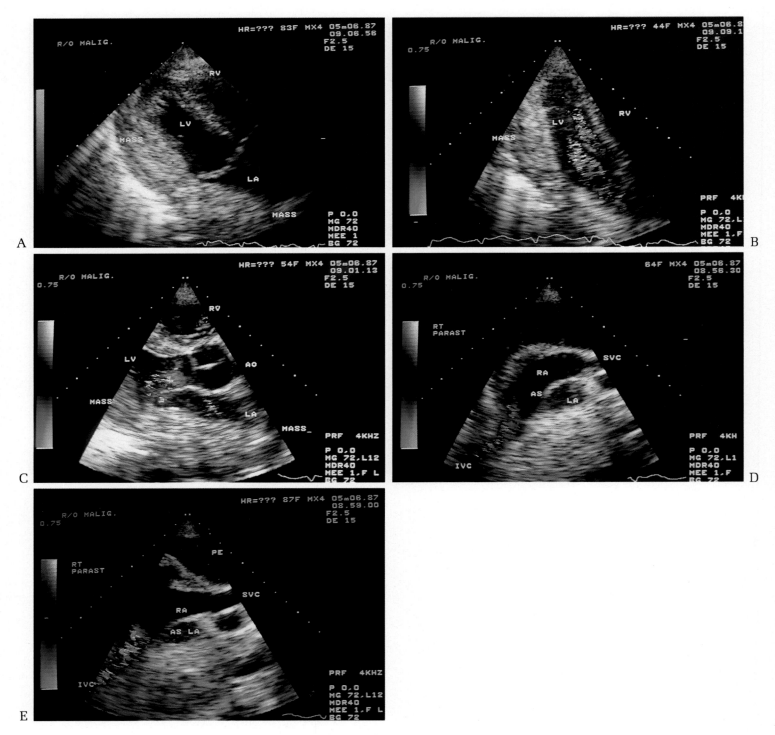

SECTION 11 MISCELLANEOUS

Figure M-4 **Mass on the anterior mitral valve leaflet.** Apical long axis view shows a small rounded echo density attached to the ventricular aspect of the anterior mitral leaflet consistent with a tumor (T) mass in a 66-year-old man who presented with multiple transient ischemic attacks (TIA's), presumably due to cerebral embolism. There was no evidence of bacterial endocarditis. The systolic frame also shows a small area of blue signals in the LA originating from the MV indicating mild MR. The bluish appearance of the echo density is related to its rapid motion, producing a "ghosting" artifact.

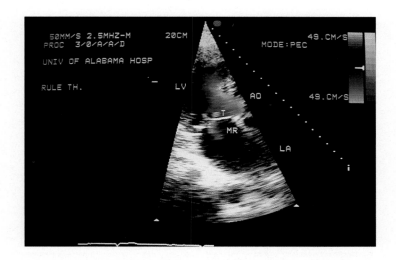

SECTION 11 MISCELLANEOUS

Figure M-5 **Left atrial myxoma.** (A) Long axis view in a 73-year-old woman presenting with chest pain shows normal LA and LV diastolic blood flow patterns, excluding the presence of obstruction to mitral inflow by the large tumor which appeared to be attached high up in the LA. (B) The systolic frame shows a small area of bluish signals in the LA originating from the MV, indicating mild MR. The patient underwent successful surgical resection of the myxoma (MYX). C is an autopsy specimen from another patient, showing an LA myxoma.

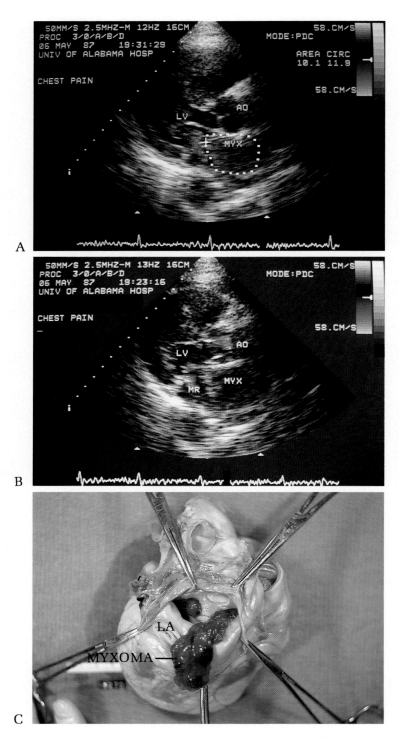

Figure M-6 **Right-sided compression by pericardial hematoma.** (A) Apical 4-chamber view in a 36-year-old man who was involved in a motorcycle accident shows narrowing of RA and proximal RV due to external compression by a hematoma (arrowhead). The mosaic-colored signals in the RV inflow suggest some obstruction to blood flow (B), and color-guided continuous wave Doppler interrogation (C) recorded a peak pressure gradient of 12 mm Hg (velocity 1.7 m/sec). Right parasternal examination (D) also shows the large hematoma (H) compressing the RA. This patient gradually improved on conservative management and did not require surgery.

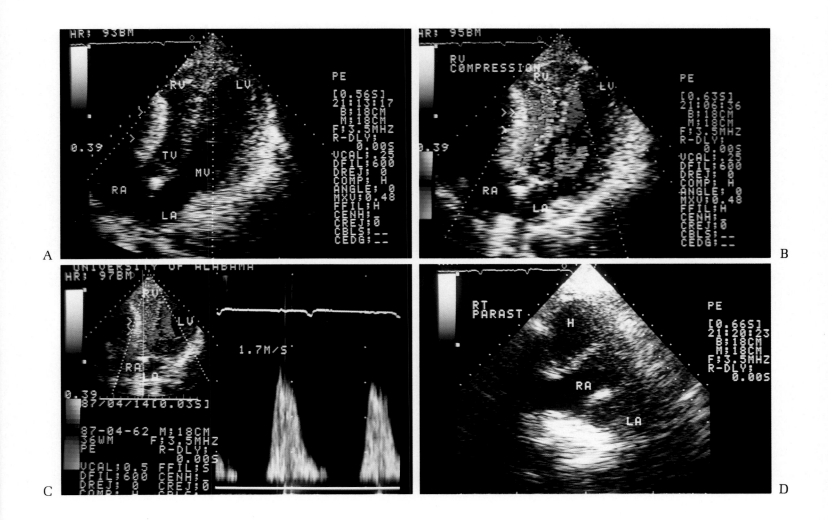

SECTION 11 MISCELLANEOUS

Figure M-7 **Right atrial myxoma.** (A,B,C,D) Apical 4-chamber views in an adult demonstrate a large right atrial myxoma (MYX) which takes up red color as it moves into the RV (and toward the transducer). (Courtesy of Dr. Rajendra Goyal, Bombay Hospital, Bombay, India.)

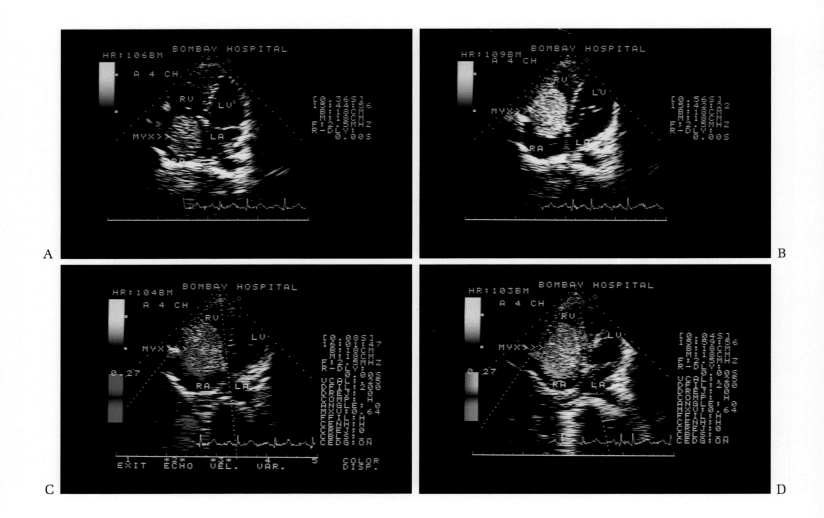

A

B

C

D

Figure M-8 **RA thrombus.** (A) Aortic short axis view in a 71-year-old man shows a circum-scribed red-colored area in the RA which represents a mobile thrombus (arrows) in this patient. The thrombus at this point in the cardiac cycle was moving toward the transducer and hence took on red color. The color helped to delineate the boundaries of the thrombus more clearly. Right parasternal examination (B) in a young woman with TV atresia shows multiple, rapidly moving circumscribed red and blue-colored areas (TH,F) representing thrombi in the markedly dilated RA. This patient subsequently died of pulmonary embolism.

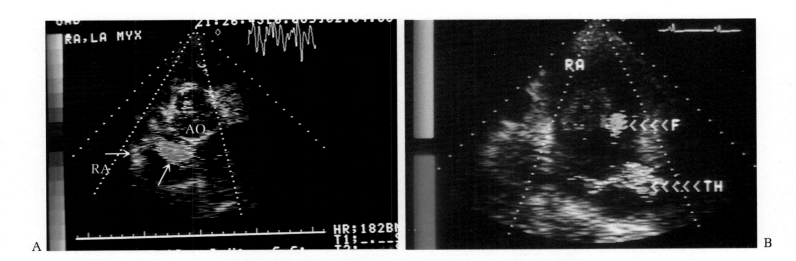

A   B

Figure M-9 **Coronary sinus hematoma.** Long axis view in an elderly man with arrhythmo-genic RV dysplasia and ventricular arrhythmia shows a large mass compressing the LA and LV. This occurred following electrophysiologic testing during which the coronary sinus was acci-dentally traumatized by catheter manipulation. The patient developed chest pain and became hypotensive, but normal color flow signals in both LA and LV excluded the presence of LV inflow obstruction and, because there was no further deterioration in the patient's clinical condition, no active intervention was undertaken. Over the next few days, the patient improved clinically, and the mass gradually decreased in size and eventually disappeared. This mass was diagnosed unanimously as an LA myxoma by several echocardiographers who were not shown the initial normal precatheterization echo study.

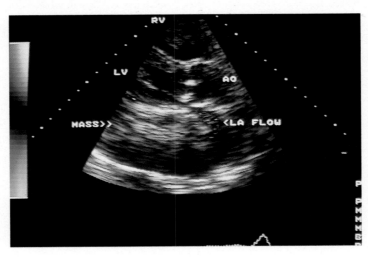

SECTION 11   MISCELLANEOUS

Figure M-10   **Arrhythmogenic RV dysplasia.** Apical examination (2D and M-mode) in a 20-year-old man shows flow signals (red) moving into the dyskinetic RV apex in both systole and diastole. The RV is dilated (A,B).

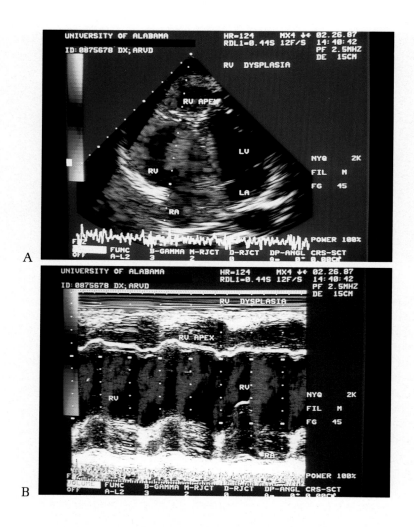

SECTION 11 MISCELLANEOUS

Figure M-11 **Bullet penetration of the heart.** (A) Short axis view at the level of the high LVO in a 23-year-old man who was shot in the back after a bar-room brawl with birdshot fired from a shotgun demonstrates a bright linear echo density (B, bullet) in the anterior VS with tail-like strong posterior reverberatory echoes (arrow) representing one of the two bullets found by 2D echo to be lodged in the VS and RV free wall. (B) Color Doppler examination shows blue and green signals in the RVO, representing aliasing and turbulent flow in the vicinity of the lodged bullet. Continuous wave Doppler examination (C) shows evidence of disturbed flow throughout the cardiac cycle (CF, continuous flow) in the RVO, but high velocities indicating LV-to-RV shunting were not detected in this patient. The large linear signals (labeled C) which correspond to loud "clicks" on the Doppler audio tones result from the Doppler ultrasonic beam encountering the bullet during cardiac motion.

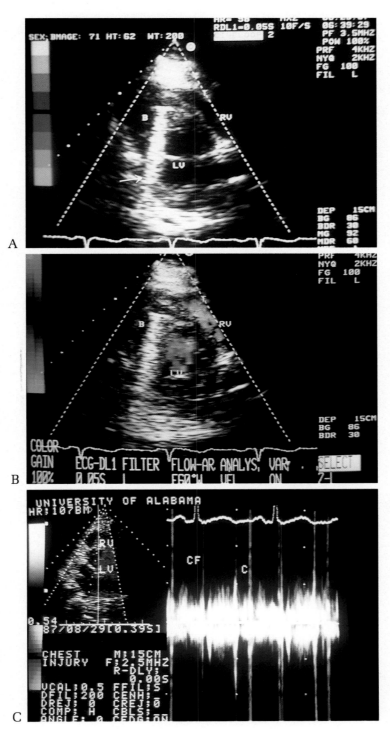

INDEX

Page numbers in italics indicate figures; numbers followed by "*t*" indicate tables.